INTERPERSONAL
COGNITION

INTERPERSONAL
COGNITION

Edited by
MARK W. BALDWIN

THE GUILFORD PRESS
New York　　London

MT

© 2005 The Guilford Press
A Division of Guilford Publications, Inc.
72 Spring Street, New York, NY 10012
www.guilford.com

Printed in the United States of America

This book is printed on acid-free paper.

Last digit is print number: 9 8 7 6 5 4 3 2 1

Library of Congress Cataloging-in-Publication Data available from the Publisher.

ISBN 1-59385-112-X

2/8/07

About the Editor

Mark W. Baldwin, PhD, received his doctorate in 1984 from the University of Waterloo and held postdoctoral fellowships at the Research Center for Group Dynamics at the University of Michigan and the Clarke Institute of Psychiatry at the University of Toronto. He then spent several years pursuing an opportunity to cowrite and cohost the award-winning children's television series *Camp Cariboo*. Returning to academia, Dr. Baldwin taught and researched psychology at the University of Winnipeg for 8 years before assuming, in 1998, his current position in the Department of Psychology at McGill University in Montreal. Along the way, he served as Chair of the Social and Personality section of the Canadian Psychological Association and Associate Editor of the *Personality and Social Psychology Bulletin*, and coauthored (with Rick Hoyle, Michael Kernis, and Mark Leary) the book *Selfhood: Identity, Esteem, Regulation*. His major research interests include interpersonal cognition, self-esteem, and adult attachment theory. Most recently, Dr. Baldwin and his students have been exploring the possibility of designing computer-based exercises to modify maladaptive automatic social cognition and have established the website *www.selfesteemgames.mcgill.ca* to report this research.

Contributors

Susan M. Andersen, PhD, Department of Psychology, New York University, New York, New York

Arthur Aron, PhD, Department of Psychology, State University of New York, Stony Brook, New York

Elaine N. Aron, PhD, Department of Psychology, State University of New York, Stony Brook, New York

Ozlem Ayduk, PhD, Department of Psychology, Columbia University, New York, New York

Jodene R. Baccus, PhD candidate, Department of Psychology, McGill University, Montreal, Quebec, Canada

Mark W. Baldwin, PhD, Department of Psychology, McGill University, Montreal, Quebec, Canada

John A. Bargh, PhD, Department of Psychology, Yale University, New Haven, Connecticut

Kimberly Burton, PhD, Department of Psychology, McGill University, Montreal, Quebec, Canada

Jessica Cameron, PhD, Department of Psychology, University of Manitoba, Winnipeg, Manitoba, Canada

Tanya L. Chartrand, PhD, Fuqua School of Business, Duke University, Durham, North Carolina

Stéphane D. Dandeneau, PhD candidate, Department of Psychology, McGill University, Montreal, Quebec, Canada

Jaye Derrick, BA, Department of Psychology, State University of New York, Buffalo, New York

Geraldine Downey, PhD, Department of Psychology, Columbia University, New York, New York

Beverley Fehr, PhD, Department of Psychology, University of Winnipeg, Winnipeg, Manitoba, Canada

Alan Page Fiske, PhD, Department of Anthropology, University of California, Los Angeles, California

Gráinne M. Fitzsimons, MA, Graduate School of Business, Stanford University, Stanford, California

Melanie Fox, MA, Department of Psychology, Graduate Faculty of Political and Social Science, New School University, New York, New York

Paul Gilbert, FBPsS, Mental Health Research Unit, Kingsway Hospital, Derby, United Kingdom

Nick Haslam, PhD, Department of Psychology, University of Melbourne, Parkville, Australia

Hubert J. M. Hermans, PhD, University of Nijmegen, Nijmegen, The Netherlands

John G. Holmes, PhD, Department of Psychology, University of Waterloo, Waterloo, Ontario, Canada

Mardi J. Horowitz, MD, Department of Psychiatry, University of California, San Francisco, California

Mark R. Leary, PhD, Department of Psychology, Wake Forest University, Winston-Salem, North Carolina

Gary Lewandowski, PhD, Department of Psychology, Monmouth University, West Long Branch, New Jersey

John E. Lydon, PhD, Department of Psychology, McGill University, Montreal, Quebec, Canada

Debra Mashek, PhD, Department of Psychology, George Mason University, Fairfax, Virginia

Tracy McLaughlin-Volpe, PhD, Department of Psychology, University of Vermont, Burlington, Vermont

Danielle Menzies-Toman, PhD candidate, Department of Psychology, McGill University, Montreal, Quebec, Canada

Mario Mikulincer, PhD, Department of Psychology, Bar-Ilan University, Ramat Gan, Israel

Sandra L. Murray, PhD, Department of Psychology, State University of New York, Buffalo, New York

Janina Pietrzak, PhD, Department of Psychology, Columbia University, New York, New York

Jeremy D. Safran, PhD, Department of Psychology, Graduate Faculty of Political and Social Science, New School University, New York, New York

S. Adil Saribay, PhD candidate, Department of Psychology, New York University, New York, New York

Polly Scarvalone, PhD, Department of Psychology, Graduate Faculty of Political and Social Science, New School University, New York, New York

James Shah, PhD, Department of Psychology, Duke University, Durham, North Carolina

Phillip R. Shaver, PhD, Department of Psychology, University of California, Davis, California

Stephen Wright, PhD, Department of Psychology, University of California, Santa Cruz, California

Preface

The human mind is profoundly attuned to the contingencies of social life. Over the past decade, we have seen an explosion of research into interpersonal cognition. The core tenet of this research is that human social cognition is not primarily about isolated social objects, such as self and other, functioning independently. Rather, social cognition is fundamentally about the dynamics of interpersonal interaction. People think about their significant relationships: about whether their loved ones love them in return, about how they fit in with the people they deal with each day, about how to meet their goals within a social network. They wonder why a new friend reminds them of their mother; they worry about the possibility of rejections and humiliations in their interactions; they seek to change the distorted expectancies that seem to lead to problems. This is the stuff of interpersonal cognition.

This volume brings together the world's leading researchers in the field, from a variety of backgrounds. All of them have developed models of the mechanisms whereby people think about their interpersonal experiences and the effects this thinking has on their subsequent interactions and sense of self. Much of the work in this area represents an attempt to integrate social-cognitive models of personality with models drawn from interpersonal, attachment, symbolic interactionist, and psychodynamic traditions. As such, the theoretical background encompasses some of the classic ideas from social and personality psychology, including *working models* (Bowlby), *transference* (Freud), the *looking-glass self* (Cooley), and so on. The recent work in this area combines these insights with current models and research techniques from the social cognition literature. Indeed, the topic of interpersonal cognition has quickly taken its place alongside person perception and self-cognition as one of the central topics in social and personality psychology.

As editor, I encouraged the contributors to devote a portion of their chapters to tracing the theoretical background of their work and outlining the major contributions they have made along the way. I asked them to devote the balance of each chapter to outlining the issues they have studied most recently and isolating the key questions for future research. I encouraged them to present a balance between theory and method, so that readers would come away with an overview of the core issues involved as well as a sense of how to go about studying them.

In the chapters that follow, several themes emerge. First, there is a focus on the basic social-cognitive processes that characterize interpersonal cognition, addressing questions of how information about interpersonal experiences is perceived, interpreted, stored in memory, and recalled. Issues related to the motivational and affective nature of interpersonal information are often front and center. Second, the social construction of identity is a central theme, and notions of the relational self and the interpersonal roots of self-esteem are included in many models presented. Third, several writers ask whether there are meaningful and identifiable constraints on the nature of interpersonal cognition, imposed by the dynamics of social life and the evolutionary history of humankind. Finally, the issue of stability versus variability and change is addressed in several chapters, particularly as clinicians examine the question of how to undo the harmful effects of distorted or maladaptive interpersonal cognition.

In the first chapter, Andersen and Saribay present their analysis of the relational self and the phenomenon of transference. They review over 15 years of research findings, demonstrating that significant-other representations can be activated via triggering cues and then applied in the perception of a novel person. This body of research shows the cognitive, self-evaluative, and, most recently, affective and motivational effects of simply being unconsciously reminded of a significant relationship.

Baldwin and Dandeneau (Chapter 2) focus on the role played by knowledge activation, which makes certain kinds of interpersonal information more or less influential in the perception of ongoing relationships and the self. They review findings linking low self-esteem and insecurity to expectations about social rejection, and then turn to recent work applying learning theory to try to modify activation patterns and thereby increase people's feelings of security.

Pietrzak, Downey, and Ayduk (Chapter 3) present their research on individual differences in rejection sensitivity, in which some people's expectations of rejection are shown to lead to a lower threshold for perceiving negative feedback from others. They combine insights from affective neuroscience with developmental and cognitive models of personality to explain the depression, hostility, conformity, and dissatisfying interpersonal dynamics that can result from anxiously anticipating rejection by valued others.

Leary (Chapter 4) considers the special case of interpersonal cognition in which a person wonders "What does this person think about me?" He reviews his sociometer theory of self-esteem, in which self-evaluative reactions are hypothesized to reflect not a freestanding need for self-esteem but, rather, a hardwired motive for inclusion, valuing, and acceptance by others. He discusses several specific questions arising from his formulation, such as why healthy self-esteem is often seen as largely independent of the opinions of others.

Fitzsimons, Shah, Chartrand, and Bargh (Chapter 5) examine the interplay between interpersonal cognition and goal striving: for example, when—and how—would being reminded of one's mother make one more motivated to achieve? Under what conditions does being in a specific goal state bring to mind one or more specific relationships? They examine questions such as these in the light of current social-cognitive work on goal representation and activation.

Lydon, Burton, and Menzies-Toman (Chapter 6) investigate motivated interpersonal cognition, specifically the sorts of illusions and biases that people often exhibit as they try to maintain a committed relationship important to their identity. The authors consider in detail the delicate calibration often evidenced between individuals' exposure to threatening information of some kind and the motivated cognitive processes that are marshaled in response.

Murray and Derrick (Chapter 7) analyze the complex and consequential process of deciding whether, and how much, to trust an intimate partner. The balance between risk-averse strategies of self-protection and relationship-promoting behaviors based in a confidence about one's partner's acceptance and love is defined by expectations and a range of motivated cognitive processes. This research demonstrates the exquisite interplay between interpersonal cognition and real-world relationship outcomes.

Fehr (Chapter 8) examines the representation and organization of interpersonal knowledge. She reviews research showing that concepts such as love, commitment, anger, and intimacy are organized as prototypes around key exemplars, and that this prototype structure shapes inferences about new interpersonal experiences. She also presents her recent work on the scripts people draw on to define an intimate friendship.

Aron, Mashek, McLaughlin-Volpe, Wright, Lewandowski, and Aron (Chapter 9) propose a form of interpersonal cognition in which a relationship partner is "included" in the self. They review and organize their past research, which has used novel experimental paradigms to show that another person's resources, perspectives, and identities can become experienced as one's own. They also introduce some more recent findings, including the discussion of what it means to feel "too close" to a relationship partner.

Mikulincer and Shaver (Chapter 10) have developed a social-cognitive model of attachment behavior, and they argue that social psychology's extensive documentation of human foibles (including defensive self-enhancement, outgroup hostility, and the like) actually best characterizes response patterns associated with insecure attachment. Their research with chronic and contextually activated attachment orientations supports their argument for a more optimistic view of human nature and grounds the positive psychology movement firmly in attachment theory and interpersonal cognition.

Fiske and Haslam (Chapter 11) review their theory that interpersonal cognition—indeed, interpersonal life—can largely be reduced to four fundamental categories, representing discrete relationship patterns. Their theory builds on anthropological observation, social-cognitive experiments, and neuroscientific explorations, and they use it to analyze phenomena ranging from personality disorders to political structures.

Gilbert's (Chapter 12) theory of social mentalities is based in evolutionary theory and the premise that interpersonal cognition is profoundly shaped by specific information-processing systems that have evolved over millions of years. He analyzes the motives and cognitive competencies that give rise to a set of familiar and influential social role enactments, including care eliciting, social alliance formation, and social ranking.

Baccus and Horowitz (Chapter 13) present a view of interpersonal cognition that is strongly influenced by psychodynamic theory and, more generally, by issues that tend to be confronted in psychotherapy. They review an approach for mapping out the interpersonal structures that define a person's personality conflicts. Then they turn to the issue of schema change, which is always central to psychotherapy, and discuss the processes and difficulties often associated with cases of spousal bereavement.

Scarvalone, Fox, and Safran (Chapter 14) present a model of interpersonal schemas that combines insights from Sullivan's interpersonal psychoanalytic and Bowlby's attachment approaches with modern social-cognitive theory. They propose that people learn implicit, procedural knowledge of how to behave in their significant relationships, and that these schemas can be problematic if they rigidly represent dysfunctional patterns. They review research relating individual variation on the Interpersonal Schema Questionnaire, which assesses expectancies on the axes of affiliation and dominance, with a range of variables including childhood trauma, depression, and transference dynamics in psychotherapy.

Hermans (Chapter 15) explores the thesis that the human mind is inherently interpersonal, a product of an imagined dialogue among a set of voices or positions that make up the individual's inner world. Likening the self to a society, he examines issues of relative power and dominance among different positions and discusses therapeutic change and the anthropological phenomenon of "shape-shifting" as representing the adoption and emphasis of new identity positions.

Holmes and Cameron, in the final chapter, examine selected developments in the field in light of their recent theoretical and empirical work on interdependence theory. For this chapter, which teams one of the field's most experienced scholars with one of its talented young researchers, I encouraged the authors to take a critical look at some of the unresolved and problematic issues they see in this still relatively young literature. Their analysis reminds us that despite the impressive progress that has been made, several thorny questions remain in our attempts to understand interpersonal cognition.

ACKNOWLEDGMENTS

It is a rare treat to have the opportunity to invite one's favorite thinkers and researchers to come together in a volume such as this, and I must say that I have enjoyed the process from start to finish. I would like to thank Seymour Weingarten, Editor-in-Chief at The Guilford Press, for his guidance and encouragement throughout this project, and all of the staff at Guilford who helped to bring the book together. Of course, I am extremely grateful to each of the authors, who replied enthusiastically to my initial requests for contributions and then delivered timely and stimulating chapters. My research has for many years been supported by the Social Sciences and Humanities Research Council of Canada, and I am grateful for that support. Finally, I thank *ma conjointe*, Patricia, for her love, her encouragement, and her immeasurably positive effect on my own interpersonal cognition.

MARK W. BALDWIN

Contents

1

The Relational Self and Transference

*Evoking Motives, Self-Regulation, and Emotions through
Activation of Mental Representations of Significant Others*

SUSAN M. ANDERSEN *and* S. ADIL SARIBAY

The notion that people hold mental representations of significant others—individuals who have been influential in their lives—in memory is not conceptually new. In some respects, it has been present in psychology since the field arose as a separate discipline. It is also central to theories of personality and clinical psychology of historical import (e.g., Freud, 1912/1958) in the discipline of psychology, across prevailing theory and empirical research in social psychology in recent years. Past relationships influence present patterns of thought, feeling, and behavior. Moreover, this is consistent with the fundamental assumption in social cognition that previous knowledge is used to give meaning to present people and situations.

Our research has focused on the social-cognitive process of transference as a way to give meaning to everyday experience in the context of everyday relations. Our work thus has its roots in early theory, while also relying very heavily on basic principles of social cognition and the experimental research methods that characterize the field. Research on transference has formed the basis of the model of the *relational self* (Andersen & Chen, 2002), which holds that people have a repertoire of relational selves in memory, each linked with a specific significant other. In this chapter, we introduce the concept of transference and give an overview of our approach with a focus on issues particularly relevant to motivation and emotion.

1

CONCEPTUALIZING THE RELATIONAL SELF

Our Theoretical Framework: An Overview

Our model of the relational self emphasizes dyadic relationships with *significant others*, individuals who have had a substantial impact on the self, whom one knows very well and cares (or has cared) deeply about (Chen & Andersen, 1999). The relationship may involve a family member or not, and may also be from the long-ago past or from one's current relational life, so long as the relationship partner is (or once was) deeply influential. One acquires particular ways of relating with the other and of experiencing the self in the context of the relationship. Aspects of the self experienced with this person thus become "entangled" in memory with knowledge about the significant other (Andersen & Chen, 2002; Andersen, Reznik, & Chen, 1997; Hinkley & Andersen, 1996). These individuals thus circumscribe the kinds of selves that are both privately experienced and publicly realized (e.g., Higgins, 1989; Higgins & Silberman, 1998). The influence of the significant other on the self can then be reexperienced with a new person, so that this past relationship pattern arises in the present, even when the significant other is not present. One becomes the relational self typically experienced in the original relationship (Andersen & Chen, 2002). For this reason, early (and also later) relationships offer a substrate for the relational selves that develop, and also underlie both resilience and vulnerability (Downey & Feldman, 1996; Gurung, Sarason, & Sarason, 2001; McGowan, 2002; Murray & Holmes, 1999; Pierce & Lydon, 1998; Shields, Ryan, & Cicchetti, 2001). Overall, our model is developmental in this respect, even though the research has not made use of a developmental paradigm.

Representations of significant others are *n*-of-1 representations or exemplars (Linville & Fischer, 1993; Smith & Zarate, 1992) in that each designates a specific, unique individual, rather than a shared notion of a social category, type, or group (e.g., Andersen & Klatzky, 1987; Brewer, 1988; Cantor & Mischel, 1979; Fiske & Taylor, 1991; Higgins & King, 1981). One aspect of significant-other representations that makes them different from representations of nonsignificant others and also different from generic constructs (e.g., specific beliefs about all people) is that they are more closely linked with the self and thus with affect, expectancies, and motives. The latter are thus likely to arise when these representations are activated and used—for example, in transference. Private experiences one has with significant others are encoded in memory and then reexperienced in relation to new persons. Close relationships are characterized by *familiarity* (e.g., Andersen, Reznik, & Glassman, 2004; Prentice, 1990), as well as by their *emotional and motivational relevance for the self*, and are based in no small measure on *exigencies of interdependence* as well. In interdependent relationships, one's outcomes are (or once were) symbolically or concretely interdependent with those of the other (e.g., Rusbult & Van Lange, 1996; see also Mills & Clark,

1994); this idea parallels our conception of a significant other. Likewise, interdependence casts acceptance or rejection by the other in a special light because of the needs that one has in this relationship, given the kind of unit relation (Heider, 1958) one has with the other, a bondedness that is not readily set aside. Needs arising in close relationships are especially important, in part because of this interdependence, especially in relation to caretakers when young, when sheer survival depends on them (Andersen et al., 1997). We discuss these issues more fully later in the chapter.

Our relational-self model is grounded in particular in the literature on transference, which itself is grounded in social cognition and in social construct theory (Bargh, Bond, Lombardi, & Tota, 1986; Higgins, 1996a; Higgins & King, 1981; see also Kelly, 1955), which focuses on transient sources of accessibility (such as priming), chronic sources of accessibility (frequency of prior use), as well as on the applicability of the construct to the stimulus. The theory of the relational self also adopts the assumptions of if–then models of personality (Mischel & Shoda, 1995). That is, it extends transference in part by proposing that the transference process underlies variability in the relational self because significant-other representations are relatively stable over time and yet contextual shifts (based on who is present in the situation) introduce shifts in the relational self across differing interpersonal contexts. In other words, within our relational-self model, we use this if–then framework from personality psychology to consider long-standing influences on the self that *people bring to situations* as "baggage." *Contemporaneous contexts* provoke differing long-standing aspects of the self, and do so because cues in these contexts overlap in some way with prior experience stored in memory. In the relational-self model, specific interpersonal cues in the situation are the "ifs" and the experiences and behaviors that result are the "thens."

Historical Context

Transference in Psychoanalytic Thought and Psychoanalysis

The clinical concept of transference has long been an essential component of psychodynamic theory, psychoanalysis, and psychotherapy (e.g., Ehrenreich, 1989; Greenson, 1965). The literature on transference has thus tended to consider transference theoretically, applying the notion to clinical case studies and in clinical practice, rather than examining it empirically using scientific methods (although see Luborsky & Crits-Christoph, 1990).

In classical Freudian theory, *transference* (Freud, 1912/1958) is said to occur when childhood fantasies and conflicts about a parent are imposed by the patient onto the analyst during psychoanalysis (Freud, 1912/1963; see also Andersen & Glassman, 1996). Freud assumed that people hold in memory "imagoes" of significant others and that they may influence relations with new individuals, both in psychoanalysis and in everyday life (Freud, 1912/1958; Luborsky & Crits-Christoph, 1990; Schimek, 1983). Although such imagoes were proposed, they also carry little causal weight in the central drive-structure model Freud proposed. The drive-structure model and the tripartite structure of mind (id, ego, superego) fueled by psychosexual drive is the bedrock of Freudian theory, embodying and accounting for unconscious conflicts and personality. In the process of transference, then, Freud assumed that the analyst should consider the transference in terms of the patient's unconscious psychosexual conflicts.

Although we do not adopt Freud's complex model or his assumptions about instincts, nor necessarily regard the transference process as irreplaceable as a focus of psychotherapy, our social-cognitive model of transference assumes that mental representations of significant others exist in memory, as do other social constructs and categories, even though they are *n*-of-1 exemplars. Likewise, we assume that it is precisely the activation and use of a significant-other representation in relation to a new person that leads one to "go beyond the information given" (Bruner, 1957) about the new person in ways that define the transference process (e.g., Andersen & Cole, 1990). That is, we assume, as Freud and others did, that transference is not limited to therapeutic settings. We also assume it is not limited to individuals suffering from psychopathology or "neurosis." We focus on transference among "normal" populations as a normal process in the contexts of everyday life, thus depathologizing the concept, even though there may be implications for psychotherapy. Our focus is daily life.

To contrast with a different clinical theory, Harry Stack Sullivan (1953) proposed that early interpersonal relations result in what he called "personifications" of the self and the significant other (i.e., the caretaker), and that "dynamisms," or dynamics, provide the link between the self and the other (as personifications) by characterizing the typical relational patterns enacted by self and other. The idiosyncratic and subjective content of each person's personifications of significant others and of their associated dynamisms then form the basis of transference. Sullivan termed the transference process *parataxic distortion.*

His notion of parataxic distortion is close to our conception and is distinct in many ways from how transference is conceptualized by Freud. Sullivan's emphasis is on models of self and other and assumed basic needs that have little to do with (go well beyond) infantile sexuality. In addition, and in particular, he assumed a fundamental need for satisfaction that includes a motive to experience tenderness and to be connected with the other, as well as motives for self-expression and effectiveness and competence in relations with significant others. To protect the self, a need for overall safety and security is also fundamental in his view. These basic needs for connection and security are also central in our thinking (Andersen et al., 1997).

Still other conceptions of transference also exist, of course (e.g.,

Horney, 1939; Horowitz, 1989, 1991; Kernberg, 1976; Kohut, 1971; Luborsky & Crits-Christoph, 1990). There is great variability among these theories. The methods of analysis used also vary widely. The most widely adopted definition of *transference* appears to be "the experiencing of feelings, drives, attitudes, fantasies, and defenses toward a person in the present which are inappropriate to the person and are a repetition, a displacement of reaction originating in regard to significant persons of early childhood" (Greenson, 1965, p. 156; see also Andersen & Baum, 1994). In our model, observed in our data, the transference we demonstrate fits this general definition reasonably well (for related theoretical work, see Singer, 1988, and Westen, 1988).

The Relevance of Attachment Theory

A theoretical model that is fundamentally integrative and relevant to how the self is bound up with important others is attachment theory. Attachment theory is integrative with respect to psychoanalytic and cognitive-behavioral theories, as well as with ethological and evolutionary psychology. It also assumes that mental models of the self and other are important and are shaped largely through early experiences with caregivers (e.g., Ainsworth, Blehar, Walters, & Wall, 1978; Bombar & Littig, 1996; Bowlby, 1969, 1973, 1980; Bretherton, 1985; Thompson, 1998). Attachment theory has generated a great deal of empirical research since Bowlby (1969, 1973, 1980) laid its foundations. Going beyond research on infants and children, the research on adult attachment has tended to focus on trait-like attachment styles and relatively little on internal working models of the self and other. Even though the latter are centrally a part of the assumptive framework of attachment theory, they were not subjected to careful experimental examination until quite recently. Fortunately, recent research has begun to fill in this gap (e.g., Baldwin, Fehr, Keedian, Seidel, & Thompson, 1993; Baldwin, Keelan, Fehr, Enns, & Koh-Rangarajoo, 1996; Mikulincer, 1998; Mikulincer & Horesh, 1999; Pierce & Lydon, 2001; Shaver & Mikulincer, 2002).

Still more work is needed to incorporate attachment theory into social-cognitive and other social-psychological models of the self and relationships. From our point of view, our model of the relational self is compatible with assumptions about internal models of self and other, and with the notion that the need for connection should make the responsiveness of caretakers particularly important in emotional suffering and resilience in the relationship (see Thompson, 1998). In our view, transference may be a mechanism underlying attachment processes, that is, underlying how internal working models in interpersonal relationships are used. This assumption is implicit in attachment theory and fits with an activation model in which specific situational cues evoke the attachment system, through activating a representation of a significant other in transference.

EVIDENCE ON THE RELATIONAL SELF AND TRANSFERENCE

To test the assumptions that follow from our conceptualization of transference and our model of the relational self, prior experimental research has
systematically examined the processes thought to underlie transference and
its consequences for social relations. We now turn to the specific findings
on which our conceptions of the relational self and transference are based.
We first describe our paradigm in brief (see Andersen & Chen, 2002, for a
more complete presentation) and then present our basic findings. The research addresses the transference process and its implications for manifestations of the relational self, including basic needs, motives, emotions, self-
evaluation, and self-regulatory efforts.

Methodology in Brief

Research on the social-cognitive process of transference involves activating
a significant-other representation through the presentation of triggering
cues. The cues themselves typically take the form of features about a new
person derived from those that the research participant in fact generated in
a previous session to describe a significant other. We begin with a preliminary session in which we ask participants to think of a significant other
and to write descriptive sentences in freehand to portray this individual.
Such features tend to include apparent habits and activities, ways of relating, physical features, attitudes, preferences, traits, and so on. The actual
experiment is presumed to be unrelated and takes place at least 2 weeks after this preliminary session. Participants arrive to a lab setting with multiple rooms and are led to believe they will meet an "interaction partner"
later in the session. They are exposed to sentence predicates about this new
person, which suggest that this person does (or does not) share a small
number of the significant other's qualities (based on the features they had
listed about their significant other). Following this exposure, their memory,
evaluation, affect, motives, expectancies, self-ratings, and behavior are assessed, depending on the purposes of the particular study. In most studies,
each participant in the control condition (i.e., the nontransference condition) is yoked on a one-to-one basis with another participant who is in the
experimental condition (i.e., the transference condition). In this way, each
pair of yoked participants is exposed to the exact same features about the
new person. This allows the content of the experimental stimuli to be perfectly controlled across conditions, and enables unequivocal conclusions
about the consequences of being exposed to significant-other resemblance
in a new person, which we show provokes the phenomenon of transference.
    In this combined idiographic–nomothetic design, the content of trans-
ference is specific to each participant but the processes we investigate are

generalizable. Moreover, the process does not require a particular standing on a predisposing individual difference factor, such as relational-interdependent self-construal (Cross, Bacon, & Morris, 2000). Though we have not tested this particular question, the process readily occurs without any such preselection. Moreover, it is not a phenomenon that occurs only for women (whom research suggests are more relationally oriented than men), nor one that occurs only in interdependent cultures (e.g., Japan), and thus does not occur in the United States. To the contrary, all our research has been conducted in the United States and most of it includes both males and females.

Inference and Memory

Initial research on the social-cognitive process of transference focused on memory and inferences about a new person, resulting from triggering a significant-other representation. This work clearly indicates that people tend to fill in the blanks about new people on the basis of their knowledge of significant others—when a particular significant-other representation is triggered. People exposed to features of a new person that are distinctively associated with a significant other have their significant-other representations activated. This is assessed through recognition memory. When tested, people indicate that they are more confident when they were exposed to significant-other features about the new person—features not actually presented—than do people in a control condition (e.g., Andersen, Glassman, Chen, & Cole, 1995; Andersen & Cole, 1990). This effect has been demonstrated repeatedly.

Several experimental controls have been used to rule out possible alternative explanations for this basic effect. For example, because the very stimuli that the participant encounters in the experiment in our paradigm are self-generated by the individual him- or herself in a previous session, one needs to be concerned about the well-known influence of self-generation, which could potentially account for the phenomenon. Both enhanced memory and other mnemonic processes result from self-generation of stimuli and can thus offer a compelling alternative explanation for transference unless ruled out. In a series of studies, we compared significant-other representations with other kinds of representations that were also self-generated by the individual before the experiment—that is, they also generated descriptors of a nonsignificant other, of a variety of public figures, and of a social category as well (e.g., a stereotype they use), such that all the stimuli in the experiment were self-generated, holding constant self-generation. Overall, our inference and memory effect turns out to be strongest when significant-other features are presented, leading to a greater tendency to go beyond the information given about the new person, which suggests that the effect simply cannot be accounted for merely by self-generation or the activation of a social stereotype (e.g., Andersen et al., 1995; Glassman & Andersen, 1999a).

Another most pressing alternative explanation that must also be ruled out (and that we thus hold constant in most of our research) involves the specific content of the features the individual lists at pretest: perhaps there is just something special about the content of the significant-other features that drives the effect. We address this issue through one-to-one yoking of research participants in the significant-other-resemblance condition with participants in the control condition. As noted, each participant in the control condition is yoked with one participant in the experimental condition so that both in the pair are exposed to exactly the same features about the new person in the experiment. Stimulus content is thus perfectly controlled.

The phenomenon has been widely demonstrated. The evidence also clearly shows that this inference and memory effect also occurs for both positive and negative significant others (e.g., Andersen & Baum, 1994; Andersen, Reznik, & Manzella, 1996), and holds across gender and individual differences such as those who have one kind of self-discrepancy as opposed to another kind from a parent's standpoint (Reznik & Andersen, 2003; this research is described below) or who happen to have been physically abused by a parent (or not abused; see Berenson & Andersen, 2003). It has also been shown that the effect can persist over time, so that once it occurs, it can remain over, say, a week's duration (Glassman & Andersen, 1999b).

It is also of interest that this inference and memory effect has been shown to occur in part due to chronic accessibility of significant-other representations. Our research has shown that even when the significant-other representation has no particular applicability to a new person (i.e., there is no applicability-based cueing), and when there is no immediately preceding prime, there is a low-level tendency to use significant-other representations more than, for example, other social category or person representations. People tend to fill in the blanks about new people in accord with what they know about significant others (Andersen et al., 1995; Chen, Andersen, & Hinkley, 1999). This chronic effect is increased, however, with the presence of cues indicating that a novel person is similar in some way to the significant other. Other interpersonal work in social psychology has also demonstrated similar additive effects of contextual cueing and chronic accessibility (e.g., Baldwin et al., 1996).

Automatic and Unconscious Activation

Perhaps the most commonly agreed upon assumption about transference as proposed by Freud, and as revised by Sullivan, is that it should arise outside of conscious awareness. Although Freud's conceptualization of conscious processes differs from ours, our assumption is and has been that one's knowledge about significant others is brought to bear on responses to new people and that this happens quite automatically—without much in the way of attention, effort, control, or conscious awareness (Andersen et al., 2004; see also Bargh, 1989).

There is also evidence supporting the idea that significant-other representations may be used with particular ease or efficiency even outside of transference. For example, research in which participants were asked to retrieve from memory and to list various features of a significant other has shown that features of these representations are retrieved from memory exceptionally quickly as compared with features of other people or categories (Andersen & Cole, 1990; Andersen et al., 1995).

To test the specific hypothesis about the unconscious activation of transference, the question was framed in terms of whether or not the significant-other representations could be activated subliminally—in a way that would lead to transference. The research involved participants in a computer game with another participant, allegedly seated elsewhere in the building, about whom they might learn something. Afterward they completed an inference task about this person. During the "computer game," significant-other features were flashed for less than 90 milliseconds in parafoveal vision and pattern-masked. In the yoked-control condition, participants were exposed to these exact same features—that is, of someone else's significant other—and were also presented with these stimuli subliminally (Glassman & Andersen, 1999a). As predicted, across two studies, the results clearly showed that participants in the significant-other condition made more inferences about the new person that derived from their own significant other than did participants in the control condition. Consciousness is not a precondition for transference. In our research, we ask participants to be accurate in their perception of the new person, and we do not ask them to compare the new person to anyone from their lives. Indeed, when participants are excluded from the experiment if they happen to spontaneously mention seeing the link between the new person's features and those listed weeks previously about a significant other, the inference and memory effect still holds (e.g., Berenson & Andersen, 2003).

Overall, the transference phenomenon and the relational self should arise relatively automatically, that is, effortlessly and even when one is unaware of it, does not intend to respond in this way, and has little control over the process. Other evidence from within this paradigm, which we review below, is also consistent with this assumption.

Evaluation and Affect

The relative immediacy with which we seem to form evaluations of new people—and the minimal information we apparently need in order to do this—are in some ways surprising. Once introduced to a stranger, we typically have an idea of how much we like the person, without devoting much (or any) effort to scrutinizing the qualities this new person has. Our research suggests that such rapid evaluations are often driven by significant-other representations. Although we discuss evaluative and affective aspects of transference in more detail later in the chapter, it is worth reviewing some basic findings here.

A central tenet of social cognition is that when a mental representation, such as a stereotype, is activated in interpersonal perception and applied to a new person, it should elicit the same positive or negative evaluation—in accordance with the theory of schema-triggered affect (Fiske & Pavelchak, 1986). We have shown that this occurs in transference. That is, when participants learn about a new person who resembles their own significant other (vs. that of a yoked participant), the new person is evaluated more positively when he or she was portrayed so as to resemble a positive significant other rather than a negative one (Andersen et al., 1996; Andersen & Baum, 1994; Berk & Andersen, 2000) or when the new person resembles the participant's own rather than another participant's positive significant other (Baum & Andersen, 1999; Reznik & Andersen, 2003). That is, under the condition of resemblance to a positive significant other, the new person comes to be particularly well liked, and this does not occur in the control condition. Even evoking a parental representation in transference associated with a self-discrepancy will also lead to the transference response as indexed by a more positive evaluation of the new person (Reznik & Andersen, 2003).

Depending on how positively one regards any particular significant other, one's most basic and immediate emotional response to the person should reflect this overall regard. If one loves a parent, then one should feel a rather primordial and simple positive affect in relation to him or her: the warm glow of familial bonding. Given this affect, it also makes sense that, when such a positive significant-other representation is activated in transference, a relatively immediate positive emotional response should be experienced. Indeed, this is exactly what occurs in the form of subtle facial expressions (Andersen et al., 1996).

That is, when learning about a new person in our standard paradigm by reading about him or her, participants' facial expressions take on the overall affect associated with the significant other—at the instance they see each feature. This affective response, coded by trained judges who viewed videotapes of participants' faces while they were in this phase of the experiment, reflected the overall evaluation of the significant other. These facial expressions are emitted rapidly, apparently with little forethought, as automatic evaluation is known to be (Bargh, Chaiken, Raymond, & Hymes, 1996). These data are thus suggestive about the relatively automatic nature of such immediate affective responses (Andersen et al., 2004), and also the likely pervasiveness of such automatic affect in everyday social encounters, including those involving transference.

It is worth mentioning as well that our treatment of emotion and affect in transference is compatible with the notion that people tend to experience a kind of "core affect" relatively instantaneously (Russell, 2003). Such core affect is thought to involve the conscious experience of neurophysiological states that are heavily defined by sheer positivity or negativity (the dimension of pleasure), but also by the dimension of arousal. Core affect is the building block of more finely tuned categories of emotional experience that should result largely from attributional and appraisal processes. A general tendency to evaluate even novel objects as positive or negative suggests that this kind of automatic evaluation is ubiquitous (Duckworth, Bargh, Garcia, & Chaiken, 2002). We argue that such core affect in the form of positive and negative affective experiences should be triggered in transference, and find that it in fact is. This research on facial affect in transference has shown the basic positive versus negative affective response based on the activation of a positive significant-other representation. In later pages, we address the question of what kinds of specific emotions are evoked in transference, and the conditions under which this occurs based on the nature of the self–other relationship.

Expectancies of Acceptance and Rejection

In line with the need for connection as a fundamental human motive, research also suggests that people are especially sensitive to contingencies of acceptance and rejection in close relationships and that they store relevant perceptions in memory as part of relationship structures (e.g., Andersen et al., 1996; Baldwin & Sinclair, 1996; Downey & Feldman, 1996). We have argued, in particular, that people's expectations for the significant other's acceptance or rejection should also come into play in the context of transference. That is, when in a transference a new person resembles a positive significant other, rather than a negative one, people should be more likely to report expecting to be accepted by the new person and not rejected by him or her. This is exactly what the evidence shows (e.g., Andersen et al., 1996; Berk & Andersen, 2000).

Likewise, when the overall view of the significant other is held constant as positive, as would typically be the case for a parent, research also shows that even those individuals who have a conflictual relationship with a particular parent—by having a self-discrepancy (see Higgins, 1987) from this parent's standpoint—still report acceptance expectancies in transference. That is, they expect to be evaluated more positively (i.e., to be more accepted) in a transference even when this transference involves a parent in whose eyes they are self-discrepant relative to a control condition in which they are exposed to control stimuli (Reznik & Andersen, 2003), which shows how robust the phenomenon can be. On the other hand, there are also limits. That is, when a parent who is reportedly loved was also physically abusive during one's childhood, one is in fact more likely to expect rejection in the transference condition relative to the control condition (Berenson & Andersen, 2003). In addition, when a significant other is someone from one's own family of origin and is positive, but is also someone with whom one tends to experience a dreaded self, one is also more likely to expect rejection in the context of transference (Reznik & Andersen, 2004). In short, anticipated acceptance or rejection from a new person arises in transference in ways that can derive from a number of different sources. One such source is how positive or negative the significant other is seen to be. Another is the degree of negativity one experiences about the self in the relationship. Expected acceptance or rejection in transference thus depends more intricately on the content and quality of the relationship than do some other indices of transference.

Other work has shown that people who are sensitive to rejection are especially vigilant to cues of disapproval from others, and that their perceptions of rejection and expectancies of more rejection are readily activated (Baldwin & Meunier, 1999; Baldwin & Sinclair, 1996; Downey & Feldman, 1996). If rejection expectancies are stored with significant-other representations, then the chronic accessibility of such representations, which we have demonstrated, suggests one way in which rejection expectancies with various significant others may generalize and be used in interpreting new social encounters.

Interpersonal Behavior

The notion that the patterns of behavior that one engages in with a particular significant other should be stored in the knowledge linking the significant other with the self in memory is central to our assumptions. Hence, another line of research has extended the paradigm into the realm of overt behavior in a brief dyadic interaction, specifically, an unstructured telephone conversation between the individual experiencing (or not experiencing) transference and another entirely naïve individual (Berk & Andersen, 2000). In this kind of behavioral confirmation paradigm (Snyder, Tanke, & Berscheid, 1977), we were thus able to examine each participant's responses in the conversation and to focus particularly on the behavior of the "target" person in the interaction when the main participant was or was not experiencing a positive or a negative transference.

The results indicated that when the new person resembled the perceiver's own significant other, and hence transference occurred, the target's own interpersonal behavior was rated as containing more of the same affect associated with the significant-other representation in memory, whether positive or negative. The ratings of independent judges, who assessed the target's contributions to the conversation without being able to hear what the perceiver was saying in the encounter, indicated more positive affect in the target's voice in the positive versus the negative transference, which did not occur in the control condition (Berk & Andersen, 2000). In short, behavioral confirmation—also known as the "self-fulfilling prophecy"—arose in the target person's behavior in transference. The target's conversational behavior took on the emotional tone of the overall affect linked with the significant-other representation and relationship.

Of course, the behavioral confirmation process is not thought to require any conscious intention to induce the other person into confirming one's expectations (see, e.g., Chen & Bargh, 1997), and hence it presumably takes place more or less outside of perceivers' awareness. In the process, the affect triggered in transference unfolds sequentially in the interaction in a way that involves it being reciprocated by the new person. Minimally, this evidence concretizes the literature on transference by tracing the transference process into its unfolding in behavior in an interaction, further attesting to the power of the phenomenon.

The Working Self-Concept and Self-Evaluation

A common thread running through many findings in the interpersonal literature is that the self is experienced and expressed in different ways according to the present interaction partner, whether this person is physically present or absent (and thus mainly psychologically present). At the simplest level, we posit that how the self is reflected upon, experienced, and expressed in a relationship is encoded as part of the general relationship structure and activated upon the activation of other elements. That is, people experience different versions of the self with differing significant others, and once reminded of a significant other, whether implicitly or explicitly, this should evoke the relational self with that other.

Supporting this idea, knowledge of the self typically experienced with a significant other comes flowing into the working self-concept when a new person activates that significant-other representation (Hinkley & Andersen, 1996). This occurs for both positive and negative significant others. That is, one becomes the self one is with this significant other in the context of transference, controlling for baseline self-definition (elicited at pretest). Beyond the fact of this change to bring the features of the relational self into the transference, it is also possible to ask about the valence of this shift in the self that occurs. Valence in the self is important because self-evaluation and self-worth are of abiding interest. Indeed, the results show that negative transference (when a negative significant-other representation is activated) provokes an influx of especially negative features into the working self-concept. A positive change in self-worth is evoked in a transference involving a positive significant other, in each case controlling for baseline self-evaluation (at pretest) (Hinkley & Andersen, 1996). Hence, shifts in self-evaluation and self-worth do occur in transference.

Moving beyond the positive–negative dichotomy in significant others, it is also possible to examine self-evaluation when holding constant significant-other evaluation and varying the nature of the self typically experienced with the significant other. That is, we examined transference with a positive significant other associated with a dreaded self (rather than a desired self; see Reznik & Andersen, 2004). It is entirely possible to like or love a significant other, and yet to repeatedly find oneself enacting a dreaded version of the self with this person. The results indicate that when a significant other is associated with a dreaded self and this significant-other representation is triggered in transference, the shift in self-evaluation that occurs in the direction of the self-with-the-significant-other becomes considerably more negative. This does not occur in the absence of transference. Moreover, it does not occur when the transference involves a significant other associated with a desired self. As another way of verifying these findings, this research has also indicated that when a dreaded self is elicited in a positive transference, the features of the dreaded self become especially accessible, as indicated by response latencies (Reznik & Andersen, 2004).

In our view, these findings suggest that transference may be a mechanism both for stability in the relational self—due to the long-standing presence of these significant others in an individual's life (and the chronic accessibility of these representations)—and for variability in the relational self, through shifts in the self provoked by triggering cues in new people. The latter—the triggering cues—are the "ifs". The "thens" are the transference process and the shifts in the self that it entails (Andersen & Chen, 2002; Mischel & Shoda, 1995). In fact, heightened accessibility of relevant relational-self features is consistent with our assumption that spread of activation from the significant-other representation to relevant self-aspects should occur when the significant-other representation is triggered in transference (see Andersen et al., 2004).

The shift in self-evaluation as a function of the relational self in transference is largely the kind of shift characterized in the model of contingent self-worth, which also adopts an if–then approach (Crocker & Wolfe, 2001). In that model, and in the research based on it, cues that are particularly relevant to contingencies of worth are the ones most likely to induce shifts in self-evaluation. Our view is comparable and specifically focused on the relational context of the self (see also Baldwin & Sinclair, 1996). Shifts in the self are evoked in transference, as are shifts in expectancies for rejection. Indeed, both kinds of shifts are also predicted to occur as a function of context and preexisting sensitivity to rejection, and this does tend to occur, as the if–then model of rejection sensitivity suggests (e.g., Downey & Feldman, 1996).

Specific Needs and Motives

We have alluded to our assumptions about basic needs and motivations in transference. In our view, motivation must be central to conceptualizing the self in relation to others because of the emotional investment people have in their relationships. As noted, motivation is also central both to attachment theory and to interpersonal psychodynamic theories. Consistent with many approaches to motivation and interpersonal functioning, we assume the need for human connection—for relatedness, tenderness, attachment, or belonging—to be central in our theory. The need for connection fuels the "significance" of significant others, and also the desire for an experience of mutual caring, respect, trust, and love. On the other hand, we acknowledge that other needs besides the basic need for connection are also important. Needs for autonomy or freedom (e.g., Deci & Ryan, 1985), for competence or control (e.g., Seligman, 1975), for meaning (e.g., Becker, 1971), and for felt security (e.g., Epstein, 1973) figure prominently in our model. Although research has yet to examine how all of these needs might arise in transference, and potentially when they might combine additively or interact in a relationship, research has demonstrated a role for the motive to be connected in transference and also a role for the motive to protect the self (or for felt security).

In our theory, we take the view that motives and goals that involve significant others are stored in memory as mental constructs linked with those significant others and, like any other construct, can be activated by contextual triggers (e.g., Bargh, 1990, 1997; Bargh & Gollwitzer, 1994). When a significant-other representation is activated in transference, it therefore influences cognition, affect, and behavior in goal-based ways—in the context of the new relations experienced. The goal-based ways in which transference influences people's interpersonal responses can be seen as falling into four classes: activating specific needs and goals; activating a self-regulatory focus; producing a self-protective regulatory response; or producing an other-protective regulatory response. We now consider each of these in turn.

First, there is the simple matter that the motives and goals one has with a significant other, which are stored with the significant-other representation in memory, should be pursued with a new person in transference. In particular, when experiencing a transference that involves a positive significant other, rather than a negative one, people tend to experience a motivation to approach the new person, in short, a motive to be emotionally open with him or her overall—rather than to withdraw and to be distant (Andersen et al., 1996; Berk & Andersen, 2000). A comparable effect also arises when the significant other is a parent and one has a self-discrepancy from that parent's perspective. In spite of the self-discrepancy, emotional closeness motivation is still evoked in transference (compared with a con-

trol condition) (Reznik & Andersen, 2003). In addition, complementing
the motivation to be close, evidence also suggests that people not only
"want" to be close to a new person who resembles a positive significant
other, but they also report that they in fact do "feel" closer to him or her
(Andersen & Strasser, 2000).

On the other hand, when the transference involves a positive significant other with whom one tends to have a goal for love and acceptance
that is chronically unsatisfied, the transference will evoke less emotional
closeness motivation, presumably due to prior disappointment (Berk &
Andersen, 2004). With a transference involving such significant others,
people report less motivation to be intimate than they do in other conditions. Hence, chronic goals with a significant other are evoked in transference, along with the significant other's typical responses to such bids.

Thus, this work links up nicely with other literatures in social cognition including research that has shown that goal states are automatically
activated (Bargh & Barndollar, 1996; Bargh & Chartrand, 1999; Bargh,
Gollwitzer, Lee-Chai, Barndollar, & Trötschel, 2001; see also Aarts &
Dijksterhuis, 2000). Recent research has now begun to extend the auto-
motive perspective into the realm of behavior in interpersonal relationships
(Fitzsimons & Bargh, 2003; Shah, 2003a, 2003b).

Self-Regulatory Focus

Beyond the activation of a need or a goal by means of activating a significant other, it is also of importance to ask about how self-regulation arises
in transference (Reznik & Andersen, 2003). To the extent that a particular
self-regulatory style or focus—that is, whether one is geared toward
obtaining positive outcomes or toward avoiding negative outcomes—is associated with the significant other, this self-regulatory focus should be activated in transference. For example, if a significant other has tended to
withhold affection or rewards based on poor performance, reaching his or
her ideals should become paramount (given the threat of the loss of love),
and should thus be triggered in transference. Likewise, if the other has
tended to threaten punishments (harsh treatment) based on poor performance, then averting or avoiding these punishments should become important, and should be triggered in transference (e.g., Andersen & Chen,
2002; also see Higgins, 1987). Self-regulatory responses should become
profoundly relevant in relation to significant others because these others
are uniquely positioned to comfort and enable an affective equilibrium.
Likewise, they are uniquely positioned to disturb one's equilibrium simply
because of one's emotional investment in their various responses.

According to self-discrepancy theory and self-regulatory focus theory,
self-discrepancies in which ideal standards are operative and discrepant
from the self are part of a broader self-regulatory system focused on promotion and on attaining positive outcomes. By contrast, self-discrepancies

in which ought standards are operative and discrepant from the self are also part of a broader self-regulatory system, in this case, focused on prevention and on detecting and avoiding negative outcomes (Higgins, 1996b, 1996c). In particular, research has examined the degree to which activation of a significant-other representation in transference would indirectly activate a self-discrepancy from the other's perspective (Reznik & Andersen, 2003). That is, participants experiencing transference involving a significant other from whose point of view they have an ideal self-discrepancy or an ought self-discrepancy should experience the activation of this particular discrepancy, which should lead to the relevant self-regulatory focus.

Indeed, the results showed just this. More motivation to avoid the new person in transference was evoked among ought-discrepant participants expecting to meet a new person relative to when they were told they would not need to do this, that is, during the precise moment that prevention was relevant (Reznik & Andersen, 2003). On the other hand, among ideal-discrepant participants, transference evoked less motivation to avoid the new person while expecting to meet him or her as compared to when no longer expecting to do so. No such pattern occurred for either group in the no-resemblance condition. Hence, activation of the significant-other representation in transference evoked the distinct self-regulatory system known to be part of having an ideal versus an ought discrepancy. We see this as an important contribution to regulatory focus research, since transference arises in the face of novel interaction partners and shows the subtle impact of significant others on the motivational system. Other recent research also supports this, as well as the notion that such processes may occur outside of awareness (Shah, 2003b, Study 3).

Self-Protective Self-Regulation

We now look at two forms of self-regulation based on the experience of threat in the context of the transference. Both forms of self-regulation depend on what exactly is threatened. Specifically, a threat to the self is likely to produce self-protective self-regulation (e.g., Hinkley & Andersen, 1996), and a threat to the other is likely to evoke other-protective self-regulation (e.g., Andersen et al., 1996). In each case, the result is that one inflates one's view or enhances one's positive emotions about whatever it is that is under attack.

When a threat to the self is experienced with reference to a significant other, then a kind of compensatory self-enhancement or self-inflation should arise to protect the self. This kind of process has been widely observed in other research literatures (e.g., Greenberg & Pyszczynski, 1985; Morf & Rhodewalt, 2001; Showers, 1992; Steele, 1988; Taylor & Brown, 1988). Hence, such a process should arise in transference when what is threatened in the transference is the self because the transference has negative implications for the self. One way in which a significant other may be experienced as a threat to the self—as negative for the self—is when he or she is disliked or not positively evaluated. As we have described, a negative transference provokes an influx of negative self-features into the working self-concept, the kind of threat to the self that ought to provoke a compensatory response, which we term "self-protective self-regulation" (Hinkley & Andersen, 1996). The results show that this is exactly what occurs. When the negative influx occurs, a parallel recruitment of positive (but transference-unrelated) features into the self-concept also occurs, which bolsters self-regard. The influx of negativity in self-evaluation provokes a complementary self-enhancement.

Indeed, this should occur not only in a transference involving a negative significant other but also in a transference involving a positive significant other—so long as this positive significant other is one with whom one tends to experience a dreaded self (Reznik & Andersen, 2004; see also Andersen et al., 2004). As described earlier, the evidence indicated that when the significant other associated with a dreaded self was activated in transference, the relevant relational-self features flowed into the self-concept that was negative in the dreaded self condition. The working self-concept shifted toward the relational self with this significant other, reflecting a threat to the self in the dreaded self condition. However, those aspects of the self that did not shift in the direction of the relational self revealed a compensatory self-enhancement. That is, when the dreaded self was evoked in transference, an influx of positive self features also flowed into the working self-concept, counteracting the threat.

Other-Protective Self-Regulation

The second form of self-regulation based on threat is other-protective. People are motivated to protect their perceptions of the significant others in whom they are invested. The interdependence one has with significant others for one's own outcomes and well-being makes it clear why one may be motivated to view a positive significant other as basically good, loving and caring, and safe in spite of flaws. Indeed, people tend to transform the flaws of their loved ones into virtues, thereby finding ways to regard shortcomings as particularly charming, funny, or endearing (e.g., Murray & Holmes, 1993). The negative aspect of the other, which might otherwise be problematic or threatening to one's view, becomes a plus. Finding a way to respond positively to negative qualities of the other may in fact be essential to maintaining a close relationship, and may thus be very well practiced. If this is well practiced, it ought to take place relatively automatically, which is what our evidence on affect regulation in transference suggests.

In short, the relatively immediate expression of facial affect in transference yields especially positive affect in a positive transference when triggering features were in fact negative (Andersen et al., 1996). In a positive transference, people actually express more positive affect in their facial expressions in response to negative characteristics deriving from their positive significant other—as these negative features are encountered about a new person. In the absence of transference, nothing of the kind occurs. The positive regard for the significant other, not the valence of the features, determines the emotion. Even though participants themselves classified these features as negative at pretest (when they listed them before the experiment), they also tended in the experiment to express positive affect to these negative features

Cast in this light, this form of self-regulation would seem to be adaptive and useful for healthy relationships. When considered differently, however, it becomes feasible that instead of minor annoyances in the behavior of a significant other, the negative qualities in question could actually be harmful. If one were to find oneself responding positively to negative behaviors that are potentially dangerous, this could be maladaptive. Registering no alarm to signals of imminent danger could be profoundly unhealthy.

In one study, for example, we asked how adults abused by a parent would respond emotionally to the parent in terms of their automatic facial affect (Berenson & Andersen, 2003). In general, when participants learned about a new person who resembled their parent and this parent was one who had been physically abusive while participants were growing up, they actually showed far more positive facial affect than did comparable participants in the control condition (who were exposed to the same triggering cues but did not experience transference). Schema-triggered facial affect emerged in their facial expressions in spite of their painful history with this parent.

Even more remarkably, this effect even obtained when we assessed responses to a negative contextual cue about the new person in transference (Berenson & Andersen, 2003). That is, because the abuse sequence in abusive relationships often begins with signs of frustration or simmering anger in the abuser, responses of this kind may be signals of trouble. This contextual cue was thus presented in the form of information that the new person seemed to be in an increasingly irritable, angry mood, and this was presented after the participant learned about the new person who resembled his or her parent (or did not). In the transference condition, participants came to express considerably more positive facial affect in response to the cue that the new person was becoming increasingly irritable and angry than they did in the nontransference condition. Moreover, this held regardless of abuse status. Even among individuals physically abused by the relevant parent (possibly even threatened with a gun or a knife), learning about the new person's increasingly irritable mood evoked more positive facial affect in the transference than in the control condition. In short, other-protective self-regulation appears to be a common response to threatening cues in the context of a positive transference.

Activating Subtle Shifts in Emotional Responses in Transference

We have shown, as noted, that a generic positive or negative affect will tend to arise in transference. As we have argued, people are deeply emotionally invested in those people in their lives whom they regard as personally significant. Because of this investment, it stands to reason that significant others would hold considerable sway in emotions. In this light, it is curious that researchers interested in interpersonal aspects of the self have focused relatively little research attention on the emotions (although see Berscheid, 1994), although there have been some major exceptions, such as self-discrepancy (Higgins, 1987) and attachment theories (e.g., Collins, 1996). We now turn to two areas where we have examined complexities in the activation of affect: the dynamics of positive mood and the influence of individual differences.

Generic Positive Mood and Its Disruption in a Positive Transference

Given that significant others are heavily laden with affect, these representations should be expected to influence, beyond the kind of relatively immediate facial affect we have mentioned, more free-floating self-reported mood as well. Evidence has in fact shown that transference may sometimes evoke mood states consistent with the overall positivity or negativity of the significant other. In one study, for example, participants experiencing a transference involving a positive, rather than a negative, significant other reported significantly less depressive mood, an effect that did not occur in the absence of transference (i.e., in the control condition; see Andersen & Baum, 1994). The effect size in this case, however, was quite small; moreover, other studies have failed to replicate the effect in these simple terms (Andersen et al., 1996).

Of course, as we have noted, research in our lab has shown that positive facial affect is evoked relatively immediately in the context of a positive transference, that is, when a positive significant-other representation is activated (Andersen et al., 1996; Berenson & Andersen, 2003). Hence, using more sensitive measures, unbiased by the influences that impinge upon self-reports, we found that transference clearly does have a relatively direct effect on emotional responses. Indeed, we have argued, based on this evidence on facial affect, that transference may evoke a kind of immediate and generic "core affect" (see Russell, 2003). Moreover, it is feasible that such subtle and immediate emotional responses may in part be the basis of the overall mood states that do (or do not) arise in transference.

This makes it even more pressing to understand exactly how it is that positive mood states do not always arise in the context of positive transference. Perhaps the explanation has to do with the fact that affective responses that arise slowly over the course of an experimental session are likely to be influenced by numerous expectancies and cognitions in the session beyond the first moments of learning about the new person. In examining this question, we thus consider a number of factors that may interfere with a positive mood in the context of a positive transference. The nature of the disruption of positive mood can stem from contextual factors with the new person, aspects of the relationship with the significant other, or aspects of the self in the relationship. We consider each in turn.

Contextually Based Expectancy Violation through Interpersonal Roles. Most significant-other relationships are defined partly by norms that derive from the particular role relationship one has with the significant other. The interpersonal role with the other involves well-developed expectations and is stored in memory with the relationship. In this respect, a role is normative and prescriptive. It specifies what is expected of each person. Hence, when the significant-other representation is activated in transference, the relevant role relationship should also be activated, along with the expectancies that are part of the role. As this implies, even though these expectancies may be (and may have been) typically fulfilled by the significant other, contextual factors may make it unlikely that the new person in the transference will be able to fulfill the expectations—for example, if he or she is in a different role. Role violations violate expectations, which in turn should provoke negative mood.

Indeed, the evidence suggests that this is exactly what occurs (Baum & Andersen, 1999). When signals indicate that a new person will not be able to adopt the complementary interpersonal relational role that the significant other adopts, positive affect is attenuated. Authority figures who are positive and significant, for example, do many things well, ranging from supporting and encouraging, to tutoring, guiding, and critiquing. When an activated significant-other representation activates the authority role and the new person then turns out not to be an authority but to be a novice, however, the role violation disrupts positive affect. This evidence is important both because it begins to show how positive affect may be compromised in a positive transference and because there is a considerable literature on interpersonal roles and norms, along with associated motives and expectancies, and the notion of role violation (e.g., Fiske, 1992; Mills & Clark, 1994; see also Bugental, 2000; Kenrick, Li, & Butner, 2003). Demonstrating the link between these literatures and research on the relational self is important and shows the further reach of the relational self.

Chronic Needs Violation and Chronically Unsatisfied Goals. In some relationships with positive significant others, of course, one's needs, wishes, and expectancies in the relationship may go unmet rather chronically, as part of the dynamic of the relationship (Berk & Andersen, 2004). This should be associated with disappointment in the relationship, even though the relationship is positive. For example, an important goal with any positive significant other is to be liked or loved and accepted, and this particular goal may chronically go unmet in the relationship, or, by contrast, may regularly be satisfied. Research thus examined such relationships in the context of transference with an eye toward understanding the limiting conditions on positive affect in the context of a positive transference.

As predicted, the results indicated that activation of chronically unsatisfied goals for acceptance and affection with a loved significant other occurs indirectly in transference when the significant-other representation is activated. Moreover, this leads to increases in negative affect, specifically in hostility, in spite of the fact that the significant other is loved. Beyond this, when the individual was actually bound to the significant other by blood, as is the case with family (i.e., of origin) members, it is specifically the case that increases in hostility in transference, presumably based on the prior disappointments, was nonetheless associated with an increased tendency to engage in overt behavior designed to get the new person to respond more positively. This suggests that a tendency to persistently pursue strategies to gain acceptance in prior relationships (even when they have not worked in that relationship) may sometimes be evoked in transference. In short, the evidence shows that positive affect is disrupted in a transference involving a relatively positive significant other when goals for love and acceptance that have chronically gone dissatisfied are triggered, based on significant-other activation. Yet, precisely to this extent, behavioral striving for this love and acceptance may persist.

Chronic Self-Violation of Own Preferences in Transference. Another way of thinking about chronic violations with significant others is to focus on the self—that is, on an individual's own responses (Reznik & Andersen, 2004). It is entirely possible to like or love a significant other, and yet to repeatedly find oneself enacting a dreaded version of the self with this person. As aversive as this may be, if one is bound to the other, for example, by blood because the person is in one's family of origin (a parent, sibling, etc.), it may not seem feasible to exit the relationship or to change patterns. When the significant-other representation is activated in transference, the dreaded self typically experienced with the other should also be activated. In turn, the emotional concomitants of this dreaded self should also be evoked in decreased positive and increased negative affect.

The results have emerged just as predicted. Activating a mental representation of a positive family-of-origin significant other associated with a dreaded self, rather than with a desired self, leads to increases in global negative mood as well as to decreases in global positive mood. In the absence of transference, no such effects occurred. Overall, one's global regard for a significant other is not sufficient to predict free-floating mood states in transference. It is important instead to take into account the specific nature of the self typically enacted with the significant other. When the aspects of self experienced with the other violate the individual's own preferences and wishes, this disrupts positive mood in a positive transference.

In sum, the weight of the evidence in the arena of global positive and negative affect in transference suggests that the violation of expectancies—of goals linked to interpersonal roles, of chronic needs with the significant other, and of preferences about which aspects of the self will and will not be expressed with a significant other—may all disrupt positive mood in an otherwise positive transference.

Specific Negative Emotions in Transference Rooted in Individual Differences

Evoking specific negative emotions (e.g., sadness/dysphoria as distinct from hostility or anxiety) in a positive transference requires, in our view, more refined conceptualization taking the self better into account. Self-discrepancy theory and self-regulatory focus theory both suggest that specific emotional vulnerabilities are associated with self-discrepancies and also that one may have a self-discrepancy from one's own perspective or from the perspective of a parent (e.g., Higgins, 1987, 1996b). People's beliefs about their parent's hopes for them (their parent's "ideals") and their beliefs about their parent's sense of their duties and obligations (their parent's "oughts") are standards that may be particularly influential for a person, and may indeed be discrepant from how the parent actually views them (i.e., their "actual self" from the parent's perspective). When the actual self is discrepant from ideal standards, it evokes depression and dejection-related affect, whereas when the actual self is discrepant from ought standards, it evokes agitation-related affect. The model implies that representations of parents are linked to representations of self, by being linked to the self-standards and self-discrepancies held from the parent's perspective. If this is correct, it should be the case that activating a parental representation will activate any self-discrepancy from the parent's standpoint, triggering the concomitant emotional vulnerabilities.

In research involving a liked or loved parent and self-discrepancies held from the parent's perspective (Reznik & Andersen, 2003), the evidence indicated that individuals with an ideal self-discrepancy from the perspective of one of their parents did in fact end up experiencing more depressed mood in transference when the representation of their parent was activated, than when not, an effect that did not occur among ought-discrepant individuals. Likewise, ought-discrepant individuals showed more agitation-related affect as indexed by resentful and hostile mood in the context of the transference condition than in the control condition (see also Strauman & Higgins, 1988), an effect that did not occur among ideal-discrepant participants. In short, the evidence shows that specific negative emotions relating to individual differences in self-discrepancy can be evoked as a function of a positive transference. The evidence (see also Andersen & Chen, 2002) thus forges a theoretical and empirical link between our work on the relational self and transference and research and theory on self-discrepancies and self-regulatory focus, thereby enabling specific affects to be predicted in transference (Reznik & Andersen, 2003; for related evidence, see also Shah, 2003b).

In our recent work, we theorize and attempt to demonstrate that transference may be a basic mechanism underlying the attachment system. Future research will show the usefulness of attachment style as yet another important individual difference allowing us to predict specific emotions arising in transference.

CONCLUDING COMMENTS

Research in our lab on the social-cognitive phenomenon of transference spans a period of more than 15 years. It springs from psychoanalytic theories, borrowing the century-old concept of transference from Freud's psychoanalysis, as later extended by Sullivan, as well as from assumptions about fundamental needs and motives, including the need for human connection and those related to attachment theory. Assumptions about social cognition also fundamentally frame the work and make it possible. The research has provided experimental evidence for the phenomenon of transference. It has also demonstrated that the phenomenon involves basic cognitive, affective, and motivational effects that occur as people make sense of novel persons in terms of those important people from their own lives whom new people tend to resemble to some greater or lesser degree. The research focuses on the activation and use of mental representations of significant others. Because of linkages between each significant other and the self, this research on transference forms the basis for the theory of the relational self (Andersen & Chen, 2002), which shows how the self shifts across differing interpersonal contexts (see also Andersen et al., 1997). Our work has thus helped address the long-standing conundrum in social psychology about whether the self is malleable or stable in its experience and expression, through highlighting the relational nature of the self.

The research has made use of an innovative methodology in a laboratory setting to overcome obstacles to a harnessing of the otherwise elusive phenomenon of transference. The conceptual and methodological tools of social cognition have been essential both in building a framework for understanding the transference process and for bringing the basic notion of transference to empirical life in social psychology. The research shows that inferences and evaluations of the new person change based on transference— when the significant-other representation is activated and used in relation to a new person—and so do feelings about the new person and motives to approach or avoid him or her, and even one's own sense of self and attempts at self-regulation in relation to him or her. The research has shown that several forms of self-regulation are evoked in transference and are a part of the operation of the relational self across varying life contexts. In short, the self fluctuates across the contexts of life in terms of which significant-other representation is activated in the transference experience.

Indeed, the evidence also suggests that emotions are evoked in transference, and that these depend on the exact nature of the self with the significant other. Emotions cannot be reduced to the global evaluation of the activated significant-other representation (such as how liked and loved vs. how disliked and detested the person is). How much one loves or detests a significant other is insufficient to fully account for emotions in transference. The relational self with this specific significant other is what is relevant in these varying emotions.

This line of research combines various methodologies and crosses bridges to different subdisciplines of psychology including clinical psychology (e.g., psychodynamic thinking), social psychology and cognitive psychology, as well as to subareas of social psychology such as those focused on the self, relationships, emotion, self-regulation, and so on (see Andersen & Saribay, in press). Beyond our specific methodological procedures, our use of a *combined idiographic–nomothetic method* has made it possible to tap the specific, idiosyncratic aspects of an individual's actual life—and this assures the meaningfulness of the stimuli used in the research. At the same time, this allows us to examine generalizable mental processes in an experimental paradigm to show the impact that transference has across a range of people. The fact that the evidence extends into the realms of motivation, self-regulation, and emotion also shows the breadth of the effect's relevance for emotional suffering and vulnerability, as well as for what may contribute to resilience. It is likely, beyond this, that specific linkages to psychopathology—as linked to interpersonal relationships—may be illuminated in future work.

More broadly, it is our view that future work in this area is especially valuable to the degree that it continues to unfold in integrative ways, invoking specific paradigms from individual subfields of personality and social psychology, as linked with the transference phenomenon, to illustrate the utility and relevance of the transference concept. Simultaneous examination of cognitive, affective, motivational, and behavioral microprocesses can also be especially valuable in yielding insights about exactly how prior relationships influence present ones and also simple, daily encounters. In addition to this level of analysis, it is also likely that research at a more macro- or superordinate level of analysis, that shows how these levels of analysis are linked to significant others, the relational self, and relationships more broadly, will be important in future research. That is, the linkages between phenomena in social and personality psychology involving social identities and social identification in the context of societal institutions and cultural context, with the relational level of analysis, deserves considerably more inquiry than they have received. Such research may begin to shed further light on the broader relevance of relational aspects of identity for social identifications (with groups), which is sorely needed (see, e.g., Andersen, Tyler, & Downey, in press; also see Sedikides & Brewer, 2001). While this was not the focus of the present chapter, pursuit of this kind of extension is ongoing among research that is likely to further trace the potential reach of the relational self. Simply put, people experience themselves in relation to those who are most significant to them, which has implications for everyday social encounters, and is likely to have broader societal implications as well.

ACKNOWLEDGMENT

This research was funded in part by Grant No. R01-MH48789 from the National Institute of Mental Health.

REFERENCES

Aarts, H., & Dijksterhuis, A. (2000). Habits as knowledge structures: Automaticity in goal-directed behavior. *Journal of Personality and Social Psychology, 78*, 53–63.

Ainsworth, M. D. S., Blehar, M. C., Walters, E., & Wall, S. (1978). *Patterns of attachment: A psychological study of the Strange Situation*. Hillsdale, NJ: Erlbaum.

Andersen, S. M., & Baum, A. (1994). Transference in interpersonal relations: Inferences and affect based on significant-other representations. *Journal of Personality, 62*, 459–498.

Andersen, S. M., & Chen, S. (2002). The relational self: An interpersonal social-cognitive theory. *Psychological Review, 109*, 619–645.

Andersen, S. M., & Cole, S. W. (1990). "Do I know you?": The role of significant others in general social perception. *Journal of Personality and Social Psychology, 59*, 383–399.

Andersen, S. M., & Glassman, N. S. (1996). Responding to significant others when they are not there: Effects on interpersonal inference, motivation, and affect. In R. M. Sorrentino & E. T. Higgins (Eds.), *Handbook of motivation and cognition* (Vol. 3, pp. 262–321). New York: Guilford Press.

Andersen, S. M., Glassman, N. S., Chen, S., & Cole, S. W. (1995). Transference in social perception: The role of chronic accessibility in significant-other representations. *Journal of Personality and Social Psychology, 69*, 41–57.

Andersen, S. M., & Klatzky, R. L. (1987). Traits and social stereotypes: Levels of categorization in person perception. *Journal of Personality and Social Psychology, 53*, 235–246.

Andersen, S. M., Reznik, I., & Chen, S. (1997). The self in relation to others: Motivational and cognitive underpinnings. In J. G. Snodgrass & R. L. Thompson (Eds.), *The self across psychology: Self-recognition, self-awareness, and the self-concept* (pp. 233–275). New York: New York Academy of Science.

Andersen, S. M., Reznik, I., & Glassman, N. S. (2004). The unconscious relational self. In R. Hassin, J. S. Uleman, & J. A. Bargh (Eds.), *The new unconscious* (pp. 421–481). New York: Oxford University Press.

Andersen, S. M., Reznik, I., & Manzella, L. M. (1996). Eliciting facial affect, motivation, and expectancies in transference: Significant-other representations in social relations. *Journal of Personality and Social Psychology, 71,* 1108–1129.

Andersen, S. M., & Saribay, S. A. (in press). Thinking integratively about social psychology: The example of the relational self and the social-cognitive process of transference. In P. A. M. Van Lange (Ed.), *Bridging social psychology*. Mahwah, NJ: Erlbaum.

Andersen, S. M., & Strasser, T. (2000). *Self-maintenance processes in transference: Dis-identifying with aspects of self to remain close to another and to regulate affect*. Unpublished manuscript, New York University.

Andersen, S. M., Tyler, T. R., & Downey, G. (in press). Becoming engaged in community: Personal relationships foster social identification. In G. Downey, C. Dweck, J. Eccles, & C. Chatman (Eds.), *Social identity, coping, and life tasks*. New York: Russell Sage Foundation.

Baldwin, M. W., Fehr, B., Keedian, E., Seidel, M., & Thompson, D. W. (1993). An exploration of the relational schemata underlying attachment styles: Self-report and lexical decision approaches. *Personality and Social Psychology Bulletin, 19,* 746–754.

Baldwin, M. W., Keelan, J. P. R., Fehr, B., Enns, V., & Koh-Rangarajoo, E. (1996). Social-cognitive conceptualization of attachment working models: Availability and accessibility effects. *Journal of Personality and Social Psychology, 71,* 94–109.

Baldwin, M. W., & Meunier, J. (1999). The cued activation of attachment relational schemas. *Social Cognition, 17,* 209–227.

Baldwin, M. W., & Sinclair, L. (1996). Self-esteem and "if . . . then" contingencies of interpersonal acceptance. *Journal of Personality and Social Psychology, 71,* 1130–1141.

Bargh, J. A. (1989). Conditional automaticity: Varieties of automatic influence in social perception and cognition. In J. S. Uleman & J. A. Bargh (Eds.), *Unintended thought* (pp. 3–51). New York: Guilford Press.

Bargh, J. A. (1990). Auto-motives: Preconscious determinants of social interaction. In E. T. Higgins & R. M. Sorrentino (Eds.), *Handbook of motivation and cognition: Foundations of social behavior* (Vol. 2, pp. 93–130). New York: Guilford Press.

Bargh, J. A. (1997). The automaticity of everyday life. In R. S. Wyer Jr. (Ed.), *Advances in social cognition* (Vol. 10, pp. 1–61). Mahwah, NJ: Erlbaum.

Bargh, J. A., & Barndollar, K. (1996). Automaticity in action: The unconscious as repository of chronic goals and motives. In P. M. Gollwitzer & J. A. Bargh (Eds.), *The psychology of action: Linking cognition and motivation to behavior* (pp. 457–481). New York: Guilford Press.

Bargh, J. A., Bond, R. N., Lombardi, W. L., & Tota, M. E. (1986). The additive nature of chronic and temporary sources of construct accessibility. *Journal of Personality and Social Psychology, 50,* 869–878.

Bargh, J. A., Chaiken, S., Raymond, P., & Hymes, C. (1996). The automatic evaluation effect: Unconditionally automatic attitude activation with a pronunciation task. *Journal of Experimental Social Psychology, 32,* 185–210.

Bargh, J. A., & Chartrand, T. (1999). The unbearable automaticity of being. *American Psychologist, 54,* 462–479.

Bargh, J. A., & Gollwitzer, P. M. (1994). Environmental control of goal-directed action: Automatic and strategic contingencies between situations and behavior. *Nebraska Symposium on Motivation, 41,* 71–124.

Bargh, J. A., Gollwitzer, P. M., Lee-Chai, A., Barndollar, K., & Trötschel, R. (2001). The automated will: Nonconscious activation and pursuit of behavioral goals. *Journal of Personality and Social Psychology, 81,* 1014–1027.

Baum, A., & Andersen, S. M. (1999). Interpersonal roles in transference: Transient mood states under the condition of significant-other activation. *Social Cognition, 17,* 161–185.

Becker, E. (1971). *The birth and death of meaning* (2nd ed.). New York: Free Press.

Berenson, K., & Andersen, S. M. (2003). *Childhood physical abuse by a parent: Transference-based manifestations in adult interpersonal relations.* Unpublished manuscript, New York University.

Berk, M. S., & Andersen, S. M. (2000). The impact of past relationships on interpersonal behavior: Behavioral confirmation in the social-cognitive process of transference. *Journal of Personality and Social Psychology, 79,* 546–562.

Berk, M. S., & Andersen, S. M. (2004). *Chronically unsatisfied goals with significant others: Triggering unfulfilled needs for love and acceptance in transference.* Unpublished manuscript, New York University.

Berscheid, E. (1994). Interpersonal relationships. *Annual Review of Psychology, 45,* 79–129.

Bombar, M., & Littig, L. Jr. (1996). Babytalk as a communication of intimate attachment: An initial study in adult romances and friendships. *Personal Relationships, 3,* 137–158.

Bowlby, J. (1969). *Attachment and loss: Vol. 1. Attachment.* New York: Basic Books.

Bowlby, J. (1973). *Attachment and loss: Vol. 2. Separation: Anxiety and anger.* New York: Basic Books.

Bowlby, J. (1980). *Attachment and loss: Vol. 3. Loss: Sadness and depression.* New York: Basic Books.

Bretherton, I. (1985). Attachment theory: Retrospect and prospect. *Monographs for the Society for Research in Child Development, 50,* 3–35.

Brewer, M. B. (1988). A dual process model of impression formation. In T. K. Srull & R. S. Wyer Jr. (Eds.), *A dual process model of impression formation* (pp. 1–36). Hillsdale, NJ: Erlbaum.

Bruner, J. S. (1957). Going beyond the information given. In H. E. Gruber, K. R. Hammond, & R. Jessor (Eds.), *Contemporary approaches to cognition* (pp. 41–69). Cambridge, MA: Harvard University Press.

Bugental, D. B. (2000). Acquisition of algorithms of social life: A domain-based approach. *Psychological Bulletin, 126,* 187–219.

Cantor, N., & Mischel, W. (1979). Prototypes in person perception. In L. Berkowitz

(Ed.), *Advances in experimental social psychology* (Vol. 12, pp. 3–52). New York: Academic Press.

Chen, M., & Bargh, J. A. (1997). Nonconscious behavioral confirmation processes: The self-fulfilling consequences of automatic stereotype activation. *Journal of Experimental Social Psychology, 33,* 541–560.

Chen, S., & Andersen, S. M. (1999). Relationships from the past in the present: Significant-other representations and transference in interpersonal life. In M. P. Zanna (Ed.), *Advances in experimental social psychology* (Vol. 31, pp. 123–190). San Diego, CA: Academic Press.

Chen, S., Andersen, S. M., & Hinkley, K. (1999). Triggering transference: Examining the role of applicability and use of significant-other representations in social perception. *Social Cognition, 17,* 332–365.

Collins, N. L. (1996). Working models of attachment: Implications for explanation, emotion, and behavior. *Journal of Personality and Social Psychology, 71,* 810–832.

Crocker, J., & Wolfe, C. T. (2001). Contingencies of worth. *Psychological Review, 108,* 593–623.

Cross, S. E., Bacon, P. L., & Morris, M. L. (2000). The relational-interdependent self-construal and relationships. *Journal of Personality and Social Psychology, 78,* 791–808.

Deci, E. L., & Ryan, R. M. (1985). *Intrinsic motivation and self-determination in human behavior.* New York: Plenum Press.

Downey, G., & Feldman, S. I. (1996). Implications of rejection sensitivity for intimate relationships. *Journal of Personality and Social Psychology, 70,* 1327–1343.

Duckworth, K. L., Bargh, J. A., Garcia, M., & Chaiken, S. (2002). The automatic evaluation of novel stimuli. *Psychological Science, 13,* 513–519.

Ehrenreich, J. H. (1989). Transference: One concept or many? *Psychoanalytic Review, 76,* 37–65.

Epstein, S. (1973). The self-concept revisited or a theory of a theory. *American Psychologist, 28,* 405–416.

Fiske, A. P. (1992). The four elementary forms of sociality: Framework for a unified theory of social relations. *Psychological Review, 99,* 689–723.

Fiske, S. T., & Pavelchak, M. (1986). Category-based versus piecemeal-based affective responses: Developments in schema-triggered affect. In R. M. Sorrentino & E. T. Higgins (Eds.), *Handbook of motivation and cognition* (pp. 167–203). New York: Guilford Press.

Fiske, S. T., & Taylor, S. E. (1991). *Social cognition* (2nd ed.). New York: McGraw-Hill.

Fitzsimons, G. M., & Bargh, J. A. (2003). Thinking of you: Nonconscious pursuit of interpersonal goals associated with relationship partners. *Journal of Personality and Social Psychology, 84,* 148–164.

Freud, S. (1958). The dynamics of transference. In J. Strachey (Ed. & Trans.), *The standard edition of the complete psychological works of Sigmund Freud* (Vol. 12, pp. 97–108). London: Hogarth Press. (Original work published 1912)

Freud, S. (1963). The dynamics of transference. In P. Rieff (Ed.), *Therapy and technique* (pp. 105–115). New York: Macmillan. (Original work published 1912)

Glassman, N. S., & Andersen, S. M. (1999a). Activating transference without con-

sciousness: Using significant-other representations to go beyond what is subliminally given. *Journal of Personality and Social Psychology, 77,* 1146–1162.

Glassman, N. S., & Andersen, S. M. (1999b). Transference in social cognition: Persistence and exacerbation of significant-other based inferences over time. *Cognitive Therapy and Research, 23,* 75–91.

Greenberg, J., & Pyszczynski, T. (1985). Compensatory self-inflation: A response to
the threat to self-regard of public failure. *Journal of Personality and Social Psychology, 49,* 273–280.

Greenson, R. R. (1965). The working alliance and the transference neurosis. *Psychoanalytic Quarterly, 34,* 155–179.

Gurung, R. A. R., Sarason, B. R., & Sarason, I. G. (2001). Predicting relationship
quality and emotional reactions to stress from significant-other-concept clarity.
Personality and Social Psychology Bulletin, 27, 1267–1276.

Heider, F. (1958). *The psychology of interpersonal relationships.* New York: Wiley.

Higgins, E. T. (1987). Self discrepancy: A theory relating self and affect. *Psychological Review, 94,* 319–340.

Higgins, E. T. (1989). Knowledge accessibility and activation: Subjectivity and suffering from unconscious sources. In J. S. Uleman & J. A. Bargh (Eds.), *Unintended
thought* (pp. 75–123). New York: Guilford Press.

Higgins, E. T. (1996a). Knowledge: Accessibility, applicability, and salience. In E. T.
Higgins & A. W. Kruglanski (Eds.), *Social psychology: Handbook of basic principles* (pp. 133–168). New York: Guilford Press.

Higgins, E. T. (1996b). Ideals, oughts, and regulatory focus: Affect and motivation
from distinct pains and pleasures. In P. M. Gollwitzer & J. A. Bargh (Eds.), *The
psychology of action* (pp. 91–114). New York: Guilford Press.

Higgins, E. T. (1996c). The self-digest: Self-knowledge serving self-regulatory functions. *Journal of Personality and Social Psychology, 71,* 1062–1083.

Higgins, E. T., & King, G. (1981). Accessibility of social constructs: Information pro-
cessing consequences of individual and contextual variability. In N. Cantor & J.
F. Kihlstrom (Eds.), *Personality, cognition and social interaction* (pp. 69–121).
Hillsdale, NJ: Erlbaum.

Higgins, E. T., & Silberman, I. (1998). Development of regulatory focus: Promotion
and prevention as ways of living. In J. Heckhausen & C. Dweck (Eds.), *Motivation and self-regulation across the life span* (pp. 78–113). Cambridge, UK: Cambridge University Press.

Hinkley, K., & Andersen, S. M. (1996). The working self-concept in transference: Significant-other activation and self change. *Journal of Personality and Social Psychology, 71,* 1279–1295.

Horney, K. (1939). *New ways in psychoanalysis.* New York: Norton.

Horowitz, M. J. (1989). Relationship schema formulation: Role-relationship models
and intrapsychic conflict. *Psychiatry, 52,* 260–274.

Horowitz, M. J. (Ed.). (1991). *Person schemas and maladaptive interpersonal patterns.* Chicago: University of Chicago Press.

Kelly, G. A. (1955). *The psychology of personal constructs.* New York: Norton.

Kenrick, D. T., Li, N. P., & Butner, J. (2003). Dynamical evolutionary psychology: Individual decision rules and emergent social norms. *Psychological Review, 110,*
3–28.

Kernberg, O. (1976). *Object relations theory and clinical psychoanalysis*. New York: Jason Aronson.

Kohut, H. (1971). *The analysis of the self*. New York: International Universities Press.

Linville, P. W., & Fischer, G. W. (1993). Exemplar and abstraction models of perceived group variability and stereotypicality. *Social Cognition, 11*, 92–125.

Luborsky, L., & Crits-Christoph, P. (1990). *Understanding transference: The CCRT method*. New York: Basic Books.

McGowan, S. (2002). Mental representations in stressful situations: The calming and distressing effects of significant others. *Journal of Experimental Social Psychology, 38*, 152–161.

Mikulincer, M. (1998). Adult attachment style and affect regulation: Strategic variations in self-appraisals. *Journal of Personality and Social Psychology, 75*, 420–435.

Mikulincer, M., & Horesh, N. (1999). Adult attachment style and the perception of others: The role of projective mechanisms. *Journal of Personality and Social Psychology, 76*, 1022–1034.

Mills, J., & Clark, M. S. (1994). Communal and exchange relationships: Controversies and research. In R. Erber & R. Gilmour (Eds.), *Theoretical frameworks for personal relationships* (pp. 29–42). Hillsdale, NJ: Erlbaum.

Mischel, W., & Shoda, Y. (1995). A cognitive-affective system theory of personality: Reconceptualizing situations, dispositions, dynamics, and invariance in personality structure. *Psychological Review, 102*, 246–268.

Morf, C. C., & Rhodewalt, F. (2001). Unraveling the paradoxes of narcissism: A dynamic self-regulatory processing model. *Psychological Inquiry, 12*, 177–196.

Murray, S. L., & Holmes, J. G. (1993). Seeing virtues in faults: Negativity and the transformation of interpersonal narratives in close relationships. *Journal of Personality and Social Psychology, 65*, 707–722.

Murray, S. L., & Holmes, J. G. (1999). The (mental) ties that bind: Cognitive structures that predict relationship resilience. *Journal of Personality and Social Psychology, 77*, 1228–1244.

Pierce, T., & Lydon, J. (1998). Priming relational schemas: Effects of contextually activated and chronically accessible interpersonal expectations on responses to a stressful event. *Journal of Personality and Social Psychology, 75*, 1441–1448.

Pierce, T., & Lydon, J. E. (2001). Global and specific relational models in the experience of social interactions. *Journal of Personality and Social Psychology, 80*, 613–631.

Prentice, D. (1990). Familiarity and differences in self- and other-representations. *Journal of Personality and Social Psychology, 59*, 369–383.

Reznik, I., & Andersen, S. M. (2003). *Individual differences and the emotions evoked in transference: Indirect triggering of self-discrepancies and self-regulatory focus through significant-other representations*. Unpublished manuscript, New York University.

Reznik, I., & Andersen, S. M. (2004). *Becoming the dreaded self: Diminished self-worth with positive significant others in transference*. Unpublished manuscript, New York University.

Rusbult, C. E., & Van Lange, P. A. M. (1996). Interdependence processes. In E. T.

Higgins & A. W. Kruglanski (Eds.), *Social psychology: Handbook of basic principles* (pp. 564–596). New York: Guilford Press.

Russell, J. A. (2003). Core affect and the psychological construction of emotion. *Psychological Review, 110,* 145–172.

Schimek, J. (1983). The construction of the transference: The relativity of the "here and now" and the "there and then." *Psychoanalysis and Contemporary Thought, 6,* 435–456.

Sedikides, C., & Brewer, M. B. (Eds.). (2001). *Individual self, relational self, collective self.* Philadelphia: Psychology Press.

Seligman, M. E. P. (1975). *Helplessness: On depression, development, and death.* San Francisco: Freeman.

Shah, J. (2003a). Automatic for the people: How representations of significant others implicitly affect goal pursuit. *Journal of Personality and Social Psychology, 84,* 661–681.

Shah, J. (2003b). The motivational looking glass: How significant others implicitly affect goal appraisals. *Journal of Personality and Social Psychology, 85,* 424–439.

Shaver, P. R., & Mikulincer, M. (2002). Attachment-related psychodynamics. *Attachment and Human Development, 4,* 133–161.

Shields, A., Ryan, R. M., & Cicchetti, D. (2001). Narrative representations of caregivers and emotion dysregulation as predictors of maltreated children's rejection by peers. *Developmental Psychology, 37,* 321–337.

Showers, C. (1992). Compartmentalization of positive and negative self-knowledge: Keeping bad apples out of the bunch. *Journal of Personality and Social Psychology, 62,* 1036–1049.

Singer, J. L. (1988). Reinterpreting the transference. In D. C. Turk & P. Salovey (Eds.), *Reasoning, interference, and judgment in clinical psychology* (pp. 182–205). New York: Free Press.

Smith, E. R., & Zarate, M. A. (1992). Exemplar-based model of social judgment. *Psychological Review, 99,* 3–21.

Snyder, M., Tanke, E. D., & Berscheid, E. (1977). Social perception and interpersonal behavior: On the self-fulfilling nature of social stereotypes. *Journal of Personality and Social Psychology, 35,* 656–666.

Steele, C. M. (1988). The psychology of self-affirmation: Sustaining the integrity of the self. In L. Berkowitz (Ed.), *Advances in experimental social psychology* (Vol. 21, pp. 261–302). New York: Academic Press.

Strauman, T. J., & Higgins, E. T. (1988). Self-discrepancies as predictors of vulnerability to distinct syndromes of chronic emotional distress. *Journal of Personality, 56,* 685–707.

Sullivan, H. S. (1953). *The interpersonal theory of psychiatry.* New York: Norton.

Taylor, S. E., & Brown, J. D. (1988). Illusion and well-being: A social psychological perspective on mental health. *Psychological Bulletin, 103,* 193–210.

Thompson, R. A. (1998). Early sociopersonality development. In W. Damon (Series Ed.) & N. Eisenberg (Vol. Ed.), *Handbook of child psychology: Vol. 3. Social, emotional, and personality development* (5th ed., pp. 25–104). New York: Wiley.

Westen, D. (1988). Transference and information processing. *Clinical Psychology Review, 8,* 161–179.

2

Understanding and Modifying the Relational Schemas Underlying Insecurity

MARK W. BALDWIN *and* STÉPHANE D. DANDENEAU

It seems obvious that people learn about relationships: about the give and take of social contact and about what can be expected when conversing, arguing, negotiating, working, playing, or sharing intimacies with another person. The effects of these learned patterns of relatedness are clear, as they guide people's behavior in later interactions and shape their experience of others and of themselves. It seems obvious, yes, and yet until recently these questions have been largely overlooked in the mainstream social-cognitive literature.

As we shall see, the powerful theoretical models and research techniques that make up the social-cognitive perspective can be, and have been, fruitfully applied to the study of interpersonal experience. People have *relational schemas*—or cognitive structures representing patterns of interpersonal relatedness—for such common interpersonal experiences as "being criticized by an authority figure" or "being unconditionally accepted by a romantic partner," as well as for specific relational patterns in specific relationships (Baldwin, 1992). These self-with-other schemas serve as filters on interpersonal experience by guiding attention to relevant information, influencing the perception and interpretation of ambiguous information, providing default values to allow people to fill in the blanks of partial information, serving as organizing frameworks for the encoding and later memory of interactions, and so on.

In this chapter we begin with a brief examination of some of the theoretical foundations of our perspective, present the assumptions of our model, and review almost two decades of research into the basic workings of relational schemas. Then we turn to our most recent research, in which we have examined the possibility of modifying relational knowledge structures. We have come to believe that the next step for the social cognitive perspective is to embrace the insights of learning theory, which from its earliest days has been focused on the processes of change in the acquisition and modification of behavior and cognition. We describe our recent efforts to apply basic learning principles, such as classical conditioning, to the issue of changing relational cognition. We have examined these questions primarily in the context of the cognitive structures underlying experiences of security and insecurity, with the goal of identifying means of decreasing the influence of insecurity-producing cognitive processes and increasing the influence of security-producing processes. Before addressing these issues of schema change, though, we begin with a review of some basic theory and research about relational schemas.

INTELLECTUAL BACKGROUND

The intellectual background to the relational schemas approach is more fully reviewed by Baldwin (1992), but it will be useful to give an overview here. Broadly speaking, these influences come from psychodynamic and interpersonal perspectives in personality theory, and from self and close relationships literatures in social psychology. These insights, combined with the now mainstream and still growing social-cognitive framework, led to our model of relational schemas.

In the personality literature, Freud wrote about the processes by which people internalize their experiences from their most significant relationships, and how they then use these representations as templates for the perception of new interpersonal experiences (i.e., in *transference*; see Andersen & Saribay, Chapter 1, this volume). He focused primarily on the internal representation of the parents, and how these come to shape mental structures and processes such as the superego and its process of evaluating, criticizing, and sometimes outright attacking the self.

Freud (1917/1957) wrote evocatively about how people "take in" a relationship and "set up" an internal version, but the empirical utility of his model of internalization was limited by the underdeveloped cognitive theory of his day. Psychodynamic and interpersonal theorists who followed made great strides, at some times refining Freud's ideas and at other times taking a fresh view (see, e.g., Greenberg & Mitchell, 1983, and Westen, 1988, for reviews). Winnicott (1975), for example, explored the complex ways in which human psychology is a deeply interpersonal affair even from the earliest days after birth, declaring that "there is no such thing as a baby" (p. 99) independent of the parent–child relationship. Sullivan (1953) examined the "me–you patterns" that children learn in interaction with their significant others, and the way these expectations shape the child's sense of security versus anxiety. Stern (1985) discussed the way children abstract across relationship experiences to learn generic patterns of interaction, which then can produce a sense of self as experienced with certain significant others. Of the psychodynamic theorists who predated modern social-cognitive theory, Bowlby was probably the most consistent in spirit. In his volumes on attachment theory (Bowlby, 1969, 1973) he proposed that people extract from their experience *working models* of the way relationships function, particularly working models of others' availability and responsiveness as well as one's own worthiness. Mitchell (1988) reviewed these and other object relational models, concluding that the basic relational unit includes "the self, the other, and the space between the two . . . in which they do things with or to each other" (p. 33).

In social psychology, interest in interpersonal cognition can be traced back at least as far as Mead, Cooley, and James. Symbolic interactionists Mead and Cooley located the roots of self-experience, and thought itself, in patterns of social communication. Cooley's notion of the looking-glass self depicted self-evaluation as a process involving three elements: "the imagination of our appearance to the other person, the imagination of his judgment of that appearance, and some sort of self-feeling, such as pride or mortification" (Cooley, 1902, p. 184). Along these same lines, James (1890) tied self-experience to interpersonal contexts, saying that a person "has as many different social selves as there are distinct groups of persons about whose opinion he cares" (p. 282). As social psychology developed, researchers explored a number of core themes involved in interpersonal cognition: humans evidently have a strong need for social belonging (see Baumeister & Leary, 1995, for a review), and in turn monitor social situations to try to maintain acceptance and avoid rejection. The result is often a tendency to present the self in socially acceptable ways, and to experience negative affects such as anxiety, depression, and low self-esteem when rejection cannot be avoided (e.g., Schlenker & Leary, 1982).

More recently, researchers studying close relationships have identified a variety of common relationship patterns that people learn to recognize and enact. For example, relationships can be characterized as more or less communal versus more or less based in quid pro quo exchange transactions, and people are keenly attentive to the cues that signal others' intentions in this regard (Clark & Mills, 1979; Fiske, 1992). Relationship partners are also very attentive to issues of relative dominance and status, and coordinate their actions based on their expectations and perceptions of others' bids for dominance (e.g., Planalp, 1985; Williamson & Fitzpatrick, 1985). Finally, an extraordinarily active research area in the past decade has involved applying Bowlby's attachment theory to the study of romantic love (Hazan & Shaver, 1987; Mikulincer & Shaver, Chapter 10, this volume), exploring the processes whereby working models of relationships shape people's understanding of their most significant interpersonal experiences.

RELATIONAL SCHEMAS: AN OVERVIEW OF THEORY AND EVIDENCE

Thinkers from a variety of perspectives, then, have converged on the principle that people internally represent their interpersonal experiences, and these representations influence their perception of subsequent interactions and themselves. The challenge over the past two decades has been to consider these processes from a social-cognitive point of view, with an eye to developing a model of the representation, activation, and application of interpersonal knowledge. This task has been undertaken in a number of different content areas by other authors and researchers, many of whom have contributed to the current volume. In our own lab we have usually focused our attention on what might roughly be termed *insecurity*—primarily, the phenomena of insecure attachment and low self-esteem. As we shall discuss, we believe this content domain gives rise to a broad range of questions about interpersonal perception, self-perception, expectation, motivation, and affect, and so is ideal as a sphere for developing a model of interpersonal cognition. At the same time, we believe the principles we derive here can readily and appropriately be applied in other content areas. We start by examining the representation of interpersonal knowledge, and then discuss an array of information-processing effects this knowledge can have.

Representation

The original formulation of the relational schemas model (Baldwin, 1992) drew heavily on the work of other writers exploring similar ideas at the time, such as Horowitz (1988) and Safran (1990) (see also Andersen & Cole, 1987; Bretherton, 1985; Crittenden, 1990; Ginsburg, 1988; Miell, 1987; Ogilvie & Ashmore, 1991; Planalp, 1985; Stern, 1985; Westen, 1988). The aim was to integrate the insights in the literature on relational cognition with developing theories of social cognition and personality more generally (e.g., Cantor & Kihlstrom, 1985).

We begin with the notion of a single cognitive structure that combines representations of the self, another person, and a prototypical pattern of interaction between self and other. Self and other are hypothesized to be represented as a self-schema and an other-schema: each is a declarative knowledge structure consisting of specific facts, memories, generic descriptors, and so on, clustered together as a "chunk of associative network" (Carlston & Smith, 1996, p. 196). In the context of insecurity, for example, self might be represented as an unworthy, inadequate loser, while other might be depicted as a powerful, rejecting criticizer.

Importantly, representations of self and other are assumed to be linked together by virtue of being embedded in an *interpersonal script* (Abelson, 1981; see also Horowitz, 1988; Safran, 1990), representing a typical pattern of interaction between self and other. The sense of self as inadequate and other as critical probably arose in the first place from repeated interactions in which self failed in some way and the other person responded negatively, and this expected pattern is reflected in the script or event schema.

We have found it useful to conceive of the interpersonal script as consisting of a series of *if–then* contingency expectations. A person might learn, for example, that "If I perform inadequately, then he will be critical of me." The ifs and thens of interpersonal scripts involve the typical behaviors of the actors, but also their inferred thoughts, goals, and feelings (Baldwin, 1992). The outcome expectancies represented in scripts have a number of functions and effects. Primarily, they allow the person to perform mental simulations of different courses of action and to anticipate their results. Then, much like a laboratory rat deciding whether to press a bar for a food pellet or pull a chain for a drink of water, the person can opt for whichever action is likely to lead to the most desired outcome. Human motivations tend to be a bit more complex than just hunger and thirst, of course, and expectations about the fulfillment or nonfulfillment of powerful goals such as social acceptance or social dominance can also produce strong emotional reactions including joy, pride, sadness, and anxiety (see Epstein, 1973, and Trzebinski, 1985, for analyses of motivational systems).

It is possible to get a rough assessment of people's social expectations in a variety of domains, simply by asking them. For example, researchers in the adult attachment literature contrast individuals having a generally secure orientation toward romantic relationships with individuals having an insecure orientation—either anxious about close relationships or avoidant of them altogether. These orientations are assumed to arise from expectancies about relationship partners' emotional availability and responsiveness, ranging from a high level of confidence (in the case of secure individuals) to uncertain, pessimistic, or even fearful views (in the case of insecure individuals). In principle, one could imagine an almost unlimited number of relevant scripts that could produce insecurity (or, conversely, security). A person might expect, for example, that any expression of anger or hostility will produce rejection by a relationship partner (Fehr, Baldwin, Collins, Patterson, & Benditt, 1999). Or a person might anticipate that being demanding or needy will lead to withdrawal by the partner (Christensen, 1987). In the adult attachment literature, issues of dependency, trust, and closeness tend to emerge as central concerns.

In one study (Baldwin, Fehr, Keedian, Seidel, & Thomson, 1993, Study 1), expectancies were identified on the basis of previous findings in the attachment literature, and formulated as if–then interpersonal scripts involving situations of dependency, trust, and closeness. Participants were asked to consider a variety of possible behaviors (e.g., "You want to spend more time with your partner") and then asked to rate the likelihood of different potential outcomes (e.g., "he/she accepts you" or "he/she rejects you"). Results showed that people with different self-reported attachment orientations tended to endorse scripts that reflected different expectancies. For example, people who reported being anxious in close relationships were more likely than others to endorse a script in which trying to be close to their partner led to negative outcomes, and self-reported avoidantly attached individuals tended to expect that trusting their partner would lead to being hurt. Securely attached individuals reported more positive expectancies, endorsing scripts that reflected the availability and responsiveness of their partner.

A similar self-report approach was taken in a study of the interpersonal expectancies associated with self-esteem. Various writers (e.g., Cooley, 1902; Rogers, 1959; Sullivan, 1953) have argued that self-evaluation and the resulting feelings of high or low self-esteem are closely tied to processes of interpersonal evaluation. People's emotional reactions to their own successes and failures, for example, are hypothesized to arise from the implications these factors are seen to have for important social motives such as attachment and social rank (see Baldwin & Baccus, 2003; Rogers, 1959). That is, a failure at a task might be particularly likely to lead to feelings of low self-esteem if the person expects that "If I fail, people will reject me" (cf. Leary, Chapter 4, this volume) or "If I fail, people will treat me as low status" (cf. Gilbert, Chapter 12, this volume). Baldwin and Keelan (1999) adopted the self-report approach developed by Hill and Safran (1994) to examine the expectancies endorsed by people of low and high self-esteem. High self-esteem was significantly associated with positive expectancies about being able to produce friendly, accepting responses from others. Low self-esteem was associated, as predicted, with a lack of confidence about producing positive social reactions.

Insecurity, then, is associated with if–then scripts in which some aspect or action of the self leads to negative social outcomes. These scripts lead the person to anticipate the thwarting of important social motives, producing the negative affective responses associated with insecurity.

Information-Processing Effects

The assumption of the relational schemas approach is that these knowledge structures function much the same way as other kinds of knowledge structures studied by social-cognitive researchers (see, e.g., Smith, 1998).

Just like stereotypes, self-schemas, or implicit personality theories, relational schemas should show a familiar set of effects on the processing of social—in this case, interpersonal—information. Attention should be drawn toward information relevant to the schema, for example. Gaps in available information should be filled in with expected or default values, and, as a result, ambiguous information ("Was she laughing *with* me or *at* me?") should be interpreted in light of the expected pattern. Memory encoding and retrieval—for example, the selection of events that are easily remembered days or months later—should show the organizing effects of the schema.

In our lab we have focused primarily on one of the most basic principles in all of social cognition: the principle of *knowledge activation*. Simply put, people have available to them an enormous array of knowledge structures: about intimate relationships, about evaluative interactions with authority figures, about rejection, about secure acceptance, about doorknobs, about elephants, and about fast-food restaurants—just to name a few. For a knowledge structure to influence the ongoing processing of information it must become activated, and this happens as a function of several interacting factors such as the salient information in the current situation; people's chronic tendencies; situational priming; spreading activation from other thoughts, feelings, or goals; and so on (we discuss these influences later when we explore our research findings; see Higgins, 1996, for a detailed discussion). The reason for our emphasis on activation is straightforward: social life is remarkably ambiguous. If a construct or schema does not get activated, it will not influence social experience. Once it does get activated, however, it can produce profound effects on the interpretation of social interaction and the self, even outside of awareness and even in the first milliseconds of perception and encoding. We start by examining the influence of relational schemas on attention to certain types of social information.

Attention

Imagine that all day long, as you walk down the street or sit in a meeting, your attention is constantly drawn to rejection feedback from others. You are vigilant for any evidence that others might be scowling at you, and if you do perceive the slightest frown (even if in reality it is just the grimace of a person who ate some bad nuts), you focus on it and find it difficult to take your attention away and concentrate on your other goals and activities. This is likely one powerful and debilitating component of insecurity. According to Posner and Petersen (1990), the attention system consists of three components: attention shifting, engagement, and disengagement. We surmise that all of these may be influenced by one's relational schemas. Several researchers (e.g., Westen, 1988; Williams, Mathews, & MacLeod,

1996), for example, have examined the hypothesis that *attentional bias*, or people's propensity to look for and be attentive to certain types of information in the environment, is a contributing cause and perpetuating factor of disorders such as social anxiety, social phobia, and depression.

Following this logic, we have studied the ability and inability to inhibit rejection information in people with low and high self-esteem. In one set of studies we used an emotional Stroop task, in which emotional words were displayed in different colors and participants had to quickly name the colors while trying to ignore the content of the words. Low and high self-esteem individuals were shown a series of rejection, acceptance, and neutral words and their color-naming responses on each trial were recorded by a microphone connected to a computer. As anticipated, people with low self-esteem, for whom rejection information is threatening and of important concern to them, experienced greater rejection interference (i.e., they were slower in their response for rejection words than for neutral words), than acceptance interference, which is indicative of their inability to inhibit rejection information. People with high self-esteem, on the other hand, did not experience a significant difference between rejection and acceptance interference (Dandeneau & Baldwin, 2004a).

Follow-up research (Dandeneau & Baldwin, 2004b) has shown similar effects using the Visual Probe Task (VPT), a measure of attentional bias that assesses attention to pictures of frowning and smiling faces rather than words. Taken together these studies confirm that insecurity, in this case indexed by low self-esteem, is associated with an attentional bias toward rejection stimuli. At the first moment of each social experience, then, people's interpersonal cognitive structures guide their attention to preferentially process certain types of information more than others.

Spreading Activation

There may be some circumstances in which insecure, low self-esteem individuals are especially sensitive to negative interpersonal information. Certain events or thoughts—such as failing in some way or making oneself vulnerable by trusting another—might increase the activation of expectations of rejection, abandonment, or other feared outcomes. Indeed, the idea that activation spreads from one element of a knowledge structure to another is held by some theorists to be a defining aspect of an organized schema (e.g., Higgins & Bargh, 1987). In the case of an interpersonal script, activation is hypothesized to spread from *if* to *then*, increasing the cognitive activation of the outcome and giving the person the subjective experience that "I can easily imagine that happening."

In an early social-cognitive examination of the interpersonal expectancies theorized to underlie adult attachment styles, Baldwin et al. (1993) reasoned that a sequential priming task could be used to assess this "wakening of associations" (James, 1890) across elements of a script. A modified version of the classic lexical decision task was created for this purpose. On each trial of this task, participants were first primed by having them read a sentence fragment that established a specific context of vulnerability (e.g., "If I trust my partner, then my partner will . . . "), then asked to quickly make word–nonword judgments on interpersonal words like *care* and *hurt* (and, on some trials, nonwords such as *blorn)*. Supporting the idea that activation spreads from *if* to *then*, avoidantly attached individuals were faster to recognize *hurt* as a word after reading a sentence describing *trusting a romantic partner*. If for these individuals thoughts of trusting a partner tend to activate thoughts of being hurt, perhaps it is not surprising they adopt an avoidant stance toward intimacy.

A similar approach was taken to study the associative links contributing to low self-esteem. Self-esteem insecurities have been theorized to arise from the sense that social acceptance is highly conditional, contingent on being successful or in some other way socially desirable (e.g., Rogers, 1959). For the insecure person, this means that any sign of failure activates the expectancy of being rejected and criticized—thwarting the profound human need for belonging and attachment. Baldwin and Sinclair (1996) used a sequential priming task to examine spreading activation across links between success and acceptance, and failure and rejection. Participants were first briefly presented with performance words (e.g., *failure, success*) then asked to make word–nonword judgments on targets consisting of social outcome words (e.g., *rejected, accepted*) or nonword letter strings. As hypothesized, people with low self-esteem showed the contingency pattern in which they were faster to identify rejection words when primed with failure and acceptance words when primed with success. A follow-up study showed that these effects could not be explained as a result of mood or the simple valence of the items since noninterpersonal targets (of positive and negative valence) showed very different effects. The interpersonal contingencies represented in these cognitive links explain why momentary self-feelings fluctuate so much for insecure persons; successes might provide some sense of being momentarily acceptable to others, but each minor failure activates the representation of being rejected and excluded by others. These findings have been replicated in several studies, most recently in a pair of studies showing that the activation effects occur within the first 250 milliseconds of being shown the prime word (Baldwin, Baccus, & Fitzsimons, 2004). Even in the first milliseconds of thinking about a social event, then, people's insecurity can be triggered by the expectancies coded in their relational schemas.

Multiple Schemas

It is customary to think of insecurity in terms of an individual's stable "attachment style" or "level of self-esteem," but this approach holds the danger of stopping at the level of description and labeling rather than proceeding to the task of explanation. From the point of view of social-cognitive models of personality (e.g., Cantor & Kihlstrom, 1985), many aspects of personality can be explained as arising from the activation of knowledge structures. This type of formulation helps to explain not only people's general behavioral tendencies but also the meaningful variability they show from situation to situation.

Consider the notion of attachment style. While there is no doubt that people differ in their approach to close relationships, and so could be said to have a "style," the tendency in the literature has often been to implicitly (or explicitly) assume that people have one attachment orientation (e.g., secure, dismissing, etc.) that they adopt in essentially all their significant relationships, and essentially across their lifespan. Baldwin and Fehr (1995) questioned this assumption following a finding that roughly 30% of participants changed their self-reported attachment "style" from one measurement to the next, even across just a 2-week period! Similar results have been reported, and explored in depth, by other researchers (e.g., Davila, Burge, & Hammen, 1997).

Baldwin, Keelan, Fehr, Enns, and Koh-Rangarajoo (1996; see also Collins & Read, 1994) hypothesized that one reason for this variability might be that most people actually have multiple relational schemas representing a wide range of relationship experiences and expectancies, including, for example, *trustworthy acceptance, unreliable attention*, and *manipulative hurtfulness*. These different patterns may be associated with different relationships (e.g., mother vs. father vs. romantic partner), but they may not; Bowlby even proposed that a person might experience multiple patterns within a single relationship. Indeed, when participants were asked to characterize their 10 most significant relationships, most people reported all three attachment "styles." Attachment orientation, then, might best be understood as a matter of which model becomes activated, as a function of partner characteristics, chronic tendencies, situational variables, and so on. Individual differences in attachment orientation, then, are largely a function of schema accessibility or the fluency with which one model versus another gets activated. When participants were asked to report on their attachment orientation with their significant others, their general self-reported attachment orientation (i.e., secure, avoidant, anxious–ambivalent) corresponded to the number of relationships in which they tended to relate to a significant other with such an orientation, and the ease with which they could generate exemplar relationships describing different attachment styles. This type of social-cognitive analysis of relationship phenomena is broadly consistent with Bowlby's original focus on internal working models. It also helps to bring work in this area back to questions of information-processing dynamics, and away from the focus on trait-like individual differences that largely defined the literature previously.

Relational Schema Priming

Our assumption is that attachment and self-esteem insecurities reflect the activation of certain kinds of relational schemas—much like the triggering that sometimes occurs when one enjoys a holiday dinner with the extended family! If so, experimentally manipulating these schemas should, logically, produce shifts in insecurity. In the late 1970s and early 1980s, the powerful cognitive technique of priming was starting to be used in the impression formation literature to show the organizing effects of schemas about personality traits. Participants who were incidentally shown the word *reckless*, for example, later perceived an ambiguous stimulus person's mountain climbing and skydiving activities more negatively than participants earlier shown the word *adventurous* (Higgins, Rholes, & Jones, 1977).

Baldwin and Holmes (1987) decided to try priming relational schemas to examine whether it might be possible to manipulate the interpersonal-cognitive roots of self-evaluation processes. In one study, female participants were instructed to spend a few moments imagining specific significant others. Some were instructed to imagine being with their parents, and others with two campus friends. The instructions went as follows:

> Focus your attention on this person. . . . Picture the person's face. Really try to get an experience of the person being with you. . . . You may want to remember a time you were actually with the person, or you may already have a clear experience of what this person is like. . . . Just try to get a good image of this person. You may find that you can see the colour of their eyes or their hair, or maybe hear their voice. . . . Imagine that this person is right there with you. . . . Now once you have an image of the person, try to zoom in and get a close-up, focused impression. . . . Hold this image for a little while. . . . Imagine talking with the person. . . . Try to feel them there with you. (Baldwin & Holmes, 1987, p. 1089)

The different relational schema primes were anticipated to activate different types of evaluative standards, and thereby influence participants' behavior in an area that might be relevant to these schemas. Ten minutes following the guided-imagery task, in an ostensibly unrelated task, participants were asked to rate their enjoyment of various written passages, one of which was a sexually permissive story describing a young woman contemplating having sex with a good-looking man whom she did not know well. As anticipated, participants instructed to imagine their parents in the guided-imagery task subsequently rated the sexually permissive story less enjoyable and less exciting that those who had imagined their (presumably more permissive) campus friends. Thus, an interpersonal prime shaped self-evaluation and self-regulation.

In a second study, Baldwin and Holmes wanted to see if it might be possible to make people momentarily more secure or insecure by priming schemas for social acceptance versus criticism, respectively. Much previous research had detailed the self-critical processes engaged in by insecure individuals, including comparing oneself negatively to others, blaming oneself for failures, and so on. From a relational schema perspective, these patterns of self-evaluation are rooted in underlying patterns of interpersonal evaluation, which theoretically should be subject to the normal laws of construct activation. In a group of male participants, half were instructed to imagine a supportive, unconditionally accepting friend who "would accept you no matter what" and the other half were instructed to imagine an evaluative, highly conditional person who liked them primarily because of the abilities and talents they had. Following the guided imagery prime, participants were given an extremely difficult task, and then asked to complete measures of self-evaluation. As anticipated, the primed relational schemas influenced the style of self-evaluation among people who were induced to self-evaluate via a standard self-awareness manipulation. For example, those who imagined a conditional person were more likely to feel badly about their failure and to attribute it to "something about me." These same participants were also more likely to overgeneralize from single negative behaviors to global conclusions about the self. Conversely, those primed with an accepting significant other became more self-accepting about their own shortcomings. In additional studies we have used these and similar manipulations (e.g., simply exposing participants to the name of a significant other who is critical or accepting; see Baldwin, 1994) to replicate and clarify these results. A study by Baldwin and Sinclair (1996, Study 3), for example, confirmed that the prime activates a set of associations linked to that relationship. That is, when primed with a conditionally accepting significant other, people's responses to a lexical decision task showed the same *if–then, failure–rejection* pattern that is chronically shown by individuals with low self-esteem.

Self-evaluative insecurity, then, arises from activated relational schemas representing critical and contingent evaluation by others. When such structures are activated, people's self-evaluations come to reflect the kinds of processes typically seen in low self-esteem or even depressed individuals, with increased levels of self-blame, overgeneralization, and so on. If secure acceptance is primed, however, evaluative processes become more self-accepting.

Baldwin et al. (1996, Study 3) applied the same logic to see if it might actually be possible to prime attachment orientations, which at that time were widely considered highly stable personality traits. Participants visualized a person with whom they felt either secure, avoidant, or anxious, and answered some bogus questions. Then they walked down the hall to participate in an ostensible "second study" about dating choices. The priming affected responses on this later task. For example, participants primed with an avoidant schema were now more drawn (than those in other conditions) toward a potential partner who desired autonomy rather than high levels of closeness and dependency, just as had already been shown with chronically avoidant people (see Frazier, Byer, Fischer, Wright, & DeBord, 1996). Thus, attachment orientations showed the influence of temporary as well as chronic accessibility effects, a finding that has been developed considerably since this initial evidence (see, e.g., Mikulincer & Shaver, Chapter 10, this volume; Pierce & Lydon, 1998).

Ifs and Thens in Relational Cognition

It is worth pausing to consider several interrelated phenomena all having an *if–then* structure, so as not to confuse one with another. Generally when we use this terminology we are referring to the behavior-outcome expectancies described by Mischel (1973), in which a person anticipates that "if I behave in such and such a way in this situation, then the other person will respond" in a specific manner. We believe that expectancies allow people to mentally simulate several possible courses of action to try to decide on the optimal choice, and we also believe that these simulations (often occurring automatically) can produce a range of affective responses from the anticipation of rewards or punishments. Other researchers (e.g., Gollwitzer, 1999) refer to a different kind of *if–then* structure, one that represents an implementation intention that a person might form, such as "If I am in a certain situation, then I will act in a certain way". Then, as Mischel and Shoda (1995) have demonstrated, people guide their behavior according to these expectancies and intentions, with the end result being an observable *if–then* behavioral signature of the kind "If this individual is in this situation, he or she tends to behave in this specific way." That is, a bully might have the behavioral signature of being aggressive with younger children, for example, because he has formed the implementation intention to act that way, having learned the behavior-outcome expectancy that bullying will produce the kind of result he desires. Thus, these three types of *if–then* formulations fit together logically.

Importantly, *if–then* structures not only relate to behavior, they also define rules for processing information. For example, Smith and Branscombe (1987) studied trait inference procedures according to which perceivers conclude "If a person helps a stranger, then she is kind." We believe that this type of *if–then* structure provides one of the main mechanisms whereby internalized relationships influence thought processes (Baldwin, 1997). Recall that interpersonal scripts are not merely behavioral, they also include assumptions about the actors' goals, intentions, beliefs, and so on. If a child internalizes a script that "If I act tough, then others will think I am important," this will establish an *if–then* link between toughness and importance that will shape his perception of the world and of himself. Internalization, then, is in part a process whereby habits of communication and interaction become habits of thought. This is a view that has its roots in the writings of Mead (1934) and Vygotsky (1934/ 1986), among others, and it is resurfacing in current analyses of children's theory of mind and how it emerges and is shaped in the context of early attachment relationships (e.g., Fonagy, 2001). An important point to remember is that, as our priming research has shown, such thought processes probably never become separated to function entirely independently of their social moorings. The human mind is intrinsically an interpersonal structure.

Implicit Processes and Subliminal Priming

We have reviewed evidence showing the importance of knowledge activation in determining people's attention to and inferences about aspects of self and relationships. Not that people are necessarily aware of the shifts that occur in their assumptions about the interpersonal world: as mentioned earlier, relational schemas are hypothesized to function automatically, producing their effects quickly (e.g., within a fraction of a second) and even outside of awareness. Indeed, it may be because their influence typically escapes notice that it is so powerful in shaping social perception (Baldwin, 1994). The implicit effects of social cognitive processes are well established now (e.g., Greenwald & Banaji, 1995), but it is worth remembering that subliminal priming, the preeminent experimental technique in this area, was considered highly suspect until some methodological and theoretical advances were published in the mid- to late-1980s (e.g., Cheesman & Merikle, 1986; although see Silverman, 1976, for some very early research on the subliminal priming of interpersonal structures).

In psychodynamic writings in particular, self-experience tends to be portrayed as strongly influenced by shadowy images of approving and disapproving others, looking on from the back of one's mind. In one study of such unconscious processes, self-criticism was subliminally primed in graduate students at the University of Michigan by briefly flashing a scowling picture of a respected and critical authority figure—the director of their department (and coincidentally a pioneer in the field of subliminal perception)—Professor Robert Zajonc. The picture was flashed four times during a bogus reaction-time task in which participants were instructed to press a button as soon as they saw a flash of light. They were then immediately asked to evaluate the quality of their own research ideas, a task that was highly ego involving for students enrolled in this empirically oriented program. As predicted, students evaluated their research ideas more negatively following the prime of their scowling department chair than following a control prime (see also Baldwin, 1994, for similar effects from a subliminal prime consisting of just a significant other's name).

A follow-up study examined this phenomenon more closely, asking whether the prime had to be of a person who was in some way significant to the participant. A group of Roman Catholic undergraduate women were first asked to read the sexually permissive passage used in our previous research, then to perform a bogus reaction-time task during which they were subliminally exposed to a disapproving picture of Pope John Paul II. This image was expected to evoke strong self-evaluative effects, given the sexually permissive passage read beforehand. As predicted, participants in this priming condition had lower ratings of self-esteem and higher ratings of anxiety than those in a no-prime control condition. Moreover, only participants who considered themselves practicing Catholics, and therefore for whom the pope was a personally significant authority figure, showed the priming effect. Finally, a third group, subliminally shown a picture of a disapproving stranger, gave self-ratings that were no different from those in the no-prime control condition. Therefore, self-evaluations were most affected by the subliminal prime when it represented a relevant and personally important authority figure.

The effects of interpersonal knowledge structures, then, can occur without any awareness of the thought processes involved. Feelings of insecurity and critical thoughts about the self may arise in consciousness without any obvious links to relational expectancies, but response time and priming research reveal the interpersonal structures that guide the mind (see also Andersen & Chen, 2002, for related research using their stimulus-applicability-based activation paradigm).

TOWARD MODIFYING THE ACTIVATION OF RELATIONAL KNOWLEDGE

We now turn to our most recent work. In the past decade, great progress has been seen in the areas of implicit psychology and motivational processes. With the advent of these developments, social cognition is beginning to revisit older frameworks such as learning theory to reincorporate them into current theory (e.g., Bargh & Ferguson, 2000). In particular, social cognition is now examining motivation and analyzing the influence of goals, from representation to automatic activation and behavioral implications. As a result, learning theories stemming from early work by Pavlov and Skinner are being called upon to help us move beyond studying the mere activation of preexisting knowledge to studying the learning of new associations. In our work on relational schemas, we have for two decades examined core social-cognitive processes such as accessibility, activation, spreading activation, attentional biases, and inhibition. For example, we already know that insecurity involves the (often automatic or unconscious) activation of negative *if–then* interpersonal scripts, producing a focus on rejection and self-criticalness. Drawing on basic cognitive learning theory principles such as classical conditioning and repetitive practice of cognitive responses, our more recent research has involved modifying these cognitive structures and processes, to alter certain detrimental cognitive processes in people who exhibit them. To the extent that this is possible, it will both provide further evidence to support the basic assumptions of the relational schemas perspective, and show the possibility of useful applications of this approach.

Previous research in the attitudes literature has shown that it is possible to change automatic attitudes. Dasgupta and Greenwald (2001), for example, demonstrated that exposure to counterstereotypical exemplars reduced participants' prejudice attitudes as measured by a racial attitudes Implicit Association Test (IAT), and that the effect was still observed during a readministered IAT 24 hours later. Modifying activation patterns cannot be assumed to be easy, however, and researchers have often highlighted the stability of the links in the associative network that has been created and maintained over the years. For example, Kawakami, Dovidio, Moll, Hermsen, and Russin (2000) had participants repeatedly negate associations with a negative stereotype in order to reduce the activation of prejudicial attitudes, and found that this training necessitated hundreds of trials in order to counter the strength of existing stereotypes. Although associative links may be strong, it seems possible, however, to modify them with proper training methods and an adequate number of trials. One of the most promising and direct approaches is classical conditioning. Olson and Fazio (2002) presented participants with random series of words and pictures, in which were embedded some key pairings between conditioned stimuli (CSs) and unconditioned stimuli (USs). Specifically, some trials paired Pokémon cartoon characters with various positive (e.g., hot fudge sundaes) or negative (e.g., cockroaches) stimuli. These Pokémon characters were then used as subliminal primes in a response-time dependent measure, and results confirmed that participants' newly formed attitudes reflected the evaluative valence of the stimulus pairings.

Learning theory is at the heart of these efforts to modify the associations and activation patterns of stereotypes and other attitudes. We have applied similar thinking to our recent research that has focused on modifying the structure and activation of relational schemas. We organize this work into the broad categories of cued activation, self-esteem conditioning, and attentional training.

Cued Activation

Simple associations pervade and structure mental life. How compartmentalized and broken would life be if you experienced every one of your sensations and every situation independently from one another without any associations to previous experience? The smell of overbuttered popcorn would not remind you of your first date at the movies with your sweetheart and your photo album would not bring back waves of emotions from your trip to Southeast Asia or your sibling's wedding. On the other hand, the sound of a siren might not also bring back feelings of guilt and humiliation associated with memories of being caught for speeding down the highway. For better or worse, our experiences, memories, thoughts, and emotions are associated together within a network that can be activated in different situations and by a range of cues.

In several studies we have capitalized on the simple phenomenon of association and examined indirect, or cued, activation of interpersonal knowledge. In these studies a novel tone (the CS) is first associated with a certain relational schema (the US), such as one representing a contingently accepting other, and then the tone is later played in the background while participants complete a task of some kind. The conditioned tone heard in the background has been shown to indirectly activate a host of cognitive processes that in turn affect a variety of behaviors and emotions.

In one version of this general paradigm (Baldwin & Main, 2001; see also Baldwin, Granzberg, Pippus, & Pritchard, 2003) participants underwent a conditioning procedure that paired one computer tone with images of social approval (smiling faces) and a second tone with images of disapproval (frowning faces). A lexical decision task confirmed that the CS approval led to slower identification of rejection words, compared with the CS disapproval. Female participants later interacted for 5 minutes with a male confederate who was trained to act in a very cool, aloof manner, to try to provoke feelings of social anxiety. During this interaction, one of the conditioned tones played repeatedly in the background, on a computer that supposedly was being used for some unrelated purpose. The conditioning had an effect. Participants exposed to the CS-approval tone during the interaction reported more positive, relaxed feelings than those exposed to the CS-disapproval tone. The effects were most pronounced for participants previously assessed as chronically highly self-conscious; these individuals reported dramatically lowered levels of social anxiety if the CS-approval tone was playing in the background. The effects of the conditioning were even evident to the confederate, as reflected in his ratings of how anxious the various participants seemed to be.

In another study (Baldwin & Meunier, 1999), we examined the influence of chronic attachment orientation on people's contingency learning. Two distinctive tones were first paired with mental representations of either a noncontingently or a contingently accepting other. This was done during a guided visualization task, in which participants were asked to visualize either a noncontingently accepting person (someone who accepted them no matter what) or a contingently accepting person (someone who accepted them only if they did well at things). A tone was played repeatedly throughout the visualization task to associate the specific relational schema to the tone. Afterward, participants completed a primed lexical decision task (taken from Baldwin & Sinclair, 1996) where one of the conditioned tones was played at the beginning of each trial. The conditioning procedure had different effects on if–then contingencies of interpersonal acceptance and rejection, depending on participants' chronic attachment orientation. When the CS for contingent acceptance was played, participants high on the preoccupied orientation showed increased evidence of failure-rejection contingencies, whereas participants high on secure attachment showed increased activation of success-acceptance contingencies. As common sense would suggest, then, cues that represent evaluation by others may be most disruptive to individuals who are particularly insecure and unsure about how others will react to them.

A third set of cued activation studies drew on recent cutting-edge research demonstrating the influence of interpersonal cognition on goal striving. We now know that relational schemas can shape the kinds of goals people pursue, the affective reactions they have when their goals are blocked, and so on (see, e.g., Andersen & Saribay, Chapter 1, this volume; Fitzsimons, Shah, Chartrand, & Bargh, Chapter 5, this volume). A fundamental aspect of motivational orientation is the feeling of autonomy, the belief that one is engaged in some activity for one's own reasons rather than being controlled by other people (Deci & Ryan, 1995). Unfortunately, the experience of being controlled by others (e.g., parents, teachers, employers) can all too easily become represented in a relational schema and then become associated with a range of contextual cues, which will then activate the same orientation toward a novel activity. A handful of lessons with a controlling piano teacher, for example, can forever turn a young student off metronomes, wooden benches, and even music in general. Ratelle, Baldwin, and Vallerand (2004) examined the generalization of motivation orientations from one situation to another. Participants first performed some engaging puzzles and periodically were given highly controlling feedback ("You did the puzzle as you should have; now you have to continue with the next one, as is expected of you."). This feedback was repeatedly paired with the presentation of a distinctive computer tone. Later, while they were working on a second enjoyable task, participants were exposed to this tone again or else to a new, different tone. Those who were exposed to the previously conditioned tone were more likely than their control condition counterparts to report feeling that they were doing this second task for controlled reasons ("Because I don't have any choice"), and were less likely to spontaneously engage in the task during a free-play session. These results demonstrate the far-reaching effects of relational schemas in shaping people's motivational orientation to their activities and pursuits. They also underscore the role of contextual cues in the process of generalizing from one activity to another.

In several studies using a range of different procedures and dependent measures, then, it has proven possible to create novel associations between a cue and an element of interpersonal knowledge. We see this as very promising evidence that basic principles from learning theory can be applied to successfully modify the associations, and resulting activation patterns, that underlie the interpersonal mind. Our research thus far has focused on rather neutral, uninspiring cues such as computer tone sequences, but our assumption is that the same principles should apply to real-life cues such as contextual features (e.g., the workplace) or affective cues (e.g., the feeling of rising social anxiety).

Self-Esteem Conditioning

But what about manipulating and modifying the activation of well-established attitudes? With the explosion of research in "implicit psychology" in the last decade, *implicit self-esteem* has become a term understood and adopted by many in the field. Most commonly conceptualized as one's automatic attitude toward the self (Greenwald & Farnham, 2001), it is considered by most as being an aspect of self-esteem largely independent of conscious, explicit self-views. We hypothesize that just as attitudes in general are formed in large part through associations among objects and valenced information, so are associations created between the self-concept and various types of social information. These associations give rise to implicit self-esteem reactions (such as, e.g., rating one's initials as more likeable than other letters of the alphabet). We therefore set out to develop a self-esteem conditioning task to reinforce positive associations to the self (Baccus, Baldwin, & Packer, 2004). Because much previous research has shown that self-esteem is largely interpersonally based, with positive thoughts about the self arising from feelings of being accepted (Baldwin & Sinclair, 1996; Leary, Tambor, Terdal, & Downs, 1995), we aimed to pair self-relevant information with acceptance in order to increase people's implicit self-esteem.

At the beginning of the computer task, participants were asked to enter self-relevant information, such as their name, birthday, and hometown. The task was then described as a reaction-time game wherein participants were to click on the word that would appear in one of four quadrants on the screen, as quickly as possible. After clicking on the word each time, a picture of a person would briefly appear. Positive associations with the self were created by pairing self-relevant information with pictures of accepting faces. That is, in the experimental condition, every time a self-relevant word, such as the participant's name or birthday, was presented in one of the quadrants, it was replaced with a picture of a smiling, accepting face, thereby pairing the self with acceptance. In the control condition, self-relevant information was randomly paired with pictures of smiling, frowning, and neutral faces. Following the conditioning procedure, participants completed two standard measures of implicit self-esteem: The Self-Esteem

Implicit Association Test (Greenwald & Farnham, 2001) and the Name Letter measure (e.g., Nuttin, 1987). Results confirmed that participants undergoing the experimental conditioning procedure showed enhanced implicit self-esteem. The conditioning procedure also showed beneficial results relating to feelings of aggression. After completing the self-esteem conditioning task, people with low explicit self-esteem reported lower aggressive thoughts and feelings compared to their counterparts in the control condition.

These findings confirm the feasibility of applying classical conditioning techniques to modify the associations underlying implicit self-esteem. They also support the analysis of implicit self-esteem as largely reflecting the activation of interpersonal knowledge—that is, when a person thinks about him- or herself, it matters whether this automatically and unconsciously activates expectations of being socially accepted, or socially rejected.

Attentional Training

In recent years, some research on personality processes has highlighted the importance of the cognitive process of attention. As we mentioned earlier in this chapter, people's habitual styles of attention deployment, such as the propensity to be hypervigilant for rejection information, seem to contribute significantly to the maintenance of insecurity and low self-esteem by focusing attention on ambiguously threatening or distressing information. Therefore, it would be useful to identify techniques to facilitate the inhibition of negative information by training an attentional bias away from (rather than toward) threatening information.

We were led to this question by one of our studies on cued activation that demonstrated differences in the inhibition of rejection as a function of people's chronic attachment orientations (Baldwin & Kay, 2003). Two computer tones were paired with either socially accepting feedback or socially rejecting feedback, and then later played as a "get ready" cue before each trial in a lexical decision task that included rejection and acceptance target words. After hearing a cue that had previously been paired with rejection, people characterized by high levels of dismissing avoidance were actually slowed down in their recognition of rejection words. In other words, they showed an inhibitory response to rejection information—this kind of response presumably allows them to maintain high self-esteem even in the face of significant rejection experiences.

We decided to explore the possibility of developing a task that would modify people's attentional bias for rejection by teaching them to inhibit rejection. Based on the well-known face-in-the-crowd paradigm (Hansen & Hansen, 1988), we developed EyeSpy: The Matrix, a game-like computer task that involves identifying as quickly as possible the one smiling/approving face in a 4 × 4 matrix of frowning pictures. In order to successfully complete the task, participants must learn to ignore frowning faces and develop an "inhibit rejection in order to find acceptance faster" mindset. Following the training task, participants completed a Rejection Stroop task that included rejection, acceptance, and neutral words. Results indicated, as we had seen in previous research, that people with low self-esteem in the control condition (who had to identify a five-petaled flower in a matrix of seven-petaled flowers) showed Stroop interference effects on rejection-related words. Low self-esteem individuals in the experimental condition that involved inhibiting frowning faces, however, exhibited significantly less interference on rejection words than their counterparts in the control condition. Therefore, the training task modified their attentional bias for rejection. There were no effects on acceptance interference, which further supports the idea that the task trains the inhibition of rejection. Also noteworthy is the fact that the task seems to have trained a response of orienting away from rejection, broadly defined, and not just a procedural habit of orienting away from frowning pictures, since the training effects transferred from pictures to the words used in the Stroop task. Thus, it seems to be possible to modify people's attentional bias for certain types of social information generally, and more specifically to teach people with low self-esteem to orient away from negative social information.

SUMMARY AND CONCLUSIONS

Human life is lived in the interpersonal spaces created by two or more people, and the psychology of those spaces is largely defined by relational schemas. We have reviewed research showing that people clearly have scripted expectations about what tends to happen in interactions, and these expectations are represented cognitively as *if–then* associations. Relational knowledge, like other social and nonsocial knowledge, functions according to the principles of activation: individual differences in personality, such as those relating to the tendency toward security or insecurity, arise from differences in the chronic accessibility of certain kinds of expectancies. These patterns of activation are largely determined by associations among elements of knowledge, so that a contextual cue of some kind (e.g., a classroom) can activate a specific relational schema (e.g., being evaluated by an authority figure), and moreover a specific event (e.g., a failure) can in turn activate an expected social outcome (e.g., critical rejection). Along the way, we reviewed research techniques we have adopted for measuring the activation of certain types of relational knowledge (e.g., lexical decision and Stroop measures) and also manipulating that activation (e.g., priming and conditioning procedures; see also Andersen & Saribay, Chapter 1, this volume, and Mikulincer & Shaver, Chapter 10, this volume, for other examples).

Although there is not space in a chapter such as this to carefully review the work of other researchers and integrate it with our own, it should be clear that we have benefited much from the efforts made by others working in this area. We find it stimulating to consider areas of overlap. In Fiske and Haslam's relational models approach (Fiske & Haslam, Chapter 11, this volume), for example, they identify four primary structures for social interaction: authority ranking, communal sharing, market pricing, and equality matching. It has occurred to us that when we and others have primed specific relational schemas, perhaps we are doing more than changing expectancies from negative (e.g., criticism) to positive (e.g., acceptance) social outcomes, for example. Perhaps what we are also doing is shifting people's construals between qualitatively different models, for example, toward an authority-ranking model, when we prime authority figures, or toward a communal-sharing model, when we prime securely accepting others. One intriguing possibility that arises out of this hypothesis is that self-esteem dynamics might be very different depending on the relational model that is activated. That is, our view is that self-esteem reactions largely reflect an expectancy-value calculation, such that high self-esteem represents a sense of confidence that one's social goals will be met, whereas low self-esteem represents a sense that one's social goals will not be met (e.g., Baldwin & Baccus, 2003; Baldwin & Sinclair, 1996). Perhaps self-esteem feelings arise from a calculation of social acceptance, as sociometer theory argues (Leary, Chapter 4, this volume), primarily when a communal sharing or equality-matching model is activated. When a market-pricing model is activated, on the other hand, self-esteem may primarily reflect an estimate of one's "market value" in the social world, based on an evaluation of one's strengths and weaknesses and the resources one brings to the table. Finally, when an authority-ranking model is activated, self-esteem might be primarily derived from an estimate of one's social rank (e.g., Gilbert, Chapter 12, this volume). That is, the impact of activated relational models may be due to an extremely complex interaction of the goals, expectancies, and self-models that tend to become activated simultaneously. These kinds of integrative hypotheses are certainly facilitated by the recognition that interpersonal cognition is at the core of many different theoretical approaches.

As we have noted, much of our research has been on insecurity, which involves expectations about meeting important social goals. We recognize that the psychodynamics of security and insecurity are undoubtedly much more complex than simple priming studies might suggest. Relational cognition is profoundly saturated with motivational concerns, as reviewed by other contributors to this volume, and the focus of social cognitive research generally has gradually shifted over the years to an examination of motivated cognition and cognition in service of goal pursuit. Much of human goal pursuit is a highly social affair: motivations can be purely social, as in needs for acceptance or belonging, or the motives for status or power. Even when the motives are not inherently social, goals are very often mediated by relations with others. At the heart of human goal structures, then, are interpersonal structures (see, e.g., Baccus & Horowitz, Chapter 13, this volume; Fitzsimons, Shah, Chartrand, & Bargh, Chapter 5, this volume). Accordingly, the *if–then* contingencies of interpersonal scripts map out a person's assumptions about how to meet goals of all kinds. One most intriguing question we see involves motivational conflict. As Horowitz (1988; Baccus & Horowitz, Chapter 13, this volume) has pointed out, people often learn problematic *if–then* scripts whereby trying to pursue certain goals with a significant other is expected to lead to dreaded or paradoxical outcomes. They also learn conflicting scripts, whereby the same *if* can lead to conflicting *thens*, or different relationships demand different behaviors for satisfying the same need. The issue of dynamic conflict in interpersonal cognition has not received adequate attention, and we are encouraged by recent efforts in this direction (see, e.g., Fitzsimons, Shah, Chartrand, & Bargh, Chapter 5, this volume).

In trying to get a handle on the dynamics of social cognition, we believe that much is to be gained by a detailed analysis of the specific contingencies making up interpersonal scripts. Sometimes it might be adequate to examine the broad strokes of relational knowledge, looking just at working models of "self" and "other," or at best, "self with other." Relational knowledge is much more complex than this, though, as various writers have suggested (see, e.g., Bretherton, 1990): People not only learn a global sense of security or trust in a relationship, they also learn about whether the other person is reliable, honest, sensitive, and so forth. In turn, each of these expectations is based in specific contingencies such as "If I express anger, she will listen to what I have to say," or "If I need emotional support, she will understand and will treat me warmly."

Attention to specific contingencies is especially required if one is interested in the question of how interventions might be designed to alter problematic relational structures. In our recent research we have begun to ask this type of applied question. We believe that drawing on learning theory has been very fruitful, and we expect to continue with this work. By experimentally modifying the cues for knowledge activation and inhibition, we can learn about how these processes work under normal circumstances. We can also start to find new and better ways to apply our knowledge of relational cognition to help people cope with and overcome feelings of insecurity. Brewin (1989, 1996) has argued compellingly that one of the major goals of psychotherapy is to reconfigure the activation patterns whereby problematic structures play the major role in people's construal of their experience. Indeed, as we have seen, insecure attachment, low self-esteem, and social anxiety all seem to involve the misapplication and overapplication of negative schemas.

The vision guiding our latest research is of a type of intervention that targets the specific activation pattern that seems to underlie the person's suffering. Problematic structures could first be identified, perhaps through clinical interview and case formulation (see, e.g., Horowitz, 1988) or via some kind of social-cognitive assessment based on the sorts of tasks developed in the experimental context. Then an intervention could be designed to address the problem identified. In some sense what we are trying to do is to modify people's internal working models of attachment, to help them experience felt security rather than insecurity on an ongoing basis. Framed this way, the specific associations and cognitive responses that need to be modified are those specifically relating to an attachment object's availability and responsiveness.

There is clearly much work to be done before the findings from the laboratory can be directly applied to the creation of psychological interventions. As we and others have found, though, people's self-esteem, sensitivity to rejection, feelings of security, motivational conflicts, and the like are all strongly influenced by the activation of some kinds of relational schemas rather than others. We now need to develop a greater scientific understanding of how those activation patterns might be modified.

ACKNOWLEDGMENTS

The preparation of this chapter was supported by a grant from the Social Sciences and Humanities Research Council of Canada to Mark W. Baldwin and a fellowship from Fondation Baxter et Alma Ricard to Stéphane D. Dandeneau. We thank Patricia Csank for her helpful comments.

REFERENCES

Abelson, R. P. (1981). Psychological status of the script concept. *American Psychologist, 36,* 715–729.

Andersen, S. M., & Chen, S. (2002). The relational self: An interpersonal social-cognitive theory. *Psychological Review, 109*(4), 619–645.

Andersen, S. M., & Cole, S. W. (1987). "Do I know you?": The role of significant others in general social perception. *Journal of Personality and Social Psychology, 59*(3), 384–399.

Baccus, J. R., Baldwin, M. W., & Packer, D. J. (2004). Increasing implicit self-esteem through classical conditioning. *Psychological Science, 15,* 498–502.

Baldwin, M. W. (1992). Relational schemas and the processing of social information. *Psychological Bulletin, 112,* 461–484.

Baldwin, M. W. (1994). Primed relational schemas as a source of self-evaluative reactions. *Journal of Social and Clinical Psychology, 13*(4), 380–403.

Baldwin, M. W. (1997). Relational schemas as a source of if–then self-inference procedures. *Review of General Psychology, 1*(4), 326–335.

Baldwin, M. W., & Baccus, J. R. (2003). An expectancy-value approach to self-esteem. In S. J. Spencer & S. Fein (Eds.), *Motivated social perception: The Ontario Symposium* (Ontario Symposium on Personality and Social Psychology, Vol. 9, pp. 171–194). Mahwah, NJ: Erlbaum.

Baldwin, M. W., Baccus, J. R., & Fitzsimons, G. M. (2004). Self-esteem and the dual processing of interpersonal contingencies. *Self and Identity, 3,* 81–93.

Baldwin, M. W., & Fehr, B. (1995). On the instability of attachment style ratings. *Personal Relationships, 2*(3), 247–261.

Baldwin, M. W., Fehr, B., Keedian, E., Seidel, M., & Thomson, D. W. (1993). An exploration of the relational schemata underlying attachment styles: Self-report and lexical decision approaches. *Personality and Social Psychology Bulletin, 19,* 746–754.

Baldwin, M. W., Granzberg, A., Pippus, L., & Pritchard, E. T. (2003). Cued activation of relational schemas: Self-evaluation and gender effects. *Canadian Journal of Behavioural Science, 35*(2), 153–163.

Baldwin, M. W., & Holmes, J. G. (1987). Salient private audiences and awareness of the self. *Journal of Personality and Social Psychology, 52*(6), 1087–1098.

Baldwin, M. W., & Kay, A. C. (2003). Adult attachment and the inhibition of rejection. *Journal of Social and Clinical Psychology, 22*(2), 275–293.

Baldwin, M. W., & Keelan, J. P. R. (1999). Interpersonal expectations as a function of self-esteem and sex. *Journal of Social and Personal Relationships, 16*(6), 822–833.

Baldwin, M. W., Keelan, J. P. R., Fehr, B., Enns, V., & Koh-Rangarajoo, E. (1996). Social-cognitive conceptualization of attachment working models: Availability and accessibility effects. *Journal of Personality and Social Psychology, 71*(1), 94–109.

Baldwin, M. W., & Main, K. J. (2001). Social anxiety and the cued activation of relational knowledge. *Personality and Social Psychology Bulletin, 27*(12), 1637–1647.

Baldwin, M. W., & Meunier, J. (1999). The cued activation of attachment relational schemas. *Social Cognition, 17,* 209–227.

Baldwin, M. W., & Sinclair, L. (1996). Self-esteem and "if . . . then" contingencies of interpersonal acceptance. *Journal of Personality and Social Psychology, 71,* 1130–1141.

Bargh, J. A., & Ferguson, M. J. (2000). Beyond behaviorism: On the automaticity of higher mental processes. *Psychological Bulletin, 126,* 925–945.

Baumeister, R. F., & Leary, M. R. (1995). The need to belong: Desire for interpersonal attachments as a fundamental human motivation. *Psychological Bulletin, 117,* 497–529.

Bowlby, J. (1969). *Attachment and loss: Vol. 1. Attachment.* New York: Basic Books.

Bowlby, J. (1973). *Attachment and loss: Vol. 2. Separation: Anxiety and anger.* New York: Basic Books.

Bretherton, I. (1985). Attachment theory: Retrospect and prospect. *Monographs of the Society for Research in Child Development, 50*(1–2), 3–35.

Bretherton, I. (1990). Communication patterns, internal working models, and the intergenerational transmission of attachment relationships. *Infant Mental Health Journal, 11*, 237–252.

Brewin, C. R. (1989). Cognitive change processes in psychotherapy. *Psychological Review, 96*, 379–394.

Brewin, C. R. (1996). Theoretical foundation of cognitive-behavior therapy for anxiety and depression. *Annual Review of Psychology, 47*, 33–57.

Cantor, N., & Kihlstrom, J. F. (1985). Social intelligence: The cognitive basis of personality. *Review of Personality and Social Psychlgy, 6*, 15–33.

Carlston, D. E., & Smith, E. R. (1996). Principles of mental representation. In E. T. Higgins & A. W. Kruglanski (Eds.), *Social psychology: Handbook of basic principles* (pp. 184–210). New York: Guilford Press.

Cheesman, J., & Merikle, P. M. (1986). Distinguishing conscious from unconscious perceptual processes. *Canadian Journal of Psychology, 40*, 343–367.

Christensen, A. (1987). Detection of conflict patterns in couples. In K. Hahlweg & M. J. Goldstein (Eds.), *Readings in social psychology* (pp. 250–265). New York: Family Press.

Clark, M. S., & Mills, J. (1979). Interpersonal attraction in exchange and communal relationships. *Journal of Personality and Social Psychology, 37*(1), 12–24.

Collins, N. L., & Read, S. J. (1994). Cognitive representations of attachment: The content and function of working models. In K. Bartholomew & D. Perlman (Eds.), *Advances in personal relationships* (Vol. 5, pp. 53–90). London: Jessica Kingsley.

Cooley, C. H. (1902). *Human nature and the social order.* New York: Schocken Books.

Crittenden, P. M. (1990). Internal representational models of attachment relationships. *Infant Mental Health Journal, 11*(3), 259–277.

Dandeneau, S. D., & Baldwin, M. W. (2004a). The inhibition of socially rejecting information among people with high versus low self-esteem: The role of attentional bias and the effects of bias reduction training. *Journal of Social and Clinical Psychology, 23*(4), 584–602.

Dandeneau, S. D., & Baldwin, M. W. (2004b). [Teaching inhibition of rejection to people with low self-esteem]. Unpublished raw data.

Dasgupta, N., & Greenwald, A. G. (2001). On the malleability of automatic attitudes: Combating automatic prejudice with images of admired and disliked individuals. *Journal of Personality and Social Psychology, 81*(5), 800–814.

Davila, J., Burge, D., & Hammen, C. (1997). Why does attachment style change? *Journal of Personality and Social Psychology, 73*, 826–838.

Deci, E. L., & Ryan, R. M. (1995). Human autonomy: The basis for true self-esteem. In M. H. Kernis (Ed.), *Efficacy, agency, and self-esteem* (pp. 31–48). New York: Plenum Press.

Epstein, S. (1973). The self-concept revisited: Or a theory of a theory. *American Psychologist, 28*(5), 404–416.

Fehr, B., Baldwin, M. W., Collins, L., Patterson, S., & Benditt, R. (1999). Anger in close relationships: An interpersonal script analysis. *Personality and Social Psychology Bulletin, 25*(3), 299–312.

Fiske, A. P. (1992). The four elementary forms of sociality: Framework for a unified theory of social relations. *Psychological Review, 99*, 689–723.

Fonagy, P. (2001). *Attachment theory and psychoanalysis.* New York: Other Press.

Frazier, P., Byer, A. L., Fischer, A. R., Wright, D. M., & DeBord, K. A. (1996). Adult attachment style and partner choice: Correlational and experimental findings. *Personal Relationships, 3,* 117–136.

Freud, S. (1957). Mourning and melancholia. In J. Strachey (Ed. & Trans.), *The standard edition of the complete psychological works of Sigmund Freud* (Vol. 14, pp. 243–258). London: Hogarth Press. (Original work published 1917)

Ginsburg, G. (1988). Rules, scripts and prototypes in personal relationships. In S. Duck (Ed.), *Handbook of personal relationships: Theory, research and interventions* (pp. 23–39). New York: Wiley.

Gollwitzer, P. M. (1999). Implementation intentions: Strong effects of simple plans. *American Psychologist, 54,* 493–503.

Greenberg, J. R., & Mitchell, S. A. (1983). *Object relations in psychoanalytic theory.* Cambridge, MA: Harvard University Press.

Greenwald, A., & Banaji, M. R. (1995). Implicit social cognition: Attitudes, self-esteem, and stereotypes. *Psychological Review, 102,* 4–17.

Greenwald, A., & Farnham, S. (2001). Using the implicit associations test to measure self-esteem and self-concept. *Journal of Personality and Social Psychology, 79,* 1022–1038.

Hansen, C. H., & Hansen, R. D. (1988). Finding the face in the crowd: An anger superiority effect. *Journal of Personality and Social Psychology, 54*(6), 917–924.

Hazan, C., & Shaver, P. R. (1987). Romantic love conceptualized as an attachment process. *Journal of Personality and Social Psychology, 52,* 511–524.

Higgins, E. T. (1996). The "Self-Digest": Self-knowledge serving self-regulatory functions. *Journal of Personality and Social Psychology, 71,* 1062–1083.

Higgins, E. T., & Bargh, J. A. (1987). Social cognition and social perception. *Annual Review of Psychology, 38,* 369–425.

Higgins, E. T., Rholes, W. S., & Jones, C. R. (1977). Category accessibility and impression formation. *Journal of Experimantal Social Psychology, 13,* 141–154.

Hill, C. R., & Safran, J. (1994). Assessing interpersonal schemas: Anticipated responses of significant others. *Journal of Social and Clinical Psychology, 13,* 366–379.

Horowitz, M. J. (1988). *Introduction to psychodynamics: A new synthesis.* New York: Basic Books.

James, W. (1890). *The principles of psychology.* Cambridge, MA: Harvard University Press.

Kawakami, K., Dovidio, J. F., Moll, J., Hermsen, S., & Russin, A. (2000). Just say no (to stereotyping): Effects of training in trait negation on stereotype activation. *Journal of Personality and Social Psychology, 78,* 871–888.

Leary, M. R., Tambor, E. S., Terdal, S. K., & Downs, D. L. (1995). Self-esteem as an interpersonal monitor: The sociometer hypothesis. *Journal of Personality and Social Psychology, 68*(3), 518–530.

Mead, G. H. (1934). *Mind, self, and society.* Chicago: University of Chicago Press.

Miell, D. (1987). Remembering relationship development: Constructing a context for interactions. In R. Burnett, P. McGhee, & D. D. Clarke (Eds.), *Accounting for relationships* (pp. 60–73). New York: Methuen.

Mischel, W. (1973). Toward a cognitive social learning reconceptualization of personality. *Psychological Review, 80,* 252–283.

Mischel, W., & Shoda, Y. (1995). A cognitive-affective system theory of personality: Reconceptualizing situations, dispositions, dynamics, and invariance in personality structure. *Psychological Review, 102,* 246–268.

Mitchell, S. A. (1988). *Relational concepts in psychoanalysis.* Cambridge, MA: Harvard University Press.

Nuttin, J. M. (1987). Affective consequences of mere ownership: The name letter effect in twelve European languages. *European Journal of Social Psychology, 17,* 381–402.

Ogilvie, D. M., & Ashmore, R. D. (1991). Self-with-other representation as a unit of analysis in self-concept research. In R. C. Curtis (Ed.), *The relational self: Theoretical convergences in psychoanalysis and social psychology* (pp. 282–314). New York: Guilford Press.

Olson, M. A., & Fazio, R. H. (2002). Implicit acquisition and manifestation of classically conditioned attitudes. *Social Cognition, 20*(2), 89–104.

Pierce, T., & Lydon, J. (1998). Priming relational schemas: Effects of contextually activated and chronically accessible interpersonal expectations on responses to a stressful event. *Journal of Personality and Social Psychology, 75,* 1441–1448.

Planalp, S. (1985). Relational schemata: A test of alternative forms of relational knowledge as guides to communication. *Human Communication Research, 12,* 3–29.

Posner, M. I., & Petersen, S. E. (1990). The attention system of the human brain. *Annual Review of Neuroscience, 13,* 25–42.

Ratelle, C., Baldwin, M. W., & Vallerand, R. (2004). *On the cued activation of situational motivation.* Manuscript submitted for publication.

Rogers, C. R. (1959). A theory of therapy, personality, and interpersonal relationships as developed in the client-centered framework. In S. Koch (Ed.), *Psychology: A study of a science* (Vol. 3, pp. 184–256). New York: McGraw-Hill.

Safran, J. D. (1990). Towards a refinement of cognitive therapy in light of interpersonal theory: I. Theory. *Clinical Psychology Review, 10*(1), 87–105.

Schlenker, B. R., & Leary, M. R. (1982). Social anxiety and self-presentation: A conceptualization and model. *Psychological Bulletin, 92,* 641–669.

Silverman, L. H. (1976). Psychoanalytic theory: The reports of my death are greatly exaggerated. *American Psychologist, 31,* 621–637.

Smith, E. R. (1998). Mental representation and memory. In G. Lindzey (Ed.), *The handbook of social psychology* (Vol. 1, pp. 391–445). New York: McGraw-Hill.

Smith, E. R., & Branscombe, N. R. (1987). Procedurally mediated social inferences: The case of category accessibility effects. *Journal of Experimantal Social Psychology, 23,* 361–382.

Stern, D. N. (1985). *The interpersonal world of the infant.* New York: Basic Books.

Sullivan, H. S. (1953). *The interpersonal theory of psychiatry.* New York: Norton.

Trzebinski, J. (1985). Action-oriented representations of implicit personality theories. *Journal of Personality and Social Psychology, 48*(5), 1266–1278.

Vygotsky, L. S. (1986). *Thought and language* (A. Kozulin, Trans.). Cambridge, MA: MIT Press. (Original work published 1934)

Westen, D. (1988). Transference and information processing. *Clinical Psychology Review, 8*(2), 161–179.

Williams, M. G., Mathews, A., & MacLeod, C. (1996). The emotional Stroop task and psychopathology. *Psychological Bulletin, 120*(1), 3–24.

Williamson, R. N., & Fitzpatrick, M. A. (1985). Two approaches to marital interaction: Relational control patterns in marital types. *Communication Monographs, 52*(3), 236–252.

Winnicott, D. W. (1975). *Through paediatrics to psycho-analysis*. London: International Psycho-analytic Library. (Original work published 1958)

3

Rejection Sensitivity as an Interpersonal Vulnerability

JANINA PIETRZAK, GERALDINE DOWNEY, *and* OZLEM AYDUK

The rejection sensitivity (RS) model posits that hypersensitivity to rejection cues, with its subsequent overreactions, is fallout from a normal learning process; rejection sensitivity is born of early, prolonged, or acute rejection experiences with caregivers and significant others. Through such experiences, children learn to expect rejection in situations involving close others, and because the relationships are significant, these expectations are emotion-laden. Thus, anxious expectations of rejection characterize the departure point of the RS dynamic. What follows are a lowered threshold for perception of negativity, an increased propensity for personalizing negative cues, and intense affective reactions. Such cognitions and affects can then lead to expressions of distress in the form of hostility or depression, creating the potential for a feedback loop that becomes a self-fulfilling prophecy. This dynamic, once acquired, can guide interpersonal perceptions and behavior throughout the life course.

The RS model was introduced to explain why some individuals appear more vulnerable to maladaptive responses to rejection experiences than do others (Downey & Feldman, 1996). In this chapter, we first describe the historical backdrop of social cognition and personality in which rejection sensitivity evolved. These two fields of research, along with research on personal relationships, intersect where cognitive and affective constructs are identified and the process by which they affect relationship behavior is delineated. The RS dynamic is one illustration of the marriage of these fields. We then describe how the recent incorporation of psychophysiological approaches to the study of social-psychological phenomena has shaped our view of RS, and provide an in-depth description of the RS model, outlining its unique contribution to work on personal relationships, and exposing the sometimes paradoxical ways in which high RS individuals cope with imminent self-threat. Finally, we take a look down avenues of current and future research.

The idea that early traumatic experiences can lead to later relationship difficulties is not novel; clinicians starting with Freud, and personality theorists starting with Horney (1937), Erikson (1950), and Sullivan (1953) proposed that interactions with parents lead to later patterns of interpersonal behavior or personality traits. Theories of why people encountered difficulties in their relationships focused on individual differences in personality attributes such as global self-esteem, attributional bias (e.g., Bradbury & Fincham, 1990; Holtzworth-Munroe & Hutchinson, 1993), and attachment style (Hazan & Shaver, 1987) as predictors of relationship success or failure. The introduction of social-cognitive paradigms provided a framework in which to examine these ideas and opened up avenues of relationship research that could be identified as psychodynamic in approach—looking at unconscious, automatic processes that led to particular relationship outcomes (Reis & Downey, 1999). Social information selection and processing began to be studied, and social phenomena gained a cognitive spin: accessibility, memory errors, and attributional biases all became valid areas of study. Drawing on notions borrowed from theories of the structure of long-term memory, interest arose in the chronically accessible scripts and processing dispositions that were activated and implemented in particular situations—for example, in close relationships. The high accessibility and availability of scripts and schemas coming from early relationships shed light on the mechanism by which previous relationships dictated new relationships.

At the same time, social cognition was affecting research in individual differences. Theorists were moving away from viewing the individual as a combination of global and consistently activated traits and toward a more dynamic vision of the individual as driven by stable cognitive–affective processing dynamics that result in systematic and coherent variability of affect, cognition, and behavior across situations (Mischel & Shoda, 1995). Emerging conceptualizations of personality drew on cognitive as well as affective phenomena to get at the unconscious processes of social information processing that underlie relationship behavior. This shift from individual differences to intraindividual processing dynamics brought a focus on the mechanisms that lead to behavior: beliefs, expectations, desires, and motivations. The strategy adopted by some researchers at the time was to observe intraindividual stability in patterns of behavior across various situations (Mischel & Shoda, 1995). This led to a focus on the cognitive and affective processing that was taking place when an individual made sense of a particular situation and decided on a course of action. Such cognitive–affective units were used to explain what made the same person behave in such different ways at different times.

Though our conceptualization of RS is rooted in attributional and attachment theories and in interpersonal approaches to personality, notably the work of Karen Horney, our approach departs from these traditional approaches in several respects. It has adopted the developments of social cognition to delineate the immediate cognitive and affective antecedents of behavior in specific situations, rather than to describe global orientations to relationships. This approach lets us look at parenting history as a determinant of personal dispositions based in mechanisms of information processing and memory, and can help us to understand the development of personality and its effects on current relationships, including cross-situational inconsistency in relationship behavior. RS can be viewed as delineating some of the key cognitive and affective subprocesses incorporated in people's working model of attachment. The RS model provides a process account of how anxious expectations of rejection lead to attributional biases and then to maladjustment through specific physiological, perceptual, and cognitive mechanisms.

This new ability to map the development of relationships through social-cognitive variables can be applied not only in a long-term sense, over an individual's lifetime, but also within a relationship, and even within a particular interaction. This approach deconstructs dispositional terms into concrete cognitions and affects, which can be independently observed, described, and then perhaps changed. Because RS is more specific and precise in its definition of the content, structure, and dynamics of insecure attachment, in our studies we have typically found it to be a better predictor of how people cope with rejection in specific situations than traditional measures of insecure attachment (for a detailed discussion of the distinction between RS and attachment style, see Ayduk, Downey, & Kim, 2000, and Downey & Feldman, 1996).

The unique contribution that the RS model makes in the context of relationship cognition is its account of the processes linking the individual's social learning history with an unfolding social situation. It is a model that embraces the social-cognitive approach and exploits its merits—focusing on dynamic processing of both cognitive and affective information—to demonstrate how these invisible factors shape relationship behavior within a specific interpersonal situation. The model focuses on the psychological (cognitive and affective) mediators of anxious expectations of rejection that lead to a hypervigilance for rejection cues, which can then affect perceptions of, attributions for, and responses to others' ambiguous behavior. Some other constructs have similar social-cognitive roots and emphases but are not as specific (e.g., transference; see Andersen & Chen, 2002), while other, more global constructs (e.g., self-esteem) lack the transparency of mechanism that leads to clear and testable predictions—as well as to viable interventions. The outcome of an interpersonal situation must involve the confluence of intermediary processes, which combine to increase the likelihood of a benign or a malevolent response. Understanding the mechanisms through which anxious attachment style, self-esteem, and other dispositions yield relationship behaviors can greatly facilitate the development of more effective intervention intended to reduce the negative consequences of interpersonal vulnerabilities (Freitas & Downey, 1998).

THE REJECTION SENSITIVITY MODEL

Extensive evidence links child maltreatment with a variety of negative outcomes (Downey, Feldman, Khouri, & Friedman, 1994; Manly, Kim, Rogosch, & Cicchetti, 2001; Widom, 1989). Researchers have long proclaimed early experiences as formative because they affect all relationships that follow. The relationships of children with parents, then with peers and teachers, form a framework of understanding and expectations for all future interactions (Sroufe, 1990). Acceptance/rejection schemas begin to develop as soon as a child is born; all human contact becomes a field for learning the rules of social interaction (Ainsworth, Blehar, Waters, & Wall, 1978; Bowlby, 1969, 1973, 1980). This framework, if confirmed time and again through interpersonal experiences, can grow stronger as the individual grows older. If a child is rejected repeatedly, close interpersonal situations in the future can essentially serve as primes for rejection: strong mental associations exist between the relevant situational cues and rejection experiences. The RS model posits that such associations, formed of prolonged or acute rejecting experiences with significant others, lead to the development of anxious expectations of rejection (Feldman & Downey, 1994; Downey, Khouri, & Feldman, 1997). Such expectations can affect the way social information is processed in later life because the perceptions and attributions people make are driven in a top-down processing manner by the expectations with which people enter an interaction (Olson, Roese, & Zanna, 1996). Anxious expectations are thus carried from one relationship to the next, and can form a stable pattern of interaction with future partners.

Because close interpersonal contexts are likely to follow automatic, routinized sequences (Berscheid, 1994) and have significance for goal attainment, they are likely to be dominated by "hot" processing. This unintentional, unconscious processing is contrasted with a rational "cool" processing system that drives deliberate action (Epstein, 1994; Metcalfe & Mischel, 1999). This "hot" processing system relies on the mental schemas and frameworks that are (chronically or temporarily) accessible, guiding perceptions and interpretations of new situations. Both Baldwin and colleagues (1992; Baldwin & Keelan, 1999; Baldwin, Keelan, Fehr, Enns, & Koh-Rangarajoo, 1996) and Andersen and colleagues (e.g., Andersen & Chen, 2002; Andersen, Reznik, & Chen, 1997) use a dual processing approach to uncover the balance of cognitive and affective processes that are activated in response to threat. The idea that cognitive responses can regulate and interact with affective responses to threat allows psychologists to draw on findings in affective neuroscience and bend the constraints of traditional methodologies, which emphasized cognitions or affects, but not their interaction.

This approach also allows us to reconcile the differences in behavioral patterns exhibited by individuals with similar social-cognitive histories of maltreatment. Why does parental maltreatment in some people lead to aggression, while in others it leads to social withdrawal? Why do some people respond to rejection with anger while others reveal anxiety? Why do some people cope with rejection through self-silencing and others with violence? These are issues that go beyond gross distinctions in developmental context, and are best answered through an uncovering of the social-cognitive processes that make individuals respond uniquely to particular interpersonal situations.

In view of the dynamic as one in which expectations of rejection are accompanied by intense affect, the questionnaire used to measure RS in adults is composed of 18 items depicting interpersonal situations wherein the respondent imagines him- or herself expressing need to a close other. To each such situation, the respondent must indicate on two separate 1–6 scales the extent to which he or she expects rejection (the need will not be met) and to what extent he or she feels anxious or concerned about this possibility. These situations were chosen through focus group interviews and extensive piloting. They demonstrate the unique trigger situations hypothesized to activate anxious expectations of rejection. The content of the request is not impersonal (the respondent is not asking the close other about the weather); rather, the respondent is requesting something, and thereby exposing him- or herself to the possibility of rejection. This rejection, if it occurred, could be interpreted in many ways, and the anxiety response is some indication of how personally important it is that it not come. Therefore, within each situation, the rating on the expectations of rejection is weighted by the anxiety rating and the product terms are then averaged over the 18 items.

Conceptualizing Rejection Sensitivity as a Defensive Motivational System

As new physiological and social-cognitive neuroscience paradigms have been introduced, the implicit nonconscious processing that occurs in relationship contexts has become more "observable." Accordingly, we have extended our social-cognitive approach to studying this dynamic into the realm of physiological and neurological underpinnings. Many aspects of an interaction with another person can determine one's comfort during and after it. Because the need for belonging/affiliation is so dominant in humans, because of the evolutionary validity of this need, it seems that assessing the basic valence of a social interaction may be the first and crucial step to take. For this reason, we have posited that acceptance–rejection is a privileged dimension of information processing, and RS has been explicitly reconceptualized as a defensive motivational system (DMS), a physiologically based mechanism that is triggered in response to threat from the environment.

In the context of RS, the DMS system is hypothesized to get activated specifically in response to acceptance–rejection cues and to function to provide a quick and effective response to threat in the environment, sheltering the self from the feared rejection. This conceptualization is rooted in work on the neurobiology of motivational systems. The understanding of how organisms defend themselves against threats in general has increased tremendously over the past decade as researchers have brought developments in cognitive, behavioral, and affective neuroscience to bear on the issue. Converging evidence from neurological and behavioral research suggests that two primary affective-motivational systems organize behavior: an appetitive system that responds to positive stimuli (i.e., rewards), motivating approach and consummatory behavior, and a defensive system that responds to negative, aversive stimuli (i.e., punishments, threat), disposing the individual toward active avoidance, and fight-or-flight (Cacioppo & Gardner, 1999; Gray, 1987; Lang, 1995; Lang, Bradley, & Cuthbert, 1990, 1995; LeDoux, 1995, 1996; Metcalfe & Mischel, 1999). Drawing from this literature, Lang and colleagues (1990) proposed a model that views human emotions as action dispositions that organize behavior along an appetitive–aversive dimension. According to this model, when negatively valenced and highly arousing stimuli are encountered, the DMS becomes activated to prepare for rapid execution of a set of automatic behaviors aimed at self-protection. What constitutes a threat can be biologically based (e.g., an inherent threat reaction to seeing a snake) or socially learned (e.g., people can learn through direct or vicarious rejection experiences to expect rejection in certain situations). Valence directs the system (i.e., approach vs. avoidance), but level of arousal determines the intensity of response.

Research on both animals and humans suggests that when this high-arousal negative-valence system is activated by the potential of danger, there is an amplification of physiological responses to newly encountered threat-congruent cues and an attenuation of physiological response to threat-incongruent cues. Thus, the organism is oriented to detect cues that are congruent with a state of threat (see LeDoux, 1996, LeDoux & Phelps,

2000, and Ohman, 2000, for reviews). The high level of arousal and negative valence also readies the organism to act when cues confirming that the
threatened outcome has occurred are detected (e.g., Lang et al., 1995;
LeDoux, Iwata, Cicchetti, & Reis, 1988). Gray (1987) has argued that
threat also activates inhibitory behaviors reflected in vigorous efforts to
freeze and remain silent. The defensive motivation that underlies this inhibitory behavioral set is to be inconspicuous, to become part of the existing context, to go "unnoticed" as a way to prevent threat from being
directed at the self. This behavioral "freeze" must be highly vigilant to
maintain a high state of readiness for action in case prevention efforts fail
(Gray, 1987, 2000). This framework thus suggests that a shift is likely to
occur from prevention-focused inhibitory tactics to intense fight-or-flight
reactions if and when a threatened outcome is perceived to be inevitable or
to have already occurred (see Figure 3.1).

Our phenomenological description of the operation of the RS system
closely parallels the operation of the DMS. According to our conceptualization of RS, in situations where rejection is a possibility (e.g., meeting a
prospective dating partner, asking one's friend to do favor), people who are
high in RS are uncertain about whether they will be accepted or rejected,
but the outcome is of critical importance to them. This view leads to
hypotheses surrounding physiological correlates of being in a rejection-
relevant situation. As mentioned above, situations where one anxiously expects rejection are threatening. The DMS should be activated, leading to a
heightened focus on and advantaged processing of threat cues (LeDoux,
1996; Ohman, 2000). Ambiguous stimuli will be more likely then to be interpreted in line with these expectations—in order to ensure survival, it is
safer to overreact than to fail to react to mild cues that might turn out to
be life-threatening. The high RS individual, then, prefers a "better safe

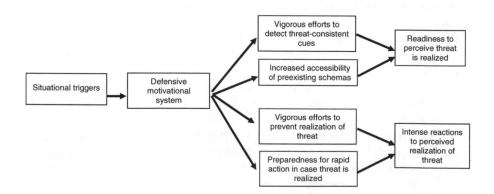

FIGURE 3.1. Rejection sensitivity as a defensive motivational system.

than sorry" strategy to protect from rejection, whereas the low RS individual might risk not detecting mild rejection cues, because such cues are less subjectively threatening to the low RS individual. Thus, for high RS individuals, situations where they anxiously expect rejection incorporate cognitive appraisals of threat under conditions of uncertainty—these are the very conditions that research in affective neuroscience as well as stress and coping suggest are likely to activate the DMS (Davis, 1992; Fanselow, 1994; Lazarus, Averill, & Opton, 1970; LeDoux, 1995; Metcalfe & Mischel, 1999; Zillman, 1993). In contrast to high RS individuals, the RS model suggests that, in the same situations, those low in RS take acceptance more for granted and are less concerned with the threat of rejection, and are thus less likely to experience heightened activation of the DMS.

We propose that, when activated, the DMS facilitates the monitoring and detection of threat-relevant cues and prepares the individual for swift response when cues of danger are detected. In situations where rejection is expected, this system is automatically activated in high RS individuals. The activation of this system can help account for the readiness with which high RS individuals perceive rejection in others' behavior and contributes to the intensity of their responses to the perceived rejection.

A recent study conducted by Downey, Mougois, Ayduk, London, and Shoda (2004) tested the hypothesis that ambiguous interpersonal situations would induce a sense of threat in high RS individuals, and activation of the DMS, wherein they would experience high negative arousal. High negative arousal can be determined in humans by measuring the *startle reflex*, the amplitude of the eye-blink response to a sudden extreme stimulus, like a burst of white noise. In this study, participants were exposed to such a stimulus while viewing various artworks depicting four kinds of themes: rejection, acceptance, noninterpersonal positivity, or noninterpersonal negativity. High RS individuals who were viewing rejection images showed a potentiation of the startle reflex; no other condition showed such an increase. This study demonstrated that indeed negative interpersonal situations put high RS people into a state of threat, wherein they responded more intensely to stimuli that could communicate interpersonal rejection.

Behavioral studies demonstrate the further links in the model. Because people are likely to interpret events in accordance with their expectations—stimuli are attended to, processed, and remembered in ways that confirm expectations—negative or ambiguous interpersonal interactions are perceived by high RS individuals to be personal affronts, attributed to others' intentional rejection of them. Accordingly, the link between anxious expectations of rejection and perceptions of intentional rejection in the negative or ambiguous behavior of close or newly encountered others was tested by Downey and Feldman (1996, Study 2). High RS individuals, when not given an alternative explanation for a negative interpersonal outcome (such as time constraints limiting a social interaction) were more likely to construe this outcome as personally motivated and intentionally rejecting. Likewise, high RS individuals reported perceiving intentional rejection in the aloof behavior of their dating partners (Downey & Feldman, 1996, Study 3). For high RS individuals, alternative explanations for seemingly rejecting behaviors are not considered; displays of acceptance might be misinterpreted or undervalued. Because of this top-down processing (i.e., processing driven more by preexisting knowledge than by proximal stimuli), and the strong affective response it engenders, reactive behavior often follows perceived rejection.

Though perceptions of rejection are likely to lead to some kind of reaction in everyone, for high RS individuals they lead to reactions that are inappropriately intense and highly defensive. For example, in a priming study, participants were asked to pronounce as quickly as they could target words that appeared on the screen following a masked prime. For high RS women, rejection primes facilitated pronunciation of hostility targets that followed. This suggests an automatic association between rejection and hostility (Ayduk, Downey, Testa, Yen, & Shoda, 1999, Study 1). Furthermore, in a daily diary study of dating couples, feelings of rejection from their romantic partners on one day elicited hostility from high RS women on the next day (Ayduk et al., 1999, Study 2). In contrast, low RS women's likelihood of getting into conflicts with their partners was not contingent on their feelings of rejection. Consistently, when discussing an unresolved relationship conflict in a lab situation, women high in RS were shown to behave more negatively and aggressively, both in terms of their verbal and this nonverbal behavior (Downey, Freitas, Michaelis, & Khouri, 1998, Study 3).

Because their partners may be surprised by strong reactions to seemingly neutral behavior, high RS people can be perceived (and responded to) as excessively sensitive and difficult, which leads to relationship dissatisfaction on both ends. Personal attributions for rejection were shown to undermine romantic relationships by increasing jealous behavior among men and increasing hostile behavior among women (Downey & Feldman, 1996, Study 4). Because intent is usually invisible and must be inferred, it is open to misinterpretation; high RS people, by overestimating the likelihood of rejection, may overestimate their partners' intent to do them harm. Partners of high RS individuals, meanwhile, may have trouble recognizing their own neutral, ambiguous, or even nonpersonally negative behavior as potentially conveying rejection.

In a daily diary study including committed dating couples, Downey, Freitas, and colleagues (1998, Study 1) showed that in days following a conflict, high RS women perceived their partners as less accepting and more withdrawn than did low RS women. High RS women's partners, meanwhile, were more likely to express relationship dissatisfaction than were low RS women's partners. Partial mediation points to partner satisfaction as the link between RS and perceptions of partner acceptance after conflict. A lab study of videotaped interactions showed that high RS women's negative behavior during conflict evoked postconflict anger in both the women and their partners (Downey, Freitas, et al., 1998, Study 2). These two studies suggest that the dynamic acts as a self-fulfilling prophecy, wherein expectations of rejection increase the probability of its occurrence (Merton, 1948; Rosenthal, 2002; Sroufe, 1990). High RS individuals are responding to rejection cues that, to them, appear all too real, in ways that a significant other may find aversive. Thus, the rejection that high RS people expect occurs, validating their cognitions and cementing them afresh. In this way, the expectations that a person brings into an interaction shape that interaction, and can create stable and destructive patterns of relational behavior. These patterns can diminish a partner's satisfaction in and commitment to the relationship, leading to breakup and a confirmation of the high RS individual's rejection expectations.

The consequences of RS are not limited to adult relationships. The dynamic is acquired early; evidence of its functioning has been observed in children as young as fifth grade. Studies conducted with middle-school children have shown that high RS children experience interpersonal difficulties including aggressive and antisocial behavior, troubled relationships with peers and teachers, and disciplinary problems leading to suspensions (Downey, Lebolt, Rincon, & Freitas, 1998).

Our findings within a social-cognitive approach provide support for the view that RS operates within a vicious cycle with rejection expectations, setting in motion actions that lead to their fulfillment. Thus, at first glance, RS appears to be a dysfunctional system that perpetuates personal and interpersonal difficulties. An alternative viewpoint is that the RS dynamic functions to defend the self against rejection by significant others and social groups. To the extent that the individual has been exposed to the pain of rejection, protecting the self from rejection while maintaining close relationships will become an important goal and a protective system such as RS will develop to serve it. The adaptive value of the DMS comes from its ability to trigger quick defensive responses under threat conditions without needing time to think (e.g., LeDoux, 1996; Metcalfe & Mischel, 1999; Ohman, 2000). Such an emergency system can become maladaptive, however, if activated indiscriminately in situations that require reflective strategic behavior, when the threat is minimal, or when efforts to prevent the realization of the threat occur at the expense of other personal goals. We propose that the initial self-protective function of the RS system does sometimes turn into this maladaptive pattern.

Though we suggest that the RS dynamic develops over time as a mechanism to protect the self, we clearly distinguish rejection expectations in the model from coping strategies. In attachment theory, beliefs and coping orientations are seen as part of an amalgamated "attachment style" consisting of cognitions and affects about the likelihood of acceptance/ rejection and strategies to cope with potential rejection. There is an assumption inherent in this approach that if you identify some aspect of a person's attachment style (e.g., what beliefs a person holds), then you know a great deal about other aspects of the person (e.g., how the person behaves and feels). Though these might be related empirically (indeed, it is common for stress and a response to stress to go hand-in-hand), it is important for our understanding of underlying mechanisms (and of high RS individuals) to separate rejection expectations from responses to them. The RS dynamic does not inevitably lead to the maladaptive behaviors described above; there is quite a bit of variability in how the expectations (and, as follows, perceptions) play out in interpersonal situations. How particular people deal with rejection expectations depends on a variety of other factors. We have looked at one of these factors, general self-regulatory abilities, which may reduce the likelihood of responding intensely and hostilely to an ambiguous behavior. In this case, responses to perceived rejection are not driven by an activated DMS alone. The more illuminating approach, then, is studying important components of processing dispositions as theoretically independent, though empirically correlated. Doing so, we can investigate how they combine together in individuals to influence behavior.

COPING WITH THE THREAT OF REJECTION VERSUS COPING WITH REJECTION

The model exposes how normal cognitive functions can develop with experience into maladaptive stable patterns of processing. In uncovering the mental steps leading to a hostile behavioral response to a seemingly innocuous comment, such as one that a distracted boyfriend might make, we seek to isolate potentially fruitful avenues of intervention. Indeed, we suggest that the dynamic can be disrupted at one of the model's links: between history and expectation, between expectation and perception, or between perception and response. Since we posit that, most commonly, the process is swift and automatic, it may seem difficult to avert the negative affective and interpersonal outcomes of RS. However, there are points that are particularly ripe for disruption. We suggest that the detection of threat cues triggers not only the RS dynamic, but also strategies designed to protect the self from the potential rejection. These strategies, however, can appear just as unmitigated and extreme as would the hostile reactions that are inhibited.

One way in which the RS process can be interrupted is through targeted behaviors intended to prevent rejection from occurring, even in the presence of threatening trigger cues—that is, when rejection is recognized as a possibility but before it occurs. Another way is through conscious and controlled efforts to self-regulate responses to rejection once it has occurred. Both of these coping strategies involve highly regulated behavior in the service of the activated DMS. We describe them more fully below.

Rejection Prevention

In addition to heightening the individual's acuity for detecting rejection cues, when activated, the DMS should trigger efforts to prevent rejection from occurring. Rejection can be prevented by avoiding social situations or fleeing from them (if rejection expectations are high, perhaps affiliation needs have to be fulfilled otherwise). However, when the desired outcome is to maintain connection with the threat source—a significant other—such avoidance is not a preferred option. Rather, anxiety about rejection can fuel efforts to prevent the loss of that relationship. Rejection-prevention efforts are therefore likely to take the form of inhibiting the actions that might elicit rejection (e.g., going "unnoticed" by keeping silent about opinions that might lead to disagreement with a partner) or active efforts to please (e.g., solicitousness and ingratiation). These activities can lead to a "loss of self"—where one's own goals, interests, and tendencies are subjugated in the interests of maintaining a relationship.

Recently, we have been examining the point in the unfolding of the RS dynamic when rejection expectations are triggered, but the irrevocable rejection is not yet perceived—for example, you've approached the girl to ask her out, but she hasn't yet said no. At such a moment, hope still exists for acceptance, and attempts can become more feverish to attain it.

Efforts to prevent rejection can involve negotiation of such dangerous turf by accommodating the self to the partner. Whereas the ability to accommodate in a relationship may be adaptive (Rusbult, Verette, Whitney, Slovik, & Lipkus, 1991), it can also become maladaptive when it occurs to the extent of subverting other important personal goals or engaging in socially harmful behavior. Indeed, Helgeson's work on communion and unmitigated communion highlights this difference (e.g., Helgeson & Fritz, 2000). While *communion* is seen as a healthy focus on and involvement in others' needs and goals, *unmitigated communion* implies a subjugation of one's own goals and needs in the service of others and predicts many of the same results as RS: negative interpersonal and physiological outcomes such as depression, self-neglect, anxiety, and poor health (Fritz & Helgeson, 1998; Fritz, Nagurney, & Helgeson, 2003; Helgeson & Fritz, 1998, 2000).

Whereas the underlying motive of individuals high in unmitigated communion is theorized to be helping partners to achieve their goals and enhancing partners' self-views, the underlying motive of high RS individuals is attaining (or maintaining) acceptance from close others (i.e., avoiding rejection). In this way, RS really is a focus on one's own goals and needs, and the activities implemented on the path toward achieving those personal goals are similar to the activities implemented by high-unmitigated-communion individuals on the path toward others' goals—leading to common affective consequences.

To date we have linked RS with two types of potentially self-defeating behavior patterns enacted to prevent rejection. First, we have shown a link between RS and risk of engagement in self- or other harmful behavior in order to maintain the relationship. A prospective study of early adolescents (Purdie & Downey, 2000) showed that, to the extent that girls were high in RS in fifth–seventh grade, they were more likely 2 years later to agree with a statement indicating that they would be willing to do things that they knew were wrong to maintain their current dating relationship (e.g., "I would do anything to keep my boyfriend with me even if it's things that I know are wrong."). Similarly, in a cross-sectional pilot study of college women, RS was associated with a heightened likelihood of reporting having actually done things that felt wrong or uncomfortable to maintain a relationship (Downey & Ayduk, 2002). Second, we have shown a link between RS and self-silencing (Jack & Dill, 1992) which is enacted to preserve a relationship (Ayduk, May, Downey, & Higgins, 2003; Downey & Ayduk, 2002). In addition, in a study of college women, RS was associated with having avoided disclosing things about one's self or one's past to prevent rejection (Downey & Ayduk, 2002). In this study, RS was also related to an unstable sense of self, consistent with the hypothesis that people who are chronically concerned with actively preventing rejection may have self-schemas that are highly contingent on perceived evaluation by important others (Downey & Ayduk, 2002). That is, in their attempts to prevent rejection, these people may align their preferences, goals, and beliefs with those of important others because they see this as a way to establish a firm interpersonal connection. When they come into contact with various important others, then, their preferences, goals, and beliefs must change with the company, and their "true" but unspoken needs are never met.

Further evidence of this tendency comes from studies involving potential rejection from Internet groups formed on the basis of attitudes that are highly salient for college students. Romero and Downey (2004) gave participants attitude questionnaires purportedly to aid in assigning them to appropriate (fictitious) established Internet groups. Participants who were high in RS were more likely to agree to do menial tasks for a group after receiving a lukewarm set of e-mails from its members than after receiving clearly rejecting messages. That is, when acceptance was still a possibility, high RS participants were more likely to perform unpleasant tasks for the group, possibly because they saw this as a strategy to ensure acceptance. In a follow-up study, Romero and Downey investigated if this strategy of subjugating one's own needs for the group's needs would translate into self-presentation of attitudes. Participants were asked to fill out a set of questionnaires designed to assess their preferences and values, allegedly to fit them into an appropriate Internet group. They then wrote a message to and received several (fictitious) replies from their group members, who either matched or mismatched with the participants' political affiliation. Participants who were high in RS actually changed their attitudes (from their background responses) in an attempt to fit better with the group norm. Thus, when acceptance was seen as possible, high RS individuals tried to change their selves in ways that they perceived would likely maximize their chance of being eventually accepted.

We argue, in line with the RS model, that such attempts to meet the needs of others are attempts to maintain relationships, and that dismissing one's own needs may be seen by individuals who are high in RS as a necessary sacrifice. In the RS model, unmitigated communion can be thought of as a behavioral strategy motivated by a desire to prevent rejection. We would argue that this strategy is implemented only under certain circumstances, when the individual believes acceptance is still possible. Although such overaccommodation may help reduce the threat of immediate rejection by the partner, it may in the long run be harmful both to self and to the relationship (e.g., Allan & Gilbert, 1997; Jack, 1991, 1999, 2003; Jack & Dill, 1992). The negative effects of overaccommodation may be direct, such that these behaviors take a toll on mood and self-concept as one makes undue sacrifices. They may also be indirect, fueling maladaptive reactions to the perception of rejection, which indicates that prevention efforts have proved futile despite one's best efforts. This is evidenced by hostile responses to rejection among high RS individuals in both lab and diary studies (Downey & Feldman, 1996; Downey, Feldman, & Ayduk, 2000; Downey, Freitas, et al., 1998).

This shift from ingratiation before rejection to hostility after rejection can be more global: it can take place over the course of a relationship. High RS individuals are presumed to come into relationships eager and enthusiastic, though anxious. In order to ensure continued acceptance from their new partner, these individuals are ready to engage in self-silencing and ingratiation, subverting their own needs and goals in the interest of maintaining the relationship they are so anxious about losing. Over time, however, as minor (or ambiguously negative) cues build up, there may be a shift toward hostile overreactions. These can be all the more surprising and apparently unmotivated, if they are made in response to behaviors that have not elicited hostility in the past (before the shift, when the high RS individual was still vying for acceptance).

If one defines one's self solely relationally, in interaction with another person (or several people, if there is more than one "relational self" to go with more than one significant other), then the self exists only to the extent that the relationship does. In this case, what does rejection signal? Does RS come from a fear of loss of self should the relationship end? Do high RS people see relationships as a source of identity that then must be discarded when the relationship ends? This inconsistent self-presentation, leading potentially to a lack of self-concept clarity, is one of the dangers of the RS dynamic that we have not yet studied thoroughly. Together, these findings suggest that high RS individuals are vulnerable to engaging in potentially self-defeating behavior in order to prevent the realization of threats to their sense of self.

Self-Regulation

The kinds of hostile and unrestrained reactions to rejection that we have found to be associated with RS may suggest the absence of effective self-control, or dysfunctional emotional regulatory systems. However, not all people who fear and expect rejection experience its negative consequences to the same degree. Though these individuals show similar physiological responses in trigger situations, indicating an activation of the DMS, they are able either to inhibit maladaptive responses or to access a repertoire of adaptive ones. How do these individuals differ from the high RS reactors? In some of our recent work, we have started to examine possible mechanisms that might moderate effect of RS on interpersonal difficulties and maladaptive personal outcomes. As we described earlier, high RS people typically overreact both in anticipation of and in reaction to rejection. At the anticipation stage, rejection cues automatically activate the DMS, leading to vigilance for rejection and making individuals susceptible to perceiving and magnifying intentional rejection even with minimally ambiguous cues. High RS people also overreact to perceived rejection because this heightened anticipatory stress appears to accentuate already active fight-or-flight or affiliation-seeking response mechanisms. The challenge for high RS individuals in rejection-related situations, then, seems to be regulating themselves so that they can restrict and modulate their automatic DMS reactivity. This conceptualization suggests that people who have the competencies to strategically down-regulate "hot" DMS activation associated with RS may be better able to cope more rationally and reflectively with rejection, and to behave in accordance with their long-term relationship goals rather than their defensive impulses, thus avoiding characteristic patterns of maladjustment.

Converging evidence from delay-of-gratification studies (Metcalfe & Mischel, 1999; Mischel, 1973, 1996) and developmental research shows that flexible and strategic attention deployment is crucial for distress and impulse inhibition (Derryberry & Reed, 2002; Derryberry & Rothbart, 1997; Thompson, 1994; Wilson & Gottman, 1996). Experimental studies of delay of gratification, for example, have shown that the child's ability to forgo immediate gratification for a delayed but preferred reward is mediated by effective attention deployment in the service of arousal reduction (Mischel, Shoda, & Rodriguez, 1989). Attention deployment strategies used to successfully delay gratification include purposeful self-distraction and cognitive reframing operations that "cool" the frustrating "hot" aspects of the delay situation (Metcalfe & Mischel, 1999).

Despite surface differences, regulation of behavior in the appetitive domain (delay of gratification) and in the defensive domain (fight-or-flight and anxiety-driven support seeking) appear to hinge on the ability to attenuate arousal by cooling the "hot" arousing and impulse-eliciting features of the situation. Maintaining the frustration inherent in these seemingly different regulatory tasks at manageable levels then enables individuals to inhibit impulsive reactions and access reflective processes that facilitate the attainment of long-term goals. Vigilance, or narrowing of attentional focus on rejection cues, adaptive in the short term (see, e.g., Ohman, 2000) but maladaptive in the long term, may mediate the relationship between anxious rejection expectations and deleterious responses.

The prototypical RS dynamic that we have described so far may characterize primarily those high RS individuals with self-regulatory difficulties. These difficulties may play out both at the rejection-anticipation phase and the reaction-to-rejection phase. In the anticipation phase, an inability to divert attention away from rejection features and from one's own internal emotional states in the face of possible rejection may hinder high RS individuals from encoding contextual information that may provide alternative explanations for others' behaviors (Arriaga & Rusbult, 1998; Dodge, 1980; Dodge & Somberg, 1987; Downey & Feldman, 1996; Holtzworth-Munroe & Hutchinson, 1993). The absence of alternative explanations may foster a readiness to perceive intentional rejection in a perpetrator's behavior (Dodge, 1980). When rejection is perceived, lack of self-regulatory ability may make high RS individuals susceptible to the "here-and-now" focus that would make them respond destructively to behavior that they perceive to be hurtful without considering the long-term impact on valued goals (Rusbult et al., 1991).

Conversely, through strategic attention deployment (i.e., purposeful avoidance of rejection cues), high RS individuals with high self-regulatory ability can dampen the activation of vigilance, better attend to situational information, and generate alternative explanations to that of intentional rejection. By making finer distinctions between intentional rejection and ambiguous behavior that may be benignly intended, they may be less susceptible to false alarms and a rapid generation of a fight-or-flight or an anxiety-driven reassurance-seeking response. Individuals high in delay-of-gratification ability also may be better at using cognitive reappraisal strategies (Gross, 1998; Kelly, 1955; Lazarus, 1999; Mischel, 1973) that transform the subjective meaning of a threatening situation (e.g., a partner's negative behavior) in such a way that it is less threatening. For example, rather than encoding an argument with a romantic partner as a globally negative event with irreversible consequences (e.g., breakup of the relationship), rejection-sensitive people high in self-regulation may be able to construe the event as simply a difference of opinions, restricting the event's negativity to the here-and-now rather than catastrophizing it. Likewise, a partner's currently negative behavior can be understood as transitory and situationally induced (e.g., due to stress), and its importance or centrality for the person's long-term goals can be attenuated by placing such behavior in a broader context. Furthermore, high RS people with greater self-regulatory ability may be better able to keep themselves focused on their long-term relationship goals. Together, these regulatory mechanisms should help high RS people to inhibit impulsive destructive behavior driven by the DMS and to activate instead reflective and effective coping strategies, thus furthering the likelihood of long-term goal attainment.

In support of these ideas, we have shown in recent work that self-regulatory competencies assessed in the delay-of-gratification paradigm (Mischel et al., 1989) moderates the link between RS and such maladaptive outcomes as aggression and low self-worth (Ayduk et al., 2000). We found that those high RS individuals who displayed an ability to delay gratification suffered relatively few of the negative outcomes (e.g., interpersonal difficulties, lower mental and physical well-being) that were experienced by high RS individuals who were unable to implement self-control strategies. This effect held true in diverse samples that differed in age, ethnicity, and socioeconomic status, suggesting that the protective role self-regulatory competencies play against RS may be relatively robust. In ongoing work, we are further investigating the mechanisms that may underlie the protective effect of self-regulatory competencies that was demonstrated in this study. Of particular interest to us is the way flexible attention shifting in the early stages of processing may affect high RS individuals' likelihood of perceiving rejection.

Although supportive of our hypothesis, these data did not clarify exactly which processes mediated the effect of delay ability (or, more generally, self-regulatory competencies) on high RS individuals' resiliency. As we suggested above, we see attentional control as a key mediator between risk and psychopathology, organizing cognitive, attributional, physiological, and motivational systems that operate for or against RS. It awaits further experimental and longitudinal research, however, to test this hypothesis more definitively.

CONCLUSION

In this chapter, we have discussed rejection sensitivity, a social-cognitive model of personal relationship behavior describing a processing dynamic whereby certain interpersonal situations trigger anxious expectations of rejection. Thanks to a defensive motivational system, these expectations lower the threshold for perceiving rejection by directing attention to and personalizing negative cues. We posit that before rejection is perceived, or while rejection is still evitable, this defensive motivational system prompts increased efforts of rejection prevention, leading to the suppression of personal goals in the interests of maintaining acceptance. After rejection is perceived, the DMS can lead to intense reactions to it, unless self-regulatory competencies are sufficient to inhibit such maladaptive "overreactions."

We hope that avenues currently under investigation will lead us to implementable interventions for high RS individuals, whose relationship behaviors can turn their rejection expectations into reality (Downey, Freitas, et al., 1998).

Many researchers have taken advantage of developments in social cognition and personality, creating a field of relationship science that delves beyond broad categorizations and global descriptions. Viewing personality as a set of processing dispositions, triggered by cues acquired from an individual's social-cognitive learning history, can demystify the personality–relationship link. This focus on psychological mediators is shared by other models that incorporate in their conceptualization some version of the notion of "mental representations" of relationships (e.g., Andersen & Chen, 2002; Baldwin, 1992). A number of attempts have been made to explain the link between relationship behavior and global personality traits through investigations of the self. While the "self" remains an elusive concept in psychology, various theories about self processes have appeared to unravel the links between, for example, low self-esteem and unsuccessful relationship histories (e.g., self-discrepancy theory; see Higgins, 1987). Many, or most, of the existing theories of individual differences in interpersonal relationships can be interpreted as social-cognitive, with at least a recognition (though not always clearly defined) of the dynamics that lead to relationship behavior. These models share a few key components.

First, though not all theories explicitly outline the process whereby cognitive–affective mediators link experience with behavior, the emphasis on them, born of new paradigms and research methodologies, is almost ubiquitous. The age of global, pan situational, stable trait characterizations is over; the tools that psychology has available to it today are leading to a more precise and more dynamic investigation of people's cognitions, affects, and behavior. One key contribution that new approaches in psychology make is to assess more definitely how theoretically and empirically related constructs (e.g., self-esteem, RS, and attachment style) differ from each other—if at all. Overall, relatively little attention has been paid to comparing the psychophysiological correlates of conceptually and empirically related personality dispositions. Yet the burgeoning interest in the neurobiological bases of psychological processes suggests the importance of this line of research. Are RS and self-esteem driven by the same neurological correlates? The new paradigms allow us to establish whether the profile of psychophysiological reactions to rejection and acceptance associated with each of these relevant constructs is similar to or different from that associated with RS.

A related idea common to current models of relationships is that individual differences in relationship behavior develop due to a social-cognitive learning history, beginning with parental interactions and developing over time. Mental representations of, and expectations and beliefs about, relationships are generated quickly and early. The contingencies of the mother–child relationship must be mastered to maintain contact (e.g., security, food) and so ensure survival. These early representations of how a relationship works affect perceptions and behavior in future relationships, potentially leading to a repeating cycle of relationship behaviors and outcomes that may appear dispositional. Though relationship cognitions are not immutable, they can be reinforced through a self-fulfilling system of attributions and inferences. This deglobalization of relationship styles mimics the decreasing popularity of using personality traits to describe individuals in favor of cognitive–affective processing dispositions (Mischel & Shoda, 1995) that are contextualized and dynamic.

Finally, the RS model, along with attachment theory and other social-cognitive models of relationships, emphasizes the dimension of acceptance–rejection in interpersonal interactions. Specifically, the focus is on interpersonal rejection as a threat, and acceptance as necessary for emotional (and possibly physical) health and well-being. Though much research has gone into exploring the causes and consequences of rejection, this unasked, unanswered question remains: Why is rejection so threatening? There is no explication in existing theories of relationships of why rejection itself is to be avoided, and why the possibility elicits such extreme and maladaptive responses. Particularly in the context of personality disorders such as borderline personality disorder, narcissistic personality disorder, and avoidant or dependent personality disorder, it is worth considering the self systems that enter into play when threat to the self is perceived. These self systems (e.g., the evaluative self, the narcissistic self, the other-directed self) differ in the meaning or implications of rejection, in the cues that convey it, and in the reactions that are likely to arise. An explanation of relationship behavior cannot be complete without an explication of the factors that convey rejection and the meaning rejection conveys and a discussion of the motivational systems that are activated to prevent or cope with it. These important issues await theoretical and empirical elaboration.

ACKNOWLEDGMENT

This research was supported by Grant No. R01-MH069703-01 from the National Institute of Mental Health.

REFERENCES

Ainsworth, M. S., Blehar, M. C., Waters, E., & Wall, S. (1978). *Patterns of attachment: A psychological study of the strange situation.* Hillsdale, NJ: Erlbaum.

Allan, S., & Gilbert, P. (1997). Submissive behavior and psychopathology. *British Journal of Clinical Psychology, 36,* 467–488.

Andersen, S. M., & Chen, S. (2002). The relational self: An interpersonal social-cognitive theory. *Psychological Review, 109,* 619–645.

Andersen, S. M., Reznik, I., & Chen, S. (1997). Self in relation to others: Cognitive and motivational underpinnings. In J. G. Snodgrass & R. L. Thompson (Eds.), *The self across psychology: Self-recognition, self-awareness, and the self-concept* (pp. 233–275). New York: New York Academy of Science.

Arriaga, X. B., & Rusbult, C. E. (1998). Standing in my partner's shoes: Partner perspective taking and reactions to accommodative dilemmas. *Personality and Social Psychology Bulletin, 24,* 927–948.

Ayduk, O., Downey, G., & Kim, M. (2001). Rejection sensitivity and depressive symptoms in women. *Personality and Social Psychology Bulletin, 27,* 868–877.

Ayduk, O., Downey, G., Testa, A., Yen, Y., & Shoda, Y. (1999). Does rejection elicit hostility in rejection sensitive women? *Social Cognition, 17,* 245–271.

Ayduk, O., May, D., Downey, G., & Higgins, E. T. (2003). Tactical differences in coping with rejection sensitivity: The role of prevention pride. *Personality and Social Psychology Bulletin, 29,* 435–448.

Ayduk, O., Mendoza-Denton, R., Mischel, W., Downey, G., Peake, P. K., & Rodriguez, M. (2000). Regulating the interpersonal self: Strategic self-regulation for coping with rejection sensitivity. *Journal of Personality and Social Psychology, 4,* 82–102.

Baldwin, M. W. (1992). Relational schemas and the processing of social information. *Psychological Bulletin, 112,* 461–484.

Baldwin, M. W., & Keelan, J. P. R. (1999). Interpersonal expectations as a function of self-esteem and sex. *Journal of Social and Personal Relationships, 16,* 822–833.

Baldwin, M. W., Keelan, J. P. R., Fehr, B., Enns, V., & Koh-Rangarajoo, E. (1996). Social-cognitive conceptualization of attachment working models: Availability and accessibility effects. *Journal of Personality and Social Psychology, 71,* 94–109.

Berscheid, E. (1994). Interpersonal relationships. *Annual Review of Psychology, 45,* 79–129.

Bowlby, J. (1969). *Attachment and loss* (Vol. 1). New York: Basic Books.

Bowlby, J. (1973). *Attachment and loss* (Vol. 2). New York: Basic Books.

Bowlby, J. (1980). *Attachment and loss* (Vol. 3). New York: Basic Books.

Bradbury, T. N., & Fincham, F. D. (1990). Attributions in marriage: Review and critique. *Psychology Bulletin, 107,* 3–33.

Cacioppo, J. T., & Gardner, W. L. (1999). Emotions. *Annual Review of Psychology, 50,* 191–214.

Davis, M. (1992). The role of the amygdala in fear and anxiety. *Annual Review of Neuroscience, 15,* 353–375.

Derryberry, D., & Reed, M. A. (2002). Anxiety-related attentional biases and their regulation by attentional control. *Journal of Abnormal Psychology, 111,* 225–236.

Derryberry, D., & Rothbart, M. K. (1997). Reactive and effortful processes in the organization of temperament. *Development and Psychopathology, 9,* 633–652.

Dodge, K. (1980). Social cognition and children's aggressive behavior. *Child Development, 51,* 162–170.

Dodge, K., & Somberg, D. R. (1987). Hostile attributional biases among aggressive boys are exacerbated under conditions of threats to the self. *Child Development, 58,* 213–224.

Downey, G., & Ayduk, O. (2002). *[Correlates of rejection sensitivity in college students].* Unpublished raw data.

Downey, G., & Feldman, S. (1996). Implications of rejection sensitivity for intimate relationships. *Journal of Personality and Social Psychology, 70*, 1327–1343.

Downey, G., Feldman, S., & Ayduk, O. (2000). Rejection sensitivity and male violence in romantic relationships. *Personal Relationships, 7*, 45–61.

Downey, G., Feldman, S., Khouri, J., & Friedman, S. (1994). Maltreatment and child depression. In W. M. Reynolds & H. F. Johnson (Eds.), *Handbook of depression in children and adolescents* (pp. 481–508). New York: Plenum Press.

Downey, G., Freitas, A., Michaelis, B., & Khouri, H. (1998). The self-fulfilling prophecy in close relationships: Rejection sensitivity and rejection by romantic partners. *Journal of Personality and Social Psychology, 75*, 545–560.

Downey, G., Khouri, H., & Feldman, S. (1997). Early interpersonal trauma and later adjustment: The mediational role of rejection sensitivity. In D. Cicchetti & S. L. Toth (Eds.), *Developmental perspectives on trauma: Theory, research, and intervention. Rochester symposium on developmental psychology, Vol. 8* (pp. 85–114). Rochester, NY: Rochester University Press.

Downey, G., Lebolt, A., Rincon, C., & Freitas, A. (1998). Rejection sensitivity and children's interpersonal difficulties. *Child Development, 69*, 1074–1091.

Downey, G., Mougois, V., Ayduk, O., London, B., & Shoda, Y. (2004). Rejection sensitivity and the defensive motivational system: Insights from the startle response to rejection cues. *Psychological Science, 15*, 668–673.

Epstein, S (1994). Integration of the cognitive and the psychodynamic unconscious. *American Psychologist, 49*, 709–724.

Erikson, E. (1950). *Childhood and society.* New York: Norton.

Fanselow, M. S. (1994). Neural organization of the defensive behavior system responsible for fear. *Psychonomic Bulletin and Review, 1*, 429–438.

Feldman, S., & Downey, G. (1994). Rejection sensitivity as a mediator of the impact of childhood exposure to family violence on adult attachment behavior. *Development and Psychopathology, 6*, 231–247.

Freitas, A. L., & Downey, G. (1998). Resilience: A dynamic perspective. *International Journal of Behavioural Development: Special issue on the development of coping, 22*, 263–285.

Fritz, H. L., & Helgeson, V. (1998). Distinctions of unmitigated communion from communion: Self-neglect and overinvolvement with others. *Journal of Personality and Social Psychology, 75*, 121–140.

Fritz, H. L., Nagurney, A. J., & Helgeson, V. (2003). Social interactions and cardiovascular reactivity during problem disclosure among friends. *Personality and Social Psychology Bulletin, 29*, 713–725.

Gray, J. A. (1987). *The psychology of fear and stress* (2nd ed.). New York: McGraw-Hill.

Gray, J. A. (2000). Three fundamental emotional systems. In P. Ekman & R. J. Davidson (Eds.), *The nature of emotion* (pp. 243–247). New York: Oxford University Press.

Gross, J. J. (1998). Antecedent- and response-focused emotion regulation: Divergent consequences for experience, expression, and physiology. *Journal of Personality and Social Psychology, 74*, 224–237.

Hazan, C., & Shaver, P. (1987). Romantic love conceptualized as an attachment process. *Journal of Personality and Social Psychology, 52*, 511–524.

Helgeson, V. S., & Fritz, H. L. (1998). A theory of unmitigated communion. *Personality and Social Psychology Review, 2*, 173–183.

Helgeson, V. S., & Fritz, H. L. (2000). The implications of unmitigated agency and unmitigated communion for domains of problem behavior. *Journal of Personality, 68*, 1031–1057.

Higgins, E. T. (1987). Self-discrepancy: A theory relating self and affect. *Psychological Review, 94*, 319–340.

Holtzworth-Munroe, A., & Hutchinson, G. (1993). Attributing negative intent to wife behavior: The attributions of maritally violent versus nonviolent men. *Journal of Abnormal Psychology, 102*, 206–211.

Horney, K. (1937). *The neurotic personality of our time*. New York: Norton.

Jack, D. C. (1991). *Silencing the self: Women and depression*. Cambridge, MA: Harvard University Press.

Jack, D. C. (1999). Silencing the self: Inner dialogues and outer realities. In T. Joiner & J. C. Coyne (Eds.), *The interactional nature of depression: Advances in interpersonal approaches* (pp. 221–246). Washington, DC: American Psychological Association.

Jack, D. C. (2003). The anger of hope and the anger of despair: How anger relates to women's depression. In J. M. Stoppard & L. M. McMullen (Eds.), *Situating sadness: Women and depressing in social context* (pp. 62–87). New York: New York University Press.

Jack, D. C., & Dill, D. (1992). The Silencing the Self Scale: Schemas of intimacy associated with depression in women. *Psychology of Women Quarterly, 16*, 97–106.

Kelly, G. A. (1955). *The psychology of personal constructs*. New York: Norton.

Lang, P. (1995). The emotion probe: Studies of motivation and attention. *American Psychologist, 50*, 372–385.

Lang, P., Bradley, M., & Cuthbert, B. (1990). Emotion, attention, and the startle reflex. *Psychological Review, 97*, 377–395.

Lang P., Bradley M., & Cuthbert B. (1995). *International Affective Picture System (IAPS): Technical manual and affective ratings*. Gainesville: University of Florida, NIMH Center for Study of Emotion and Attention.

Lazarus, R. S. (1999). *Stress and emotion: A new synthesis*. New York: Springer.

Lazarus, R. S., Averill, J. R., & Opton, E. M. Jr. (1970). *Towards a cognitive theory of emotion*. New York: Academic Press.

LeDoux, J. E. (1995). Emotion: Clues from the brain. *Annual Review of Psychology, 46*, 209–235.

LeDoux, J. E. (1996). *The emotional brain*. New York: Touchstone.

LeDoux, J. E., Iwata, J., Cicchetti, P., & Reis, D. J. (1988). Different projections of the central amygdaloid nucleus mediate autonomic and behavioral correlates of fear. *Journal of Neuroscience, 1*, 238–243.

LeDoux, J. E., & Phelps, E. A. (2000). Emotional networks in the brain. In M. Lewis & J. M. Haviland-Jones (Eds.), *Handbook of emotions* (pp. 157–172). New York: Guilford Press.

Manly, J. T., Kim, J. E., Rogosch, F. A., & Cicchetti, D. (2001). Dimensions of child maltreatment and children's adjustment: Contributions of developmental timing and subtype. *Development and Psychopathology, 13*, 759–782.

Merton, R. (1948). The self-fulfilling prophecy. *Antioch Review, 8*, 193–210.

Metcalfe, J., & Mischel, W. (1999). A hot/cool-system analysis of delay of gratifica-
    tion: Dynamics of willpower. *Psychological Review, 106,* 3–19.
Mischel, W. (1973). Toward a cognitive social learning reconceptualization of per-
    sonality. *Psychological Review, 80,* 252–253.
Mischel, W. (1996). From good intentions to willpower. In P. M. Gollwitzer & J. A.
    Bargh (Eds.), *The psychology of action: Linking cognition and motivation to be-
    havior* (pp. 197–218). New York: Guilford Press.
Mischel, W., & Shoda, Y. (1995). A cognitive–affective system theory of personality:
    Reconceptualizing situations, dispositions, dynamics, and invariance in person-
    ality structure. *Psychological Review, 102,* 246–268.
Mischel, W., Shoda, Y., & Rodriguez, M. (1989). Delay of gratification in children.
    Science, 244, 833–938.
Ohman, A. (2000). Evolutionary, cognitive, and clinical perspectives. In M. Lewis &
    J. M. Haviland-Jones (Eds.), *Handbook of emotions* (pp. 573–593). New York:
    Guilford Press.
Olson, J. M., Roese, N. J., & Zanna, M. P. (1996). Expectancies. In E. T. Higgins & A.
    W. Kruglanski (Eds.), *Social psychology: Handbook of basic principles* (pp.
    211–238). New York: Guilford Press.
Purdie, V., & Downey, G. (2000). Rejection sensitivity and adolescent girls' vulnera-
    bility to relationship-centered difficulties. *Child Maltreatment, 5,* 338–349.
Reis, H. T., & Downey, G. (1999). Social cognition in relationships: Building essential
    bridges between two literatures. *Social Cognition, 17,* 97–117.
Romero, R., & Downey, G. (2004). *[Rejection sensitivity as a predictor of intragroup
    behavior].* Unpublished raw data.
Rosenthal, R. (2002). Covert communication in classrooms, clinics, courtrooms, and
    cubicles. *American Psychologist, 57,* 839–849.
Rusbult, C. E., Verette, J., Whitney, G. A., Slovik, L. F., & Lipkus, I. (1991). Accom-
    modation processes in close relationships: Theory and preliminary empirical ev-
    idence. *Journal of Personality and Social Psychology, 60,* 53–78.
Sroufe, L. A. (1990). An organization perspective on the self. In D. Cicchetti & M.
    Beeghly (Eds.), *The self in transition: Infancy to childhood. The John D. and
    Catherine T. MacArthur Foundation Series on Mental Health and Development*
    (pp. 281–307). Chicago: University of Chicago Press.
Sullivan, H. S. (1953). *The interpersonal theory of psychiatry.* New York: Norton.
Thompson, R. A. (1994). Emotion regulation: A theme in search of definition. *Mono-
    graphs of the Society for Research in Child Development, 59,* 25–52.
Widom, C. S. (1989). The cycle of violence. *Science, 244,* 160–166.
Wilson, B. J., & Gottman, J. M. (1996). Attention—the shuttle between emotion and
    cognition: Risk resiliency, and physiological bases. In E. M. Hetherington & E.
    A. Blechman (Eds.), *Stress, coping and resiliency in children and families. Fam-
    ily research consortium: Advances in family research* (pp. 189–228). Hillsdale,
    NJ: Erlbaum.
Zillmann, D. (1993). Mental control of angry aggression. In D. M. Wegner & J. W.
    Pennebaker (Eds.), *Handbook of mental control* (pp. 370–392). Englewood
    Cliffs, NJ: Prentice-Hall.

4

Interpersonal Cognition
and the Quest for Social Acceptance

Inside the Sociometer

MARK R. LEARY

During the 1980s and much of the 1990s, social psychology was dominated by an interest in *social cognition*, the processes by which people perceive, draw inferences about, and think about other individuals and social groups. Literally thousands of studies focused on the processes that guide people's inferences about one another and the consequences of those inferences for phenomena such as person perception, attribution, stereotyping, intergroup behavior, attraction, conflict, aggression, and emotion. This emphasis on social cognition was certainly not misplaced—after all, human beings devote a great deal of thought to discerning the characteristics, feelings, and intentions of other people, and how people think about others obviously affects their own feelings and behaviors. Yet, in exploring the nature, determinants, and consequences of social cognition, researchers have largely ignored a broad portion of interpersonal thought that deals with the reflexive process by which people think specifically about what other people might be thinking about them.

When people think about other individuals, they are at least as interested in trying to determine how those individuals perceive and evaluate them as they are in trying to draw inferences about the others' personal traits or motives, if not more so. A man and a woman on a first date undoubtedly want to get to know one another, but they are also acutely interested in determining the other's impressions of and feelings about him- or herself. An employee desires to understand the boss's personality and preferences but also wants to know how the boss perceives him or her. Members of two conflicting groups draw inferences about each others' intentions, but also wonder about how members of the other group see them. In many, if not most social encounters, people desire to know how they are viewed by others.

Furthermore, the conclusions that people reach regarding others' impressions and evaluations of them have dramatic effects on their emotions and behavior, and often lead them to behave in ways that they hope will elicit particular perceptions, evaluations, and behaviors from others. Aside from a few spontaneous reactions based on evolutionary adaptations (such as reactions to frowns and stares; see Ohman, 1986) and conditioned emotional responses rooted in previous experience (Baum & Andersen, 1999), most of our reactions to other people—and their reactions to us—are determined by the impressions that we have of each other. People respond to one another largely in terms of their inferences about each other's characteristics, attitudes, intentions, roles, beliefs, and so on. Furthermore, because people realize that others' reactions to them are based partly on these impressions and evaluations, they recognize that it is in their own best interests to pay attention to how they are being perceived and evaluated and, occasionally, to try to control the nature of the impressions that others form (Leary, 1995; Schlenker & Pontari, 2003). Knowing how one is viewed by other people is an important determinant of people's behavior and emotion and contributes to their success in social life.

The ability to engage in this sort of *reflexive thinking*—to imagine how we are perceived through others' eyes—is a unique and remarkable human characteristic. Although other great apes—chimpanzees, bonobos, and gorillas, for example—show some evidence of being able to take others' viewpoints and to infer what others might be thinking (for a review, see Mitchell, 2003), we have little evidence that any animal other than *Homo sapiens* can think consciously about what others are thinking about it. In fact, archeological evidence suggests that even human beings did not possess their current level of reflexive thinking until relatively recently in the evolutionary past. The earliest testament to such an ability is found in the first bodily adornments, dating to approximately 50,000 years ago, which indicate that people were able to imagine how they were perceived by others and engaged in symbolic actions to affect others' impressions of them in desired ways (Leary & Buttermore, 2003). The emergence of this ability was an important evolutionary milestone because it allowed human beings to monitor how others saw them, allowing them to manage their impressions in others' eyes to influence how others treated them.

People may think about how others perceive them on a very large number of dimensions, wondering, for example, whether others view them as intelligent, attractive, bigoted, overly cautious, arrogant, shy, motivated, ethical, successful, unhappy, or whatever. However, in a large proportion of the instances in which people try to infer other people's perceptions of them, they are ultimately interested in discerning whether others evaluate them positively or negatively—that is, as possessing socially desirable or socially undesirable characteristics that may have implications for interpersonal acceptance and rejection. This does not suggest that people are not concerned with other people's judgments of them on other dimensions as well. Occasionally people wish to know whether they are perceived as powerful, helpless, or intimidating, for example, and such characteristics may be more relevant to dominating other people than to being accepted by them. As we will see, however, being accepted by other people is a pervasive motive in social life. Indeed, people spend a good deal of effort trying to determine the degree to which others value and accept them. Thus, this chapter focuses on how people monitor and think about interpersonal evaluations that have implications for their acceptance and rejection by others.

MONITORING RELATIONAL VALUE

People appear to have an evolved need to form ongoing, supportive relationships with others. The failure to develop and maintain some minimum number of supportive relationships not only leaves people without tangible support and protection but also predisposes them to a number of psychological and physical problems (Baumeister & Leary, 1995). Being accepted by other people is a fundamental necessity of social life; no matter what other material or social outcomes people may desire, they will be unlikely to attain them without being accepted by at least a few other people somewhere along the way. Certainly, during most of human evolution, human beings would have found it virtually impossible to survive without the benefits associated with social acceptance.

Given the importance of interpersonal acceptance and the negative consequences of interpersonal rejection, people monitor their relational value to other people on an ongoing basis. "Relational value" refers to the degree to which a person regards his or her relationship with another individual, whatever that relationship might be, as valuable or important. People regard some of their relationships as exceptionally valuable, as essentially vital to their well-being, but regard other relationships as of only limited value or of no value or importance whatsoever. Relational value is reflected differently in different kinds of relationships; it means something quite different to be relationally valued by a romantic partner than by a nextdoor neighbor than by a colleague at work, for example.

But, in each case, people monitor their relational value in other people's eyes because it is a central determinant of how others treat them. Being valued as a friend, a partner, an employee, a team member, or whatever means that others have a stake in one's well-being, and thus will provide desired social and material outcomes commensurate with one's relational value to them. The failure to be relationally valued—or, worse, to have a negative relational value—means that others will be indifferent to one's well-being or perhaps even antagonistic to it. To the relationally valued go the spoils, so people can not afford to disregard their relational value in other people's eyes.

Being relationally valued is so important in human life that people appear to possess a dedicated psychological system that monitors and responds to events in terms of their implications for the individual's relational value. Deborah Downs and I called the system that monitors a person's relational value (or, more colloquially, his or her social acceptance by other people) the "sociometer" (Leary & Downs, 1995). The sociometer has three essential functions: (1) it monitors the social environment for cues that are relevant to the individual's relational value to other people; (2) it responds with negative affect (and, typically, lowered self-esteem) when it detects that one's relational value is low or declining, thereby prompting a conscious assessment of the situation; and (3) it motivates behaviors intended to enhance relational value or at least to forestall further declines. Thus, the sociometer consists of three separate but interrelated processes that involve a monitor, the output from the monitor, and a motivator, each of which we discuss in the following sections.

The Monitor

Charles Horton Cooley (1902), best known for his description of the "looking-glass self," was perhaps the first to observe that people monitor others' reactions to them at an automatic and nonconscious level, writing that people "live in the minds of others without knowing it" (p. 208). Consistent with Cooley's hunch, research has shown that people are very good at detecting cues that are relevant to their relational value—cues that connote liking/disliking, approval/disapproval, and acceptance/rejection. Although they only occasionally think consciously about how others are perceiving and evaluating them, people seem exquisitely attuned to cues that others are evaluating them, and they process such cues preattentively. The classic cocktail party phenomenon—in which a person nonconsciously detects his or her name spoken amid the chaotic chatter of a lively party (Cherry, 1953)—attests to the fact that people automatically monitor their environments for information that is relevant to what others are thinking about them. The person who is brought up short by hearing his or her name in the hubbub of a party can not help but wonder what the other people are thinking and saying. In fact, Baldwin, Carrell, and Lopez (1990) showed that people are affected by stimuli that are relevant to their relational value (such as the faces of important evaluative figures) that are presented below the threshold of awareness. People seem to be prepared to detect evaluative reactions from other people.

In fact, not only is the sociometer highly sensitive to cues that are relevant to others' evaluations, but it sometimes seems more sensitive to evaluative feedback than it needs to be. For example, people sometimes react strongly to the judgments of people whose evaluations, from an objective point of view, should be of little or no concern to them. Even a rebuff by a stranger in another city can sometimes hurt one's feelings, momentarily diminish self-esteem, or lead one to ponder the other person's perceptions. Although having strong reactions to seemingly unimportant indications of one's relational value sometimes reflects nothing more than an insecure sensitivity to others' evaluations, there are three functional reasons why people sometimes respond to social evaluations that, from all appearances, should not matter.

First, in the ancestral environment in which the sociometer evolved, virtually everyone with whom an individual interacted was a member of his or her own small group, an important source of support, and thus someone whose opinion mattered. Therefore, the sociometer would have evolved to respond to evaluations from everyone and would not have distinguished between people whose judgments were versus were not important. Of course, in modern society, making such a distinction would be quite useful, but in the ancestral environment it was not, as most people's evaluations of the individual were potentially consequential. As a result, people today seem overly concerned with others' judgments of them. As I discuss momentarily, people today may consciously override the sociometer's automatic response and decide to ignore a particular person's evaluation of them, but the sociometer itself responds automatically to indications of low relational value regardless of the identity of the evaluator.

Second, many systems that monitor the environment for threats to an organism's well-being are biased toward false positives (Rozin & Royzman, 2000). Because failing to detect a potential threat is usually more disastrous than attending to a false alarm, the sociometer may be overly sensitive to cues that connote low relational value. A single failure to realize that one's behavior has angered or alienated other people may be far worse than many false alarms in which a person needlessly worries that he or she has been evaluated negatively.

Third, as described in detail later, even when negative evaluations by a particular person have absolutely no tangible implications for the individual's well-being, they may nonetheless raise the specter of similarly negative evaluations by people whose judgments do matter. So, when a stranger in another city indicates that we are incompetent, unattractive, or otherwise of low relational value, such feedback may portend the reactions of those who are important to us, and the sociometer may alert us to consider this possibility.

Importantly, the sociometer responds not only to actual cues in the immediate social environment but also to remembered, anticipated, and imagined stimuli in the person's own mind. Thus, mentally replaying past rejections can re-create many of the feelings of the original event, and anticipating or imagining negative evaluations can trigger the sociometer's "alarm." These internally elicited reactions sometimes produce unnecessary distress (as when a person needlessly replays a past rejecting event or worries over a potential rejection that ultimately may not occur), but they also serve to alert the individual when he or she contemplates actions that may jeopardize his or her relational value. By imagining how people may respond to a particular behavior, the individual can make judicious behavioral choices. Thus, in addition to reacting to real social cues that signal low relational value, the sociometer helps people to anticipate others' potential reactions (see Haupt & Leary, 1997).

The sociometer is an inherently imperfect mechanism for detecting threats to relational value because it often relies on symbolic inputs that have many possible interpretations. Aside from extreme expressions of displeasure—such as obvious nonverbal expressions of anger, displeasure, or disgust, or explicit verbal indicators of low relational value ("You're worthless, I hate you, and I never want to see you again!")—the cues from which people judge their relational value are typically symbolic, and thus ambiguous, emerging from facial expressions, nonverbal behavior, and paralanguage. Perhaps this is part of the reason that people have difficulty inferring what specific other individuals think about them. Research by Depaulo, Kenny, Hoover, Webb, and Oliver (1987) suggested that people have a rough idea of how they are perceived by other people in general, but they are not very accurate in assessing how particular individuals perceive them.

The Output

When the sociometer detects cues that connote that one's relational value to another person is low or declining, it alerts the individual through negative affect, much like other systems that function to detect threats to well-being. The negative feelings interrupt ongoing cognition and behavior to prompt a conscious assessment of the situation (Simon, 1967) and induce the person to take steps to solve the problem (and thereby eliminate the negative feelings). Given the importance of interpersonal acceptance, particularly in the environment in which human beings evolved, it would have been essential to ensure that threats to one's value to other members of the group were addressed as quickly and fully as possible. The sociometer achieves this goal by providing immediate aversive feedback when cues suggest that one's relational value is low or declining or, as noted, even when one contemplates behaving in ways that might endanger one's interpersonal bonds.

Several affective states arise from the perception of low or declining relational value. Depending on the circumstances, perceiving that other people do not adequately value their relationships with us may be associated with hurt feelings, sadness, anxiety, jealousy, anger, loneliness, and other negative emotions (Baumeister & Tice, 1990; Buckley, Winkel, & Leary, 2004; Leary & Buckley, 2000; Leary, Koch, & Hechenbleikner, 2001; Leary & Springer, 2000; Snapp & Leary, 2001). The specific emotions that people experience depend heavily on the nature of the existing relationship between them and the person's attributions for the rejecting event. For example, rejections that involve the loss of a real or hoped-for relationship tend to elicit sadness; rejections that seem unwarranted and that interfere with the attainment of desired goals cause anger; and those that result from the real or imagined intrusion of a third party lead to jealousy (Leary et al., 2001).

The sociometer is also intimately linked to people's state self-esteem, which can be viewed as another output of this system (Leary, 1999; Leary & Baumeister, 2000; Leary & Downs, 1995). Self-esteem has traditionally been conceptualized as a person's private self-evaluation. Many theorists have suggested that healthy self-esteem ought not to be affected by other people's evaluations of the individual (e.g., Bednar, Wells, & Peterson, 1989; May, 1983). Sociometer theory turns this conceptualization on its head by suggesting that self-esteem is actually a psychological gauge of other people's real, potential, and imagined evaluations of the individual, particularly on dimensions that are relevant to the person's relational value. As such, it is naturally affected by other people's evaluations (Leary & Baumeister, 2000). This functional perspective on self-esteem helps to explain why self-esteem is so strongly affected by interpersonal feedback (its function is to help monitor others' reactions vis-à-vis acceptance and rejection), why public events affect self-esteem more strongly than private events, why the predictors of self-esteem involve attributes and events with potential implications for relational value, and why people seem to have a motive to seek self-esteem even though it has been difficult for researchers to determine why self-esteem is useful (in reality, people are trying to increase their relational value in other people's eyes rather than their self-esteem per se). (See Leary & Baumeister, 2000, for a review of the relevant literature.)

A good deal of research supports sociometer theory's description of the role of self-esteem in monitoring relational value (for reviews, see Leary, 1999, and Leary & Baumeister, 2000). First, laboratory manipulations that convey low relational value (e.g., rejection, disapproval, disinterest) consistently lower participants' state self-esteem (Leary, Cottrell, & Phillips, 2001; Leary, Haupt, Strausser, & Chokel, 1998; Leary, Tambor, Terdal, & Downs, 1995, Studies 3 and 4; Nezlek, Kowalski, Leary, Blevins, & Holgate, 1997; Snapp & Leary, 2001), and rejecting events in everyday life are associated with negative self-feelings (Baumeister, Wotman, & Stillwell, 1993; Leary et al., 1995, Study 2; Leary, Springer, Negel, Ansel,

& Evans, 1998). Furthermore, the effects of performing certain actions on people's self-esteem closely mirror how they believe those behaviors will affect others' reactions to them vis-à-vis acceptance and rejection (Leary et al., 1995, Study 1), and longitudinal research shows that perceived relational value prospectively predicts changes in self-esteem (Srivastava, 2003).

Data also show that the relationship between self-assessment and self-esteem is moderated by the degree to which people believe that a particular attribute is important for social acceptance. MacDonald, Saltzman, and Leary (2003) asked participants to rate themselves on each of five domains (competence, physical attractiveness, wealth and possessions, sociability, and morals) and to indicate the degree to which other people view each domain as important for social acceptance and rejection. Results showed that the more participants thought that a domain was relevant to interpersonal acceptance or rejection, the more strongly their self-appraisals on that domain predicted their self-esteem.

Occasional examples may be found in which self-esteem is affected by events that appear to have no real or potential implications for the person's relational value. For example, a person may feel badly about him- or herself for a failure or shortcoming on a dimension that no one else appears to value. Such instances appear to be rare, however, representing an extremely small proportion of the events that affect self-esteem. Even so, such cases have been raised to refute the hypothesized role of self-esteem in monitoring relational value, and thus deserve attention. Importantly, to function as a sociometer, self-esteem must be sensitive not only to real relational evaluation occurring in the immediate situation but also to the potential implications of that evaluation for acceptance and rejection in other situations in the future. Just as a student may become distressed when she obtains a low score on a practice version of the SAT even though the practice test does not matter whatsoever, a person may feel badly about him- or herself when rejected by someone whose acceptance does not really matter. Although of no importance itself, such a rejection may nonetheless activate the sociometer to warn the individual of potential problems down the road that perhaps may be avoided. It also may be the case that concerns with social acceptance may become functionally autonomous so that personal deficiencies on any dimension lower self-esteem even if those deficiencies have no immediate interpersonal consequences.

One question regarding the sociometer theory of self-esteem that has not been previously addressed is why the sociometer is linked to people's feelings *about themselves*. On the surface, other psychological warning systems seem to function quite effectively via negative affect without invoking self-relevant processing, as when fear elicits one's retreat from a poisonous snake in the woods or disgust leads one to avoid contact with putrid material. However, the case is not as clear as it first seems. Even in the case of physical threats to well-being (such as confronting a coiled and hissing snake), one's cognitions involve the relation of the threat to oneself, and the self-relevant conclusion is that something about oneself is not as it should be (in the case of the snake, the conclusion is that one is in the wrong place). Such a conclusion is not much different from inferring that another person does not like, value, or accept us because something about us is not as it should be (e.g., we lack certain desirable attributes or possess undesirable ones). Emotions arise in response to information about the relationship between the individual and his or her environment (Frijda, 1986), and thus always convey information about both the environment and the person. In the case of events that connote low or declining relational value, people generally consider the possibility that the rejection occurred because they behaved inappropriately or possess undesirable characteristics. Given the attributional ambiguity surrounding rejecting events, it is almost always possible for people to attribute other people's rejecting reactions to themselves. Thus, it is only a short step from perceiving that other people do not value us to suspecting, if not concluding, that the others' reactions are due to our own shortcomings or misbehaviors. Thus, perceptions of low relational value invariably induce self-relevant processing.

Of course, people may devalue us not because of any shortcoming or misbehavior on our part but rather because they have different preferences, interests, and values than we do. However, this was not likely to have been the case during the long span of human evolution in which the sociometer evolved. Given that virtually all of one's interactions were among the same members of a small, homogeneous clan, interpersonal rejection most likely signaled that the individual needed to correct his or her actions rather than that the rejector was using idiosyncratic criteria for judgment. Today, people's reactions to us are as likely to say something about *them* as they do about *us*, yet we tend to assume, at least when we first feel devalued, that we may be at fault. We may later consciously decide that a particular rejection does not reflect negatively on us, but the automatic default response seems to be that the rejection stemmed from our own personal characteristics or behavior. Thus, most rejections implicate the individual him- or herself and lower self-esteem, at least initially.

Motivation

When people have detected that their relational value is low or declining, they often take steps to bolster their relational value or at least to make sure that it doesn't fall any lower. Thus, the sociometer seems to induce a motive to deal with threats to one's relational value.

Many of these efforts to restore relational value involve self-presentational attempts to demonstrate that one possesses attributes that make one a valuable social interactant or relationship partner. A great deal of research shows that events that lower one's relational value in others' eyes—such as public failures, embarrassments, and disclosures of negative information—lead people to engage in remedial actions to repair their tainted image (Baumeister & Jones, 1978; Gonzales, Pederson, Manning, & Wetter, 1990; Schlenker, 1980; Scott & Lyman, 1968). Although people may engage in facework for other reasons, in most cases they believe that their public image has been damaged in a way that may lead others to value them less positively.

Sometimes, people's behaviors following rejection do not, on the surface, appear to increase their social value, approval, or acceptance from others. For example, people who feel unaccepted often withdraw or express anger, neither of which typically endear them to other people. However, such reactions may sometimes stem the tide of rejection even if they do not restore the person's relational value. People who feel rejected often have no viable options for improving their social image and relational value and, in fact, their continued efforts to do so would lead others to reject them even more emphatically. Thus, the best that a rejected person can sometimes do is to withdraw from interaction, lick his or her wounds, assess the situation, and perhaps reemerge later after sufficient time has passed. Even anger is sometimes beneficial by showing that one regards the other person's acceptance and relationship as highly important or by signaling that one will not tolerate future rejection. And, once a person realizes that rejection is permanent, there is often nothing more to lose by aggressing anyway.

Many writers have attributed face-saving behaviors to a motive to preserve self-esteem, arguing that people who try to put their best foot forward following a rejection or self-presentational predicament (or even who withdraw or lash out) are trying to repair their self-image and feelings about themselves. Sociometer theory disputes this explanation, and indeed the underlying notion that people have a need for self-esteem. When people perceive that their relational value is low or declining, their self-esteem also declines because, as noted, state self-esteem is an aspect of the sociometer's output. When they then behave in ways to improve their image, they are not trying to raise their self-esteem per se but rather to enhance their relational value. If they are successful in doing so, their self-esteem will indeed rise but only because it reflects their improved relational value. Of course, people sometimes do things simply to feel good about themselves, just as they do things to experience a variety of other positive emotions. But these behaviors do not arise from a "need" for self-esteem.

OVERRIDING THE SOCIOMETER

Sociometer theory does not suggest that people are concerned with what everyone thinks of them or are always concerned with other people's evaluations. People do not seek relational value from everyone they meet, partly because they have only a limited number of relational niches (Tooby & Cosmedes, 1996). Seeking more and more acceptance not only does little good, but it can harm people's existing relationships by spreading them too thin, interpersonally speaking, and leaving them unable to devote the time and effort needed to sustain their most important relationships. Furthermore, other considerations sometimes take precedence over being relationally valued. Social acceptance is fundamentally important to people's well-being, but it would be a strange psychological system that continuously overrode all other concerns in a quest for acceptance.

Not only do people not always actively seek acceptance, but they can override the sociometer when it alerts them to possible problems with their relational value by consciously and deliberately deciding to disregard certain interpersonal evaluations. Although I know of no evidence on this phenomenon, my sense is that an initial indication of low relational evaluation typically (if not inevitably) induces, just for a moment, a pang of negative affect (e.g., unease, hurt) and, if not lowered self-esteem, at least the thought that the other person's reaction might be due to undesirable aspects of one's personal characteristics or behavior. In such cases, the sociometer has detected a potential threat to the person's relational value in a particular target's eyes and automatically alerted the person as it is designed to do.

However, almost immediately, a controlled appraisal of the situation quickly determines whether the target is, in fact, an individual whose judgment of one's relational value is of importance. If the answer is "yes," then the person assesses the situation more fully, consciously considers the other person's impressions and evaluations, judges the likely consequences of the relational evaluation, and makes attributions for why his or her relational value is unacceptably low. Depending on the outcome of these deliberations, the person may or may not decide to react.

If, however, the target is judged to be someone whose relational evaluation is not (or should not be) important in the immediate interpersonal context, the negative affect quickly abates and the person is not motivated to enhance his or her relational value. Essentially, the person has consciously and deliberately overridden the sociometer's automatic response, akin to switching off or ignoring the smoke alarm once one has ascertained that the smoke in the kitchen is from a piece of burnt toast and not from a fire. Many warning systems possess this two-stage character in which an automatic process that is calibrated to be highly sensitive to threats is reevaluated by a second, controlled process. Just as the strange noise in the house at night automatically evokes fear until reasoned consideration reassures one that it is only the cat, another's expression of displeasure or disinterest makes one uneasy until one decides that the person's evaluation is not important anyway.

People seem to differ in their ability to override their sociometer's automatic responses to perceived low relational value. Some people seem able to brush off all but the most momentous indications that they are not valued, whereas others agonize over minor rebuffs and slights by people whose judgments have no real consequences for them. For example, people who are rejection-sensitive (Downey & Feldman, 1996), socially anxious (Leary & Kowalski, 1995), or low in self-esteem (Leary & MacDonald, 2003) may be more strongly affected by indications that other people do not like and accept them because they do not easily override the automatic warnings of their sociometers.

Another variable that may reflect people's ability to override the sociometer is *sociotropic breadth*, a term that Nicole Panicia and I coined to refer to the number of people about whose relational evaluation (i.e., acceptance and rejection) an individual is concerned. A person with a wide sociotropic breadth wishes to be valued and accepted by a large number and array of people, both those whose evaluations objectively matter and those whose evaluations should be of little import. A person with narrow sociotropic breadth is concerned primarily about the acceptance of only a relatively small group of individuals and generally disregards the judgments of those who are outside this circle. We measured sociotropic breadth by asking respondents to imagine interacting with each of 24 individuals who varied in social distance from the respondent, ranging from close others about whose acceptance people are rightfully concerned (e.g., friend, mother, favorite professor) to targets whose acceptance most people would probably not seek (e.g., sales clerk, homeless person, fellow airplane passenger). Respondents rated how much they would want the other person to "like and accept" them (or, conversely, how much it would bother them to be disliked and rejected by this person). We have only begun to understand the implications of sociotropic breadth, but preliminary findings suggest that sociotropic breadth predicts people's concerns with social acceptance in interpersonal interactions and the degree to which they try to forestall rejection—for example, by conforming to a group's opinion. Our sense is that people with a wide sociotropic breadth find it more difficult to override their sociometer's initial response than those with a narrow breadth. As a result, they find themselves frequently reacting to the relational evaluations of people whose judgments objectively do not matter.

Although certain people are less strongly affected by indications that they are not relationally valued than other people are, virtually everyone reacts to cues that connote rejection at least occasionally. Yet some individuals claim that they are totally unconcerned with other people's evaluations of them and that, contrary to a central premise of sociometer theory, their feelings about themselves are not affected by other people's judgments of their social acceptability (Harter, Stocker, & Robinson, 1996).

Such claims obviously offer a challenge to the idea that people are inherently motivated to be accepted and that they react emotionally (and with lowered self-esteem) when they believe others do not value them.

Cooley (1902) characterized the claims of people who purport to be unconcerned with others' evaluations of them as "illusion" (p. 208), and research has borne him out. Our retrospective studies of rejection episodes have not revealed a single individual who did not indicate that the episodes he or she described had pronounced effects on his or her feelings (Leary et al., 1998), and our research on sociotropic breadth did not reveal anyone whose score indicated that he or she was totally unperturbed by the prospect of rejection by at least a few individuals. More to the point, in two experiments, we studied people who were preselected because they adamantly claimed that their self-feelings were unaffected by social approval and acceptance. After allowing participants to share information about themselves, we provided them with bogus feedback indicating that they were accepted and approved of or rejected and disapproved of by other participants and measured their emotions and state self-esteem. In both studies, acceptance–rejection feedback affected the self-esteem of participants who claimed to be unaffected by approval and acceptance just as much as people who acknowledged that approval and acceptance do affect how they feel about themselves (Leary et al., 2003). These data do not show that people who are impervious to acceptance and rejection do not exist, but they do suggest that most people who claim to be unaffected by acceptance and rejection are mistaken. People can not function in interpersonal life without paying attention to how they are perceived and evaluated by others, particularly with regard to their relational value in others' eyes. Those who are oblivious or indifferent to others' evaluations are likely to behave in ways that lead everyone to shun them.

Why, then, do some people claim that they do not care what other people think about them when data suggest that they are clearly do? Setting aside the fact that people generally underestimate the impact of social influences on their behavior (Sabini, Siepmann, & Stein, 2001) and the possibility that some people ironically present themselves as unconcerned with social evaluations in order to be seen as independent, autonomous, and confident, I see two possible reasons. The first is that people who generally feel accepted (and thus acceptable) may experience relatively few acute instances of rejection that would show them that they are, in fact, concerned with what other people think of them. Just as it is much easier for a rich man than a poor man to believe that he's not interested in money, it is easier for people who generally feel acceptable to deny that acceptance is important to them. The fact that people who claim to be unaffected by acceptance and rejection tend to have higher trait self-esteem than those who admit to being affected supports this explanation (Harter et al., 1996; Leary et al., 2003). Given that people with high trait self-esteem believe that they are more valuable and acceptable (Leary et al., 1995; Leary & MacDonald, 2003), they may have fewer experiences that show them otherwise.

A second reason that some people underestimate their sensitivity to rejection is that they are better at overriding their sociometers. People who quickly and effectively override the sociometer's initial response to events that connote low or declining relational evaluation will subjectively feel that they are relatively unaffected by others' evaluations. In contrast, people who rarely override their sociometers will be more aware that they are sensitive to others' acceptance and rejection. People who do not engage in a secondary analysis of events that trigger the sociometer, who are unable to dismiss other people's evaluations of them no matter how unimportant, or who generally conclude after the secondary appraisal that they should, in fact, be concerned about the individual's acceptance of them will subjectively experience more frequent rejections, and thus more easily see how rejection affects them.

CORRECTING PROBLEMS WITH RELATIONAL VALUE

When people have detected that their relational value is low or declining and they believe that maintaining relational value in the evaluator's eyes is important, they become motivated to improve their relational value, or at least to be sure that it doesn't fall any lower. As noted, most of their efforts along these lines involve self-presentational tactics designed to demonstrate that they possess attributes that warrant a higher level of relational value than they believe they have at present. So, for example, they may excuse or justify undesired actions that portrayed them in a negative light (Schlenker, 1980), tout positive attributes that may compensate for their shortcomings (Baumeister & Jones, 1978), conform to other people's opinions in the hope that similarity will promote relational value (Leary, 1995), or do favors to ingratiate themselves (Jones & Wortman, 1973).

Whatever tactics people employ, they will try to assess whether their efforts to improve their relational value are successful. Unfortunately, even under the best of circumstances, people have trouble judging other people's impressions of them (DePaulo et al., 1987), and the task is even more difficult in the throes of an interpersonal predicament with implications for one's relational value. As a result, it is extremely difficult to know when one has performed sufficient interpersonal penance to rectify an interpersonal predicament. In many cases, the person has surmised that his or her value in another's eyes is low on the basis of minimal cues, and thus has no solid basis for knowing whether his or her social image has been repaired and relational value reestablished. Even when the other individual has explicitly expressed displeasure with the person, it will be difficult to know whether one's remedial efforts have been effective. To make matters worse, other people are often under normative pressure to act as if the individual's social image and relational value are restored whether or not this is the case. People sometimes brush off such events ("It's no big deal, no hard feelings") when, in fact, the person's value in their eyes remains seriously damaged.

The problem is further compounded by the fact that, as Goffman (1955) suggested, people tend to assume the worst about the effects of events on other people's impressions of them. Although a "worst-case reading" of the situation is sometimes beneficial because it assures that the person takes the problem seriously and engages in adequate remedial actions, it also leads people to worry excessively and sometimes needlessly about the effects of their misbehaviors on their relational value and to go overboard to correct the situation. The negatively biased processing of interpersonal feedback in these situations may explain why people often overapologize for even minor infractions and sometimes obsess about interpersonal encounters that went badly.

CONCLUSIONS

People think a great deal about how they are perceived and evaluated by others, and about the degree to which others value having relationships with them. The sociometer appears to process cues regarding relational value automatically at a preattentive level, triggering negative emotions and conscious analysis of the situation when the possibility of low or declining relational value is detected. People whose sociometer detects lower-than-desired relational value find themselves in the unenviable position of trying to discern whether a true threat (rather than a false alarm) is present and, if so, how to counteract it. The person often has scant information to judge other people's evaluations and whether his or her remedial actions have helped to rectify the situation.

Although researchers in social cognition have studied the processes involved in drawing inferences about other people's attributes, motives, and intentions, we know virtually nothing about how people draw inferences about others' evaluations of them, test their hunches about what other people are thinking about them, or determine whether their social image and relational value have been restored after events have threatened them. A few pockets of research—on stigmatization, self-presentation, the "spotlight effect," metaperception, and stereotype threat, for example—touch upon people's thoughts about others' perceptions of them, yet how people make inferences about their social image and relational value is not understood. This is obviously a ripe topic for future research.

REFERENCES

Baldwin, M. W., Carrell, S. E., & Lopez, D. F. (1990). Priming relationship schemas: My advisor and the pope are watching me from the back of my mind. *Journal of Experimental Social Psychology, 26,* 435–454.

Baum, A., & Andersen, S. M. (1999). Interpersonal roles in transference: Transient mood effects under the condition of significant-other resemblance. *Social Cognition, 17,* 161–185.

Baumeister, R. F., & Jones, E. E. (1978). When self-presentation is constrained by the target's knowledge: Consistency and compensation. *Journal of Personality and Social Psychology, 36,* 608–618.

Baumeister, R. F., & Leary, M. R. (1995). The need to belong: Desire for interpersonal attachments as a fundamental human motivation. *Psychological Bulletin, 117,* 497–529.

Baumeister, R. F., & Tice, D. M. (1990). Anxiety and social exclusion. *Journal of Social and Clinical Psychology, 9,* 165–195.

Baumester, R. F., Wotman, S. R., & Stillwell, A. M. (1993). Unrequited love: On heartbreak, anger, guilt, scriptlessness, and humiliation. *Journal of Personality and Social Psychology, 64,* 377–394.

Bednar, R. L., Wells, M. G., & Peterson, S. R. (1989). *Self-esteem: Paradoxes and innovations in clinical theory and practice.* Washington, DC: American Psychological Association.

Buckley, K. E., & Winkel, R. E., & Leary, M. R. (2004). Reactions to acceptance and rejection: Effects of level and sequence of relational evaluation. *Journal of Experimental Social Psychology, 40,* 14–28.

Cherry, E. C. (1953). Some experiments on the recognition of speech, with one and with two ears. *Journal of the Acoustical Society of America, 25,* 975–979.

Cooley, C. H. (1902). *Human nature and the social order.* New York: Scribner.

DePaulo, B. M., Kenny, D. A., Hoover, C., Webb, W., & Oliver, P. (1987). Accuracy of person perception: Do people know what kinds of impressions they convey? *Journal of Personality and Social Psychology, 52,* 303–315.

Downey, G., & Feldman, S. (1996). Implications of rejection sensitivity for intimate relationships. *Journal of Personality and Social Psychology, 70,* 1327–1343.

Fridja, N. (1986). *The emotions.* New York: Cambridge University Press.

Goffman, E. (1955). On facework. *Psychiatry, 18,* 213–231.

Gonzales, M. H., Pederson, J. H., Manning, D. J., & Wetter, D. W. (1990). Pardon my gaffe: Effects of sex, status, and consequence severity on accounts. *Journal of Personality and Social Psychology, 58,* 610–621.

Harter, S., Stocker, C., & Robinson, N. S. (1996). The perceived directionality of the link between approval and self-worth: Liabilities of a looking glass self-orientation among young adolescents. *Journal of Research on Adolescence, 6,* 285–308.

Haupt, A. H., & Leary, M. R. (1997). The appeal of worthless groups: Moderating effects of trait self-esteem. *Group Dynamics: Theory, Research, and Practice, 1,* 124–132.

Jones, E. E., & Wortman, C. B. (1973). *Ingratiation: An attributional approach.* Morristown, NJ: General Learning Press.

Leary, M. R. (1995). *Self-presentation*. Boulder, CO: Westview Press.

Leary, M. R. (1999). The social and psychological importance of self-esteem. In R. M. Kowalski & M. R. Leary (Eds.), *The social psychology of emotional and behavioral problems: Interfaces of social and clinical psychology* (pp. 197–221). Washington, DC: American Psychological Association.

Leary, M. R., & Baumeister, R. F. (2000). The nature and function of self-esteem: Sociometer theory. *Advances in Experimental Social Psychology, 33*, 1–62.

Leary, M. R., & Buckley, K. (2000). Social anxiety as an early warning system: A refinement and extension of the self-presentational theory of social anxiety. In S. G. Hofman & P. M. DiBartolo (Eds.), *Social phobia and social anxiety: An integration* (pp. 128–145). New York: Allyn & Bacon.

Leary, M. R., & Buttermore, N. (2003). The evolution of the human self: Tracing the natural history of self-awareness. *Journal for the Theory of Social Behavior, 33*, 365–404.

Leary, M. R., Cottrell, C. A., & Phillips, M. (2001). Deconfounding the effects of dominance and social acceptance on self-esteem. *Journal of Personality and Social Psychology, 81*, 898–909.

Leary, M. R., & Downs, D. L. (1995). Interpersonal functions of the self-esteem motive: The self-esteem system as a sociometer. In M. Kernis (Ed.), *Efficacy, agency, and self-esteem* (pp. 123–144). New York: Plenum Press.

Leary, M. R., Gallagher, B., Fors, E. H., Buttermore, N., Baldwin, E., Lane, K. K., & Mills, A. (2003). The invalidity of disclaimers about the effects of social feedback on self-esteem. *Personality and Social Psychology Bulletin, 29*, 623–636.

Leary, M. R., Haupt, A., Strausser, K., & Chokel, J. (1998). Calibrating the sociometer: The relationship between interpersonal appraisals and state self-esteem. *Journal of Personality and Social Psychology, 74*, 1290–1299.

Leary, M. R., Koch, E., & Hechenbleikner, N. (2001). Emotional responses to interpersonal rejection. In M. R. Leary (Ed.), *Interpersonal rejection* (pp. 145–166). New York: Oxford University Press.

Leary, M. R., & Kowalski, R. M. (1995). *Social anxiety*. New York: Guilford Press.

Leary, M. R., & MacDonald, G. (2003). Individual differences in self-esteem: A review and theoretical integration. In M. R. Leary & J. P. Tangney (Eds.), *Handbook of self and identity* (pp. 401–418). New York: Guilford Press.

Leary, M. R., & Springer, C. (2000). Hurt feelings: The neglected emotion. In R. M. Kowalski (Ed.), *Behaving badly: Aversive behaviors in interpersonal relationships* (pp. 151–175). Washington, DC: American Psychological Association.

Leary, M. R., Springer, C., Negel, L., Ansel, E., & Evans, K. (1998). The causes, phenomenology, and consequences of hurt feelings. *Journal of Personality and Social Psychology, 74*, 1225–1237.

Leary, M. R., Tambor, E. S., Terdal, S. K., & Downs, D. L. (1995). Self-esteem as an interpersonal monitor: The sociometer hypothesis. *Journal of Personality and Social Psychology, 68*, 518–530.

MacDonald, G., Saltzman, J. L., & Leary, M. R. (2003). Social approval and trait self-esteem. *Journal of Research in Personality, 37*, 23–40.

May, R. (1983). *The discovery of being*. New York: Norton.

Mitchell, R. W. (2003). Subjectivity and self-recognition in animals. In M. R. Leary & J. P. Tangney (Eds.), *Handbook of self and identity* (pp. 567–593) . New York: Guilford Press.

Nezlek, J. B., Kowalski, R. M., Leary, M. R., Blevins, T., & Holgate, S. (1997). Personality moderators of reactions to interpersonal rejection: Depression and trait self-esteem. *Personality and Social Psychology Bulletin, 23,* 1235–1244.

Ohman, A. (1986). Face the beast and fear the face: Animal and social fears as prototypes for evolutionary analyses of emotion. *Psychophysiology, 23,* 123–145.

Rozin, P., & Royzman, E. B. (2001). Negativity bias, negativity dominance, and contagion. *Personality and Social Psychology Review, 5,* 296–320.

Sabini, J., Siepmann, M., & Stein, J. (2001). The really fundamental attribution error in social psychological research. *Psychological Inquiry, 12,* 1–15.

Schlenker, B. R. (1980). *Impression management: The self-concept, social identity, and interpersonal relations.* Monterey, CA: Brooks/Cole.

Schlenker, B. R., & Pontari, B. A. (2000). The strategic control of information: Impression management and self-presentation in daily life. In A. Tesser, R. Felson, & J. Suls (Eds.), *Perspectives on self and identity* (pp. 199–232). Washington, DC: American Psychological Association.

Scott, M. B., & Lyman, S. (1968). Accounts. *American Sociological Review, 33,* 46–62.

Simon, H. A. (1967). Motivational and emotional controls of cognition. *Psychological Review, 74,* 29–39.

Snapp, C. M., & Leary, M. R. (2001). Hurt feelings among new acquaintances: Moderating effects of interpersonal familiarity. *Journal of Social and Personal Relationships, 18,* 315–326.

Srivastava, S. (2003). *How self-evaluations relate to being liked by others: Integrating interpersonal processes and individual differences.* Unpublished manuscript, Dept. of Psychology, Stanford University.

Tooby, J., & Cosmedes, L. (1996). Friendship and the banker's paradox: Other pathways in the evolution of altruism. *Proceedings of the British Academy, 88,* 119–143.

5

Goals and Labors, Friends and Neighbors

Self-Regulation and Interpersonal Relationships

GRÁINNE M. FITZSIMONS, JAMES SHAH,
TANYA L. CHARTRAND, *and* JOHN A. BARGH

Where there is great love, there are always wishes.
—WILLA CATHER

The goals that individuals pursue in daily life shape and influence the course of their interpersonal relationships. Just as importantly, relationship partners—friends, family members, romantic partners, and colleagues—influence the goals individuals choose to pursue, their success at attaining them, and the consequences of those goal pursuits. Recognizing the important interplay between self-regulatory processes and social relationships, a burgeoning number of researchers have recently set out to examine goal pursuit in interpersonal contexts (e.g., see upcoming volumes by Shah & Gardner, in press, and Vohs & Finkel, in press).

This chapter presents one theoretical perspective on this integration of interpersonal and motivational approaches. Combining theories on the nature of interpersonal representations (e.g., Andersen & Chen, 2002; Baldwin, 1992) with recent theorizing about the cognitive properties of goals (e.g., Bargh, 1990; Kruglanski, 1996), we propose a model of interpersonal cognition that focuses on the essential role that goals play in the links between self and other. In this chapter, we outline our ideas about how the self's goals are cognitively linked with representations of significant others, and the interpersonal and motivational factors that may moderate the effects of these associations.

In particular, we are interested in how these goal–person associations can affect both goal pursuit and interpersonal relationships in a dynamic and interactive fashion. First, we suggest that significant others can act as both objects and triggers of the self's important goals, eliciting automatic perceptual, affective, and behavioral changes in the self. Whether we want intimacy or independence, romance or revenge, fun or friendship, other people are often the *objects* of the self's most powerful desires and needs. Significant others can also act as *triggers* of the self's goals, eliciting motives that go on to automatically lead the self to engage in goal-directed cognition and behavior. For example, for a college student, just thinking about one's judgmental mother can elicit a strong desire to impress her (even if she isn't around), causing studying to seem more attractive and club hopping to seem less attractive (at least temporarily).

Second, we propose that active goals can also have powerful influences on perceptions of and behaviors toward significant others, depending on the nature of the relationship between the goal and the significant other in question. The way we think about and act toward our relationship partners depends on how instrumental they are for our goal pursuit—for example, if we are committed to achieving a given goal, we will feel more warmly toward friends who can actually help us achieve that goal. When exam time rolls around, the average college student values those friends who actually went to class during the semester, and devalues his or her class-skipping friends, much more than during the middle of the semester, when his or her preferences may even have been reversed.

Before discussing our model and evidence in detail, we describe the research and theory from which this model emerges. First, our ideas fit into an innovative research area examining the cognitive properties of motivational constructs (Bargh, 1990; Kruglanski, 1996). This background provides core principles that the current research depends on, theorizing in novel ways about the meaning and nature of goal pursuit. Second, our findings contribute to research on goals within interpersonal relationships and on the effects of other people on the self regulatory process. Finally, our ideas are shaped by theories of "the relational self," which suggests that the self-concept has strong associative links to representations of other people, such as friends and family members (Andersen & Chen, 2002; Baldwin, 1992). We briefly describe each of these background areas before turning to our model.

GOALS AS MENTAL REPRESENTATIONS

According to *goal systems theory*, goals are represented as a network of cognitive associations imbued with unique functional and structural features (see Shah, Kruglanski, & Friedman, 2002). Goals are mental representations of desired end states that are governed in a joint fashion by motivational and cognitive principles (see Chartrand & Bargh, 2002; Shah et al., 2002). Because of their status as mental structures, goals can be beneficially studied with the same social-cognitive tools and theories that have been applied to constructs like traits and stereotypes. If goals are indeed represented cognitively, they should share the features that characterize these other constructs, and be guided by the same principles of accessibility, activation, and organization (Bargh, 1990; Bargh, Gollwitzer, Lee-Chai, Barndollar, & Troetschel, 2001; Hull, 1931; Kruglanski, 1996; Shah & Kruglanski, 2003).

In goal systems theory, goals are linked to both higher and lower order goals within a hierarchy (e.g., the goal *to lose weight* could be linked to a higher order goal *to be healthy*, as well as to a lower order goal *to eat carefully*), as well as laterally to goals from other hierarchies. That is, goals share excitatory links with other goals that are facilitative (e.g., *to have an active social life* and *to meet new people*), and inhibitory links with competing or alternative goals (e.g., *to meet new people* and *to master crossword puzzles*). Recently, evidence has begun to accrue in support of these links among goals (Shah, Friedman, & Kruglanski, 2003; Shah & Kruglanski, 2003). For example, the activation of one goal has been shown to positively or negatively impact pursuit of another goal, depending on the nature of the link (i.e., excitatory or inhibitory) between the two goals (Shah & Kruglanski, 2003).

Goals are also thought to be linked to a variety of other knowledge structures, such as the means that individuals may use to obtain a specific goal (e.g., *coupons* can become linked to a goal *to save money*, and *running shoes* can become linked to a goal *to exercise more*), as well as features of situations in which that goal is commonly used (e.g., *the library* may become linked to a goal *to get good grades*). Indeed, studies have found evidence for both directions of this kind of link. That is, means can activate associated goals: the word *reading* causes the goal *to be knowledgeable* to become more accessible (Shah & Kruglanski, 2003); similarly, goals can activate associated means: a *transportation* goal activates *bicycle* for those people who commonly use bicycles to get from place to place (Aarts & Dijksterhuis, 2000).

Automatic Goals

Of particular importance to our current model, goals—as mental representations—should be governed by the same rules of temporary and chronic accessibility that govern other knowledge structures. That is, the accessibility of goals should vary with the situational or social context (Bargh, 1990; Higgins, 1996). Depending partly on the level of accessibility, some active goals will reach conscious awareness, while others will become activated but operate outside of consciousness. Importantly, even these nonconsciously operating goals can exert powerful effects on an individual's thoughts, feelings, and behaviors (Bargh, 1990; Bargh et al., 2001; Chartrand & Bargh, 1996).

How does a goal become active without the intervention of consciousness? According to Bargh's (1990) auto-motive theory, associations develop between a goal and features of the situations in which the goal is often consciously initiated. Eventually, the presence of the associated situational features is sufficient to activate the goal automatically, and once activated, the goal is theorized to operate to guide perception and behavior without need for conscious guidance or intervention (see Chartrand & Bargh, 2002).

Thus, although goal pursuit can be activated by deliberate intent and guided with conscious awareness (Bandura, 1986; Carver & Scheier, 1998; Deci & Ryan, 1985), the complete sequence of goal pursuit—from activation to operation—can also occur entirely outside of consciousness (Bargh, 1990; Chartrand & Bargh, 2002). Although the study of nonconscious goal pursuit has emerged only recently within social cognition, there already exists substantial empirical support for the hypothesis that goals can be activated and pursued nonconsciously (Aarts & Dijksterhuis, 2000; Bargh et al., 2001; Chartrand & Bargh, 1996; Fischbach, Friedman, & Kruglanski, 2003; Fitzsimons & Bargh, 2003; Moskowitz, Gollwitzer, Wasel, & Schaal, 1999; Shah, Friedman, & Kruglanski, 2003; Shah, 2003).

For example, in a set of experiments, goals were activated through priming manipulations and shown to guide subsequent social behavior in a purposeful, though nonconscious, fashion (Bargh et al., 2001). After being exposed to words related to achievement (e.g., *achieve, succeed*) in a word search game, participants performed significantly better on a subsequent verbal achievement task than did those who received neutral primes, with participants displaying no awareness of how they were affected by the primes. In this and other experiments examining social goals like cooperation as well as goals like achievement, primed goals were shown to influence behavior over extended periods of time (10–15 minutes), and in complex interaction with the changing demands and informative qualities of the situation. Participants' behavior also displayed the hallmark qualities of conscious goal pursuit: (1) resuming pursuit of the goal after interruption, (2) manifesting an increase in goal strength after a delay, and (3) persisting in the face of obstacles. Thus, the behaviors primed by the goal-related words did possess qualities of motivated behavior, not simply rote behavioral sequences or trait-mimicking behaviors (see Bargh et al., 2001).

LINKS BETWEEN GOALS AND INTERPERSONAL STRUCTURES

Thus, goals are theorized to be mental representations, linked to other goals and cognitive constructs. Beyond the straightforward associations created among related goals, as well as goals and means, we have recently hypothesized that goals may actually become associated with *interpersonal* structures (Fitzsimons & Bargh, 2003; Shah, 2003). Because other people play such an essential role in our day-to-day lives, in both the personal and the professional domains, it is critical to understand how their existence "within our minds" can affect the self. In particular, we hypothesize that as the objects of powerful motives and needs, significant others likely have direct and uninterrupted associations with the self's goals.

Namely, we propose that goals may be embedded in the associative links between self and other, with connections created between the self's goals and the self's representation of important relationship partners. For example, if Gary has a goal *to become a great snowboarder*, this goal could become linked to representations of people in his life who are targets of a higher order goal (e.g., learning to snowboard will impress Gary's brother-in-law), are role models for the snowboarding goal, are pursuing that same goal themselves, are competitive in that goal domain (e.g., an old sports rival), or are facilitative of goal pursuit (e.g., a friend who baby-sits so Gary can have a day on the slopes).

Of course, most models of goal pursuit have emphasized the independent nature of self-regulation: goal selection, pursuit, and attainment are thought to be guided by the self's own desires, willpower, and executive control processes (Carver & Scheier, 1998; see Gollwitzer & Bargh, 1996). However, if we are correct in positing that goals are embedded in or associated with interpersonal structures, then the consideration of interpersonal factors could contribute much to the understanding of goal pursuit, as interpersonal theorists have frequently noted (e.g., Andersen & Chen, 2002; Berscheid, 1994; Trzebinski, 1989).

Others as Objects of the Self's Goals

The most obvious way that significant others influence self-regulation is through their role as the desired objects of individuals' goal pursuits. Many of the most important goals that people pursue in everyday life are goals in which the desired outcome is inherently interpersonal. Some examples of these interpersonal goals are (1) intimacy goals, (2) goals to perceive one's partner positively, and (3) goals for attachment and security. The goal for intimacy is theorized to be a fundamental driving force in everyday life and a characteristic of healthy psychological functioning, promoting not only relationship satisfaction (Cantor & Malley, 1991; Clark & Reis, 1988), but also positive health outcomes (e.g., Atkins, Kaplan, & Toshima, 1991; Cohen, 1988; Glanz & Lerman, 1992). Beyond intimacy, successful relationships require relationship-protecting goals to maintain commitment in the face of conflicts and partner transgressions. The most extensively researched of such goals is the goal to perceive significant others in the most positive light possible, especially relative to alternative partners (Johnson & Rusbult, 1989; Murray & Holmes, 1997; also see Murray & Derrick, Chapter 7, this volume). Individuals also have powerful motivations for attachment bonds and relationship security. Goals have recently emerged as an important focus in the study of adult attachment relationships (e.g., Collins & Read, 1994; Mikulincer, 1998; Rom & Mikulincer, 2003) which examines how individual differences in attachment anxiety and avoidance are manifested in different interpersonal goals and behavioral strategies (see Shaver & Mikulincer, 2002).

Significant others play an important role in self-regulation as the objects or targets of essential goals, leading individuals to pursue and maintain close relationships, to protect those relationships through altering their own perceptions, and to seek security and attachment bonds. The roles that other people play as objects or targets of powerful motivations should not be undervalued: certainly these overarching needs for relationship security and satisfaction influence a wide range of important relationship phenomena.

Others as Triggers of the Self's Goals: A Relational-Self Perspective

Beyond the domain of the relationship context, significant others play a key role in self-regulation more generally, affecting the goals that individuals choose to pursue, at what time, and to what degree of success. Indeed, there has been a long-standing emphasis in psychology on how our internal representations of other people may come to influence our sense of self and efforts at self-regulation through, for instance, role taking (Mead, 1934), reflected self-appraisals (Cooley, 1902/1964), identification (Freud, 1937), or the process of internalization (Schaffer, 1968).

We suggest that significant others can elicit these wide-ranging effects on goal pursuit at least partly because of the direct links that we theorize to exist between representations of others and the self's goals. Certainly, when significant others are objects or targets of goals, as discussed in the previous section, an association likely exists between the goal and the significant other. However, goal–person associations may develop for a variety of other reasons as well, with the common thread simply being the existence of an association that permits the significant other to act as a trigger of the self's goals.

A variety of theoretical models have presented related ideas about how significant others are mentally represented and also about how such representations can have automatic influences on perception and behavior (Andersen & Chen, 2002; Andersen & Cole, 1990; Aron, Aron, Tudor, & Nelson, 1991; Baldwin, 1992, 1995; Chen, 2001; Hazan & Shaver, 1987; Holmes, 2000; Miller & Read, 1991; Park, 1986; Planalp, 1987). These theories propose that individuals have complex, detailed, and multifaceted mental representations of their relationships with significant others, consisting of interrelated representations of the self, the significant other, and the relations between the two.

Importantly, once these representations of significant others become activated—by seeing, interacting with, or somehow being reminded of the significant other—they can lead to automatic influences on a wide range of phenomena. Much of that evidence comes from research conducted by Andersen and her colleagues on the "transference" phenomenon, in which an activated significant-other representation is applied nonconsciously to a new individual who reminds the self of an important relationship partner (e.g., Berk & Andersen, 2000; Hinkley & Andersen, 1996). This research program has convincingly demonstrated that many of the qualities of an important relationship partner—and qualities of the self when with that other—can become activated outside of consciousness and guide perception and behavior (Andersen, Reznik, & Manzella, 1996; Glassman & Andersen, 1999).

In a now classic set of studies examining the effects of activated significant other constructs on self-evaluation, Baldwin, Carrell, and Lopez (1990) found that practicing Catholics who were subliminally exposed to a photograph of a scowling pope subsequently rated themselves more negatively than they did when presented with a picture of a scowling unknown other. That the effect was not observed for nonpracticing Catholics suggested that the effects of primed relational representations do indeed depend on the relevance of the other person and the unique associations formed between the self and the other.

Although the inclusion of goals in relationship representations has not yet received a great deal of empirical attention, several theorists have suggested that significant-other representations may indeed have motivational components—including information about needs, goals, and plans involving the relationship (Miller & Read, 1991; Moretti & Higgins, 1999; Park, 1986; Trzebinski, 1989). There is preliminary evidence for the inclusion of motivation in significant-other representations as well. For example, when representations of significant others are activated, people approach a new acquaintance who resembles a positive significant other and avoid a new acquaintance who resembles a negative significant other, in comparison to a yoked participant's positive and negative significant other (Andersen et al., 1996).

A TRIANGULAR MODEL OF ASSOCIATIONS:
THE SELF, GOALS, AND SIGNIFICANT OTHERS

In sum, we have reviewed theory and research suggesting that goals are cognitive representations governed by rules of accessibility and activation, and have theorized that they may be linked to representations of significant others, embedded in the relational associations between self and other. Borrowing from theories of the relational self, we hypothesize that these links may elicit automatic effects on perception and behavior.

We have recently proposed a triangular model of implicit associations that seeks to detail both the bidirectional and implicit relations between mental representations of our significant others and our goals, also highlighting the importance of considering how both representations relate to the self. The model can be used as a framework for generating predictions about how significant others can affect goal-directed behavior and how goals can affect interpersonal perception and behavior.

Specifically (see Figure 5.1), the model suggests that representations of the self, significant others, and goals are cognitively associated, and that these associations may have implicit effects on behavior. First, the model proposes an implicit path through which the mental construal of others may impact the self's everyday behavior because of the self's association with significant others and their close association with various goals.

Moreover, as with other cognitive links, such associative effects may occur quite spontaneously, without conscious intervention or control. The mere activation of one's internal representation of a close other may be enough to invoke the goals with which this individual is associated. Goals, as cognitive constructs like any other, will thus become activated whenever the relational representation is activated, in an all-or-none fashion (see Hayes-Roth, 1977). Unlike other forms of goal priming, however (in which goals are activated automatically, without any moderating variables; see Bargh et al., 2001), goal priming via the activation of significant-other representations may depend on the nature of one's relationship to the sig-

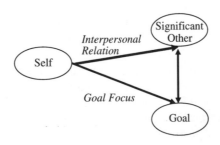

FIGURE 5.1. Triangular model of significant other–goal associations.

nificant other in question, as well as to the nature of the link between the self and the goal construct (e.g., goal commitment, goal focus, and perceived self-efficacy; see Bandura, 1986).

First, we predict that activating a significant-other representation should lead to heightened accessibility of associated goals, and should cause the goals to influence the self's perception and behavior. Second, that mechanism should be moderated by qualities of the association between the goal and the significant other, the self and the significant other, and the self and the goal.

Beyond the effects of how significant others affect goal pursuit, the model also speaks to the influence of active goal constructs on interpersonal perception and behavior. If the links between goals and significant-other representations are bidirectional in nature, as the model presupposes, then our third hypothesis is that activating goal constructs may lead to heightened accessibility of associated significant-other representations. Finally, this effect should also be moderated by qualities and features of the associations among the three elements of the model: the self, the goal, and the significant other. We next describe evidence for each of the hypotheses generated by the model, and elaborate on some related new research that addresses how active goals can elicit automatic effects on interpersonal perception and behavior.

Effects of Significant Others on Automatic Goal Pursuit

The research described below investigates the hypothesis that the activation of significant-other (SO) representations (through thinking of or seeing a significant other) can activate associated goals, and that these goals can then operate outside of awareness to influence subsequent behavior in line with the goal content of the SO representation. Furthermore, this research discusses moderating variables that have been shown to alter the effects of primed SO representations.

Others as Triggers of Self's Goals

SOs have been found to elicit nonconscious effects on self-regulation by serving as triggers for the goals that the individual commonly pursues with that SO (Andersen et al., 1996; Baldwin, 1992; Fitzsimons & Bargh, 2003). Over time, goals that an individual frequently pursues with an SO are hypothesized to become automatically associated with the SO representation.

In several experiments, just thinking about an SO for a few minutes initiated goal-directed behavior in line with the goals that individuals reported associating with that SO (Fitzsimons & Bargh, 2003). For example, at the beginning of the semester, college students reported the goals they pursued with their mother, with approximately half of the participants reporting a goal to please their mother by achieving academically. Students returned for an experiment several months later, and completed a priming task disguised as a memory test, in which participants either answered questions about their mother (e.g., list vacations your mother has taken, describe her appearance), or neutral, noninterpersonal questions (e.g., describe the path you walk to school). We hypothesized that priming participants with their mother activated all goals that they associated with her, including the goal to achieve academically. Next, participants completed a "verbal achievement task." As predicted, participants primed with their mother outperformed control participants on the verbal achievement task. Most importantly, the priming manipulation only affected participants who had previously reported a goal to please their mother by achieving academically, emphasizing the importance of the active goal constructs in mediating these SO priming effects.

Others as Triggers of the Significant Other's Goals for Self

The second route through which SOs have been shown to exert a nonconscious effect on self-regulation is by activating the self's representation of the SO's goals for the self, rather than the self's goals toward the SO (Moretti & Higgins, 1999; Shah, 2003). SOs, once represented mentally, can in a sense "watch us from the back of our minds" (Baldwin & Holmes, 1987), causing individuals to be more likely to behave in line with the wishes, standards, and goals that the SO has for them. By functioning as an inner audience, SOs can evoke goals and evaluative standards that individuals then feel motivated to meet, affecting behavior in line with the SO's desires (Baldwin & Holmes, 1987; Moretti & Higgins, 1999; Shah, 2003).

Thus, activating SO representations should also activate goals that the SO has for the self (e.g., Sam's mother wants him to become a pianist), as well as goals the self has when with the SO (e.g., Sam wants to gain independence from his mother, so he wants to become a guitarist instead). Of course, in many relationship contexts, the goals the self has with the SO and the goals the SO has for the self are likely to be related—for example, the reason someone wants to please his mother by achieving is likely because the mother wants him to achieve. However, these are evidently distinct processes within an interpersonal relationship: individuals have many goals with a SO (e.g., manipulate the SO, impress the SO, analyze the SO's behavior) that are not the goals the SO would have for the self. To assume these would always lead to the same outcome is to assume that the self and the SO have identical desires and plans.

To elucidate the effects of activating an SO's goals for the self, Shah (2003) asked participants to nominate an SO who would want them to perform well on a certain task, as well as one who would not care whether they performed well. As predicted, subliminally priming participants with the names of these Sos affected self-reported goal commitment, goal accessibility, and task performance, in line with the motivations of their SOs. For example, being primed with the words *father* and *dad* led participants to report more commitment to an achievement goal, to have that goal made more accessible (as demonstrated by facilitated responses in a reaction-time task; see Bargh & Chartrand, 2000, for details), and to pursue that goal to a greater degree, to the extent that they felt close to their father and perceived him to care about their achievement on that task.

In a stronger and more conservative test of the accessibility effects, Chartrand and Shah (2004) used a somewhat different paradigm. In a pretest earlier in the quarter, participants were asked to name the SOs who most strongly had various goals for them (e.g., the SO had a goal for the self to achieve, relax, or cooperate, etc.). In a lexical decision task, individuals were subliminally primed with the name of an SO before each trial. Results revealed that individuals were faster to recognize goal words after being primed with the name of the SO who had that particular goal for them (versus an SO who had a different goal for them). On a trial-by-trial basis, then, participants demonstrated heightened accessibility for goals that they associated with recently primed SOs.

Moderators of the Significant Other–Goal Link

One unique aspect of priming goals via the activation of SO representations is that the intensity (and even the direction) of the effect depends heavily on the nature of the various associative links between the self and the SO, the self and the goal construct, and the SO and the goal construct. There are many associations that likely moderate the influence of SOs on goal-directed behavior. First, one's goal pursuits are more readily influenced by an SO to the extent that one feels particularly close to that SO or that the relationship is particularly important (see Aron et al., 1991; Brewer & Gardner, 1996; Read & Miller, 1989). In a series of studies, Shah (2003) found that relationship closeness and importance moderated the extent to which SO priming led to goal-directed behavior. That is, the closer and more important participants felt to a given SO, the more they behaved in line with the goals that SO had for them.

Closeness is not the only relationship quality that may influence the SO–goal priming link. Another possible moderator is the extent to which relationship partners are perceived as controlling—that is, as placing external pressure on the self to do what the relationship partner wants him or her to do. When individuals perceive an SO to be controlling or authoritative (see Deci & Ryan, 2000; Ryan & Deci, 2000), they may respond in a unique fashion to that person's goals and wishes. In particular, they may respond with "reactance," doing the exact opposite of what the SO wants them to do (Brehm & Brehm, 1981). In terms of our model, individuals responding with motivated reactance would be likely to inhibit the goal that was primed by the SO, and possibly even activate and pursue an opposing goal.

In a preliminary study examining reactance in nonconscious goal pursuit, participants were subliminally primed with the name of a controlling SO who wanted them to work hard, or a controlling SO who wanted them to relax and have fun (Chartrand, Dalton, & Fitzsimons, 2004). As predicted, participants responded to the controlling SO primes by directing their behavior away from the SO's goal for them. Those primed with a controlling SO who wanted them to work hard performed worse on a verbal achievement test than those primed with a controlling SO who wanted them to relax.

Another association that has been shown to moderate the SO–goal priming effect is the complexity of the relationship between the SO's and the self's goals, as indicated by the number of different goals associated with the SO (Shah, 2003). That is, the greater the number of goals an SO has for the self, the less likely that the SO will cause any given one of those goals to become active and guide the self's behavior. One possible explanation for this finding stems from research on the "fan effect" (Anderson, 1974, 1983), in which the higher the number of specific facts linked to a general mental construct, the less likely any particular fact will be remembered. Another explanation of this effect is "response competition" (see Macleod, 1991): even when an SO is strongly associated with multiple goals, the goals may compete with or inhibit each other, reducing the effect of any of the goals. For example, the more goals participants reported associating with an SO who also wanted them to succeed at an achievement task, the less that their performance on that task was affected by being primed with that SO (Shah, 2003).

Summary of Effects of Others on Automatic Goal Pursuit

In sum, the above-mentioned sets of research suggest that mental representations of the SOs in one's life are associated with both the goals that the self pursues toward the other and the goals that the SO has for the self. Thus, thinking of or interacting with an SO will activate these associated goals, and can lead to either of these kinds of automatic goal-directed behavioral responses, without a person necessarily being aware of the source of those responses. Taken together in a complementary fashion, the studies propose that behavior can be automatically influenced by both people's own interpersonal goals—that may or may not be linked to a partner's standards or wishes—and people's mental representations of the partner's goals for the self. Which of the two kinds of goals (self's vs. other's) will guide behavior in a given situation is likely to depend on multiple factors, from temporary aspects of the situation to more long-term characteristics of the relationship (see Shah & Kruglanski, 2002). Elucidating the features that determine the source of the influence—the self's goals with those of the SO, or the SO's goals for the self—is an important avenue for future research in this area.

Further research will undoubtedly uncover other implicit mechanisms of interpersonal influence on goal pursuit, as well as further specify the nature and consequences of the currently observed routes through which SOs can guide nonconscious self-regulation. Given the frequency with which people think about and interact with SOs, they are likely to be a frequent source of nonconscious self-regulatory actions.

Automatic Effects of Goals on Interpersonal Perception

According to our triangular model, associations exist among representations of the self, the self's goals, and SOs. In the prior section, we described research examining the hypothesis that associations between goals and SOs should lead to implicit effects on goal pursuit. In particular, we focused on how activated SO representations could affect the self's goal-directed behavior.

In examining the implicit link between SOs and goals, Figure 5.1 details another effect of the linkages between goals and SOs that may have important interpersonal implications. If associations do exist between the self's goal constructs and representations of SOs, as we have suggested, then these associations should also elicit effects in the opposite causal direction. That is, accessible goals should also automatically invoke associated SO representations, bringing to mind those SOs who are role models, or who facilitate goal progress, or who are somehow connected to the active goal.

The importance of these associations may extend beyond accessibility effects to real interpersonal perception and behavior. Combining our associative model with theories of automatic goal-driven evaluations (Ferguson & Bargh, in press; Moors, De Houwer, & Eelan, 2004; Smith & Lazarus, 1990), we further propose that when a goal is automatically activated, evaluations of and behavior toward associated SOs will be affected, depending on the specific nature of the SO–goal link.

There are many theoretical and empirical forerunners to the study of goal effects on interpersonal perception, too many to describe succinctly here. Ever since the "New Look" era in psychological research (e.g., Allport, 1955; Bruner, 1957), psychologists have taken for granted that motivational states act as a filter for perceiving the social world, directing focus onto goal-relevant targets, guiding interpretations, and imbuing social situations with meaning (e.g., Bruner, 1957; Bruner & Postman, 1948; Jones & Thibaut, 1958; Kelly, 1955). For example, research on person memory has supported the New Look theorizing about the effects of active motivational states on information processing in the interpersonal domain (e.g., Hamilton, Katz, & Leirer, 1980; Hastie & Kumar, 1979). They way we evaluate and perceive other people depends on the kinds of information-processing goals we bring into an interpersonal situation, whether we are conscious of those goals or not (Chartrand & Bargh, 1996).

The current research on the effects of goals on the accessibility of interpersonal structures, as well as on evaluations of SOs, aims to contribute to these past findings by emphasizing the implicit and interpersonal nature of these effects, as well as by elucidating the mechanisms by which active goals affect interpersonal phenomena.

Effects of Goals on Accessibility of Significant-Other Representations

As generated by the model presented in Figure 5.1,we have hypothesized that activating a given goal will automatically heighten the accessibility of associated SOs. There are multiple ways by which SOs could become associated with one's goals, each of which has different implications for the interpersonal effects of goal pursuit. For example, SOs could become associated with a given goal if the self perceived them to be role models for goal attainment (see Johnson, Chartrand, Norton, & Nelson, 2004). Similarly, they could become associated with goal constructs by sharing the same goal as the self, or by being similar to or identified with the self. Another possibility, and the one that we focus on here, is that SOs who facilitate the self's goal achievement in one way or another can become associated with the goal construct itself (see Shah & Kruglanski, 2003). Such SOs may actively help one attain goals or may simply constitute social mirrors that reflect one's various desired attributes, serving as comparison standards to assess—and possibly to facilitate—progress. Indeed, as mentioned earlier, goals (like the goal to achieve) can become activated by attainment means in a bottom-up fashion, whether these means constitute situations (like the library) or behaviors (like study) (Shah & Kruglanski, 2003). Individuals who facilitate an individual's goal pursuit may thus become linked with the goal because of their role as a *means* to goal attainment.

In a first test of these ideas, Fitzsimons and Shah (2004) predicted that when a goal is active, representations of SOs who facilitate goal progress will become temporarily more accessible, and representations of nonfacilitating SOs will become temporarily less accessible. We obtained prior information from our participants about the names of friends who did and did not facilitate a list of goals. In a subsequent experimental session, half of the participants were primed with the goal "have an active social life" via a scrambled sentence task (Srull & Wyer, 1979), and all were then asked to list the names of all of their friends. Following Higgins, King, and Maven's (1982) work on "primacy of output," we used this list measure as a rough index of accessibility, with names generated earlier in the list thought to be higher in accessibility that those lower in the list. As predicted, we found that participants primed with a sociability goal listed the names of facilitating friends earlier in the list—and those of nonfacilitating friends later in the list—than did unprimed participants. These findings provide initial evidence that goals will automatically affect the accessibility of associated interpersonal structures, in line with the specific contents of the links between the goal and the SO in question. Just as goals activated instrumental means in earlier studies (Shah & Kruglanski, 2002), goals also appear to activate representations of instrumental SOs, and possibly even inhibit representations of noninstrumental others.

Effects of Goals on Perceptions of Significant Others

Thus, initial evidence suggests that facilitative SOs come to mind more readily, and nonfacilitative SOs come to mind less readily, when a goal is activated. We further suggest that activating a goal may have an automatic influence on *perceptions* of SOs, depending on the content of the links between those SOs and the currently active goal. According to appraisal theory (e.g., Smith & Lazarus, 1990) and new findings on goal-driven automatic evaluations (Ferguson & Bargh, in press; Moors et al., 2004), active goals can have automatic effects on evaluations of objects in the environment, such that goal-instrumental objects are evaluated more positively than are goal-noninstrumental objects.

When a goal is active, then, we predict that SOs will be evaluated depending on the information embedded in the links between the goal construct and the SO—specifically, information relating to the SO's goal instrumentality will be used as a basis for evaluation. That is, an active goal will cause goal-facilitative SOs to be evaluated more positively than nonfacilitative SOs, relative to when a different goal (or no particular goal) is active.

To examine this idea, Fitzsimons and Shah (2004) had participants nominate close friends who were facilitative and not facilitative for a list of important goals. After a number of filler tasks, participants completed a scrambled sentence task (Srull & Wyer, 1979) designed to activate an achievement goal. After the goal-priming task, participants were asked to answer questions about their relationships with friends, with the first two friends being those whom participants had earlier nominated as being particularly facilitative and nonfacilitative of the goal to achieve at school.

As predicted, the currently accessible goal to achieve at school affected how participants evaluated their friendships to facilitating and nonfacilitating friends. Participants in the control condition, who had no primed goal to achieve, did not report feeling any differently about their facilitating and nonfacilitating friends. In contrast, participants primed with a nonconscious achievement goal felt closer to facilitating friends, reported their relationships as more important, and planned to spend more time with facilitating than nonfacilitating friends. Participants did not report any awareness of the influence of the primed goal on their evaluations of their friends, nor were they aware that the goal was made accessible. In sum, these findings suggest that perceptions of friends and other close others likely depends in part on the nature of one's currently active goals, and that the influence of activated goals can result automatically, without any conscious awareness of the process.

Thus, primed goals can have the predicted influence on shaping interpersonal perceptions. What about goals that are more chronically active in daily life: Do they have the same effects on interpersonal perceptions? According to our hypotheses about the associations between goals and SO constructs, we would expect that changes in goal accessibility over time will affect interpersonal perceptions in a similar fashion. As goal accessibility increases, perceptions of closeness should be more affected by the extent to which SOs facilitate goal progress.

In an experiment designed to test this idea (Fitzsimons & Shah, 2004), participants did a number of tasks that measured goal accessibility, SO facilitation, and relationship closeness at two time points, separated by 2 weeks. As predicted, changes in goal accessibility significantly interacted with ratings of SO facilitation to positively predict change in closeness ratings. When goals were more accessible at Time 2 than at Time 1, participants used facilitation ratings as a basis for evaluating their closeness to SOs, much like they did when a goal was made temporarily more accessible through priming techniques in the previous study. In contrast, when goals were less accessible at Time 2, participants were less likely to use facilitation ratings as a basis for evaluating their friendships.

Thus, the findings from these two studies provide evidence that the automatic activation of goals does affect interpersonal perceptions, depending on the nature of the particular association between SOs and the goals that are currently active. When a goal is active, other people in the social environment may be evaluated as they relate to the active goal: people who are "goal-congruent" (Lazarus, 1991) are evaluated more positively, while those who are "goal-incongruent" are evaluated more negatively. These evaluations depend on the information embedded in the links between the goal construct and the SO, such as the individual's beliefs about the SO's traits, skills, goals, or general helpfulness.

Furthermore, the nature of the association between the self and the SO is also likely to moderate the interpersonal effects of goal priming, just as it did in Shah's (2003) SO priming studies. For example, the nature and quality of the relationship between the self and the SO—relationship closeness, importance, or identification between the self and the SO—will likely be important in predicting the kinds of interpersonal effects that result from active goal states. Moreover, these effects will also be influenced by the nature of the relationship between the self and the particular goal pursuit, such as how committed individuals feel to achieving a goal and how important the goal is to their identity. The nature of the associations between the constructs may alter the kinds of behavioral and perceptual results of activating any other of these constructs, and will have an important effect both on self-regulation and on interpersonal relationships.

CONCLUSIONS

We have suggested that the way we construe and mentally represent our SOs can greatly impact our everyday behavior through their close association to various goals. Furthermore, just as with the effects of other cognitive associations, we hypothesize that these associative effects may occur without need for conscious guidance. These automatic effects may also occur in a bidirectional fashion that emphasizes the dynamic and complex relationship between SOs and the self's motives, needs, and desires. First, SOs (especially close ones) can trigger nonconsciously operating goals that subsequently guide perception and behavior. Second, active goal states—whether conscious or not—are likely to trigger associated SOs and affect the way individuals perceive and behave toward SOs. Through these bidirectional paths, goals and SOs can affect each other and elicit strong, important, and automatic effects on our perception and behavior, both inside and outside of the interpersonal domain.

There is one caveat that we must mention. For the sake of generating testable hypotheses in this initial version of our model, we have examined the effects of goal–SO associations as though they are independent routes through which SOs and goals affect each other. However, as Figure 5.1 suggests, various interrelations may exist between the mental representations of the self, the self's goals, and SOs, and these interactions will determine how any one element influences perception and behavior. Interactions among associations in the model may make it more or less likely that an SO will prime a given goal, or that a goal will affect interpersonal behavior. For example, if an individual is highly committed to a given goal *and* very close to a given SO who is linked to that goal, then the SO may have even stronger and more powerful effects on behavior. Thus, we hypothesize that these associations are interrelated and interdependent: they affect each other in a dynamic fashion, and they interact automatically to guide behavior.

As our initial focus on these associations as independent (rather than interdependent) demonstrates, this research is still very new, and there remain many issues to explore, questions to answer, and avenues for future research. We would like to mention a few such avenues here, as examples of the kind of work we believe would shed light on some of the complex relationships we are discussing. First, we'd like to examine how active goals influence real *relationship behavior* within friendships and romantic relationships. For example, we would like to study overt acts of trust and commitment, provision of social support, as well as accommodative behaviors in response to partner transgressions (Rusbult, Verett, Whitney, Slovik, & Lipkus, 1991). We suspect that these behaviors may also be influenced by the extent to which current friends or romantic partners are perceived as instrumental to goal progress. That is, partners who can help us with the goals that are currently important to us may receive some relationship benefits beyond being evaluated more positively. We may also be willing to accept more flaws, and give more back to our friends and partners, when they can help us with our goals.

Second, we are currently investigating the ways that active goals may change the way individuals categorize their social and interpersonal world. We hypothesize that SOs may be categorized according to their usefulness for our current goals, and thus be more "interchangeable" or "substitutable" to the extent that they are similar with regards to their instrumentality for the self's active goals. These categorizations would be likely to shift frequently, depending on the nature of the temporarily activated goals and motivations of the individual.

Finally, we are very interested in examining the effects of SOs on goal pursuit in real interpersonal interactions. In our studies, we have activated the representation of an SO and measured goal-directed behavior in what is otherwise an interpersonal vacuum. Of course, in natural interactions, both partners have goals, and we expect that the interdependence and interactions of the self's goals with the SO's goals will profoundly—and automatically—shape each partner's behavior.

Thus, we will continue to emphasize the role that significant others can play in automatically guiding goal pursuit, and the role that goals can play in determining the quality of interpersonal relationships. Overall, we aim to highlight the importance of significant others in the self-regulatory process. Contrary to Simon and Garfunkel's legendary claims, we believe that no man is an island—we are all strongly shaped by the significant others in our lives (and in our minds).

REFERENCES

Aarts, H., & Dijksterhuis, A. (2000). Habits as knowledge structures: Automaticity in goal-directed behavior. *Journal of Personality and Social Psychology, 78,* 53–63.

Allport, G. W. (1955). *Becoming: Basic considerations for a psychology of personality.* New York: Yale University Press.

Andersen, S. M., & Chen, S. (2002). The relational self: An interpersonal social-cognitive theory. *Psychological Review, 109,* 619–645.

Andersen, S. M., & Cole, S. W. (1990). "Do I know you?": The role of significant others in general social perception. *Journal of Personality and Social Psychology, 59,* 384–399.

Andersen, S. M., Reznik, I., & Manzella, L. M. (1996). Eliciting facial affect, motivation, and expectancies in transference: Significant-other representations in social relations. *Journal of Personality and Social Psychology, 71,* 1108–1129.

Anderson, J. R. (1974). Retrieval of propositional information from long-term memory. *Cognitive Psychology, 6,* 451–474.

Anderson, J. R. (1983). *The architecture of cognition.* Cambridge, MA: Harvard University Press.

Aron, A., Aron, E. N., Tudor, M., & Nelson, G. (1991). Close relationships as including other in the self. *Journal of Personality and Social Psychology, 60,* 241–253.

Atkins, C. J., Kaplan, R. M., & Toshima, M. T. (1991). Close relationships in the epidemiology of cardio-vascular disease. In W. H. Jones & D. Perlman (Eds.), *Advances in personal relationships* (Vol. 3, pp. 207–231). London: Jessica Kingsley.

Baldwin, M. W. (1992). Relational schemas and the processing of social information. *Psychological Bulletin, 112,* 461–484.

Baldwin, M. W. (1995). Relational schemas and cognition in close relationships. *Journal of Social and Personal Relationships, 12,* 547–552.

Baldwin, M. W., Carrell, S. E., & Lopez, D. F. (1990). Priming relationship schemas: My advisor and the pope are watching me from the back of my mind. *Journal of Experimental Social Psychology, 26,* 435–454.

Baldwin, M. W., & Holmes, J. G. (1987). Salient private audiences and awareness of the self. *Journal of Personality and Social Psychology, 52,* 1087–1098.

Bandura, A. (1986). *Social foundations of thought and action: A social-cognitive theory.* Englewood Cliffs, NJ: Prentice-Hall.

Bargh, J. A. (1990). Auto-motives: Preconscious determinants of social interaction. In E. T. Higgins & R. M. Sorrentino (Eds.), *Handbook of motivation and cognition: Foundations of social behavior* (Vol. 2, pp. 93–130). New York: Guilford Press.

Bargh, J. A., & Chartrand, T. L. (2000). The mind in the middle: A practical guide to priming and automaticity research. In H. T. Reis & C. M. Judd (Eds.), *Handbook of research methods in social and personality psychology* (pp. 253–285). New York: Cambridge University Press.

Bargh, J. A., Gollwitzer, P. M., Lee-Chai, A., Barndollar, K., & Trotschel, R. (2001). The automated will: Nonconscious activation and pursuit of behavioral goals. *Journal of Personality and Social Psychology, 81,* 1014–1027.

Berk, M. S., & Andersen, S. M. (2000). The impact of past relationships on interpersonal behavior: Behavioral confirmation in the social-cognitive process of transference. *Journal of Personality and Social Psychology, 79,* 546–562.

Berscheid, E. (1994). Interpersonal relationships. *Annual Review of Psychology, 45,* 79–129.

Brehm, S. S., & Brehm, J. W. (1981). *Psychological reactance: A theory of freedom and control.* New York: Academic Press.

Brewer, M. B., & Gardner, W. L. (1996). Who is this "we"?: Levels of collective identity and self representations. *Journal of Personality and Social Psychology, 71,* 83–93.

Bruner, J. S. (1957). Going beyond the information given. In H. Gulber (Ed.), *Contemporary approaches in cognition* (pp. 257–271). Cambridge, MA: Harvard University Press.

Bruner, J. S., & Postman, L. (1948). Symbolic value as an organizing factor in perception. *Journal of Social Psychology, 27,* 203–208.

Cantor, N., & Malley, J. (1991). Life tasks, personal needs, and close relationships. In G. J. O. Fletcher & F. D. Fincham (Eds.), *Cognition in close relationships* (pp. 101–125). Hillsdale, NJ: Erlbaum.

Carver, C. S., & Scheier, M. F. (1998). *On the self-regulation of behavior.* New York: Cambridge University Press.

Chartrand, T. L., & Bargh, J. A. (1996). Automatic activation of impression formation and memorization goals: Nonconscious goal priming reproduces effects of explicit task instructions. *Journal of Personality and Social Psychology, 71*(3), 464–478.

Chartrand, T. L., & Bargh, J. A. (2002). Nonconscious motivations: Their activation, operation, and consequences. In A. Tesser, D. A. Stapel, & J. V. Wood (Eds.), *Self and motivation: Emerging psychological perspectives* (pp. 13–41). Washington, DC: American Psychological Association.

Chartrand, T. L., Dalton, A., & Fitzsimons, G. J. (2004). *Evidence for automatic reactance: When controlling significant others automatically activate opposite goals.* Manuscript in preparation, Duke University.

Chen, S. (2001). The role of theories in mental representations and their use in social perception: A theory-based approach to significant-other representations and transference. In G. B. Moskowitz (Ed.), *Cognitive social psychology: The legacy and future of social cognition* (pp. 125–142). Mahwah, NJ: Erlbaum.

Clark, M. S., & Reis, H. T. (1988). Interpersonal processes in close relationships. *Annual Review of Psychology, 39,* 609–672.

Cohen, S. (1988). Psychosocial models of social support in the etiology of physical disease. *Health Psychology, 7,* 269–297.

Collins, N. L., & Read, S. J. (1994). Cognitive representations of attachment: The structure and function of working models. In K. Bartholomew (Ed.), *Attachment processes in adulthood* (pp. 53–90). Bristol, PA: Jessica Kingsley.

Cooley, C. H. (1964). *Human nature and the social order.* New York: Schocken Books. (Original work published 1902)

Deci, E. L., & Ryan, R. M. (1985). *Intrinsic motivation and self-determination in human behavior.* New York: Plenum Press.

Deci, E. L., & Ryan, R. M. (2000). The "what" and "why" of goal pursuits: Human needs and the self-determination of behavior. *Psychological Inquiry, 11,* 227–268.

Ferguson, M., & Bargh, J. A. (in press). Liking is for doing: The effect of goal pursuit on automatically activated attitudes. *Journal of Personality and Social Psychology.*

Fishbach, A., Friedman, R. S., & Kruglanski, A. W. (2003). Leading us not into temptation: Momentary allurements elicit overriding goal activation. *Journal of Personality and Social Psychology, 84*(2), 296–309.

Fitzsimons, G. M., & Bargh, J. A. (2003). Thinking of you: Nonconscious pursuit of interpersonal goals associated with relationship partners. *Journal of Personality and Social Psychology, 84(1), 148–163.*

Fitzsimons, G. M., & Shah, J. W. (2004). *Effects of active goals on interpersonal evaluations.* Manuscript in preparation.

Freud, A. (1937). *The ego and the mechanisms of defense.* New York: International Universities Press.

Glanz, K., & Lerman, C. (1992). Psychosocial impact of breast cancer: A critical review. *Annals of Behavioral Medicine, 14,* 204–212.

Glassman, N. S., & Andersen, S. M. (1999). Activating transference without consciousness: Using significant-other representations to go beyond subliminally given information. *Journal of Personality and Social Psychology, 77,* 1146–1162.

Gollwitzer, P. M., & Bargh, J. A. (1996). *The psychology of action: Linking motivation and cognition to behavior.* New York: Guilford Press.

Hamilton, D. L., Katz, L. B., & Leirer, V. O. (1980). Cognitive representation of personality impressions: Organizational processes in first impression formation. *Journal of Personality and Social Psychology, 39(1, Suppl. 6),* 1050–1063.

Hastie, R., & Kumar, P. A. (1979). Person memory: Personality traits as organizing principles in memory for behaviors. *Journal of Personality and Social Psychology, 37(1),* 25–38.

Hayes-Roth, B. (1977). Evolution of cognitive structures and processes. *Psychological Review, 84,* 260–278.

Hazan, C., & Shaver, P. (1987). Romantic love conceptualized as an attachment process. *Journal of Personality and Social Psychology, 52, 511–524.*

Higgins, E. T. (1996). Knowledge activation: Accessibility, applicability, and salience. In E. T. Higgins & A. W. Kruglanski (Eds.), *Social psychology: Handbook of basic principles* (pp. 133–168). New York: Guilford Press.

Higgins, E. T., King, G. A., & Mavin, G. H. (1982). Individual construct accessibility and subjective impressions and recall. *Journal of Personality and Social Psychology, 43(1),* 35–47.

Hinkley, K., & Andersen, S. M. (1996). The working self-concept in transference: Significant-other activation and self change. *Journal of Personality and Social Psychology, 71(6),* 1279–1295.

Holmes, J. G. (2000). Social relationships: The nature and function of relational schemas. *European Journal of Social Psychology, 30,* 447–495.

Hull, C. W. L. (1931). Goal attraction and directing ideas conceived as habit phenomena. *Psychological Review, 38,* 487–506.

Johnson, C. S., Chartrand, T. L., Norton, M. I., & Nelson, L. (2004). *Beyond inspiration: The effect of role models on performance.* Manuscript under review.

Johnson, D. J., & Rusbult, C. E. (1989). Resisting temptation: Devaluation of alternative partners as a means of maintaining commitment in close relationships. *Journal of Personality and Social Psychology, 57,* 967–980.

Jones, E. E., & Thibaut, J. W. (1958). Interaction goals as bases of inference in interpersonal perception. In R. Tagiuri & L. Petrullo (Eds.), *Person perception and interpersonal behavior* (pp. 151–178). Stanford, CA: Stanford University Press.

Kelly, G. A. (1955). *The psychology of personal constructs. Vol. 1: A theory of personality.* New York: Norton.

Kruglanski, A. W. (1996). Goals as knowledge structures. In P. M. Gollwitzer & J. A.

Bargh (Eds.), *The psychology of action: Linking cognition and motivation to behavior* (pp. 599–618). New York: Guilford Press.

Lazarus, R. S. (1991). *Emotion and adaptation.* New York: Oxford University Press.

MacLeod, C. M. (1991). Half a century of research on the Stroop effect: An integrative review. *Psychological Bulletin, 109,* 163–203.

Mead, G. H. (1934). *Mind, self, and society.* Chicago: University of Chicago Press.

Mikulincer, M. (1998). Adult attachment style and affect regulation: Strategic variations in self-appraisals. *Journal of Personality and Social Psychology, 75,* 420–435.

Miller, L. C., & Read, S. J. (1991). On the coherence of mental models of persons and relationships: A knowledge structure approach. In G. J. O Fletcher & F. D. Fincham (Eds.), *Cognition in close relationships* (pp. 69–100). Hillsdale, NJ: Erlbaum.

Moors, A., De Houwer, J., & Eelen, P. (2004). Automatic stimulus-goal comparisons: Support from motivational affective priming studies. *Cognition and Emotion, 18,* 29–54.

Moretti, M. M., & Higgins, E. (1999). Internal representations of others in self-regulation: A new look at a classic issue. *Social Cognition, 17,* 186–208.

Moskowitz, G. B., Gollwitzer, P. M., Wasel, W., & Schaal, B. (1999). Preconscious control of stereotype activation through chronic egalitarian goals. *Journal of Personality and Social Psychology, 77,* 167–184.

Murray, S. L., & Holmes, J. G. (1997). A leap of faith?: Positive illusions in romantic relationships. *Personality and Social Psychology Bulletin, 23,* 586–604.

Park, B. (1986). A method for studying the development of impressions of real people. *Journal of Personality and Social Psychology, 51,* 907–917.

Planalp, S. (1987). Interplay between relational knowledge and events. In R. Burnett & P. McGhee (Eds.), *Accounting for relationships: Explanation, representation and knowledge* (pp. 175–191). New York: Methuen.

Read, S. J., & Miller, L. C. (1989). Inter-personalism: Toward a goal-based theory of persons in relationships. In L. A. Pervin (Ed.), *Goal concepts in personality and social psychology* (pp. 413–472). Hillsdale, NJ: Erlbaum.

Rom, E., & Mikulincer, M. (2003). Attachment theory and group processes: The association between attachment style and group-related representations, goals, memories, and functioning. *Journal of Personality and Social Psychology, 84,* 1220–1235.

Rusbult, C. E., Verette, J., Whitney, G. A., Slovik, L. F., & Lipkus, I. (1991). Accommodation processes in close relationships: Theory and preliminary empirical evidence. *Journal of Personality and Social Psychology, 60,* 53–78.

Ryan, R. M., & Deci, E. L. (2000). Intrinsic and extrinsic motivations: Classic definitions and new directions. *Contemporary Educational Psychology, 25,* 54–67.

Schaffer, R. (1968). *Aspects of internalization.* New York: International Universities Press.

Shah, J. Y. (2003). Automatic for the people: How representations of significant others implicitly affect goal pursuit. *Journal of Personality and Social Psychology, 84*(4), 661–681.

Shah, J. Y., Friedman, R., & Kruglanski, A. W. (2003). Forgetting all else: On the antecedents and consequences of goal shielding. *Journal of Personality and Social Psychology, 83*(6), 1261–1280.

Shah, J. Y., & Gardner, W. (in press). *Handbook of Motivation Science*. New York: Guilford Press.

Shah, J. Y., & Kruglanski, A. W. (2002). Priming against your will: How goal pursuit is affected by accessible alternatives. *Journal of Experimental Social Psychology, 38*, 368–383.

Shah, J. Y., & Kruglanski, A. W. (2003). When opportunity knocks: Bottom-up priming of goals by means and its effects on self-regulation. *Journal of Personality and Social Psychology, 84*(6), 1109–1122.

Shah, J. Y., Kruglanski, A. W., & Friedman, R. (2002). A goal systems approach to self-regulation. In M. P. Zanna, J. M. Olson, & C. Seligman (Eds.), *The Ontario Symposium on Personality and Social Psychology* (pp. 247–276). Hillsdale, NJ: Erlbaum.

Shaver, P. R., & Mikulincer, M. (2002). The psychodynamics of social judgments: An attachment theory perspective. In J. P. Forgas, K. D. Williams, & W. von Hippel (Eds.), *Responding to the social world: Implicit and explicit processes in social judgments and decisions* (pp. 85–114). London: Cambridge University Press.

Smith, C. A., & Lazarus, R. S. (1990). Emotion and adaptation. In L. A. Pervin (Ed.), *Handbook of personality theory and research* (pp. 609–637). New York: Guilford Press.

Srull, T. K., & Wyer, R. S. (1979). The role of category accessibility in the interpretation of information about persons: Some determinants and implications. *Journal of Personality and Social Psychology, 37*, 1660–1672.

Trzebinski, J. (1989). The role of goal categories in the representation of social knowledge. In L. A. Pervin (Ed.), *Goal concepts in personality and social psychology* (pp. 363–411). Hillsdale, NJ: Erlbaum.

Vohs, K. D., & Finkel, E. J. (Eds.). (in press). *Intrapersonal processes and interpersonal relationships*. New York: Guilford Press.

6

Commitment Calibration with the Relationship Cognition Toolbox

JOHN E. LYDON, KIMBERLY BURTON,
and DANIELLE MENZIES-TOMAN

In Canada and the United States it is much easier to obtain a divorce today than it was 50 years ago. An implicit assumption in easing the constraints on marriage was that people would remain in marriages that were highly satisfying and leave ones that were less so. Moreover, a social concern about relaxing divorce laws was that people would terminate relationships at the first sign of distress or even boredom. Yet, as social psychologists could have predicted, we now know that some people stay in chronically dissatisfying relationships and that not everyone terminates a relationship as soon as he or she experiences a drop in satisfaction. Conversely, it appears that some people in rewarding relationships nevertheless end their relationships. The explanation for this, of course, is psychological commitment.

Commitment is the motivation to maintain and sustain a relationship even in the face of adversity. For some time now researchers have recognized the inextricable link between motivation and cognition (Sorrentino & Higgins, 1986; Kunda, 1990). Consequently, in this chapter, we focus on how commitment promotes relationship survival and devote special attention to commitment's motivational effects on perception and cognition. First, we review the four theoretical foundations of our work. Then we describe why, when, and how commitment promotes relationship survival. Finally, we discuss important theoretical issues to be addressed with couple data and examine the developmental trajectories of commitment in close relationships. Although thoroughly interpersonal in our attention to the ways in which relationship commitment motivates relationship-maintaining perceptions and cognitions, we outline a theoretical framework that has identification at its origin. Identity and commitment provide a nexus between the self and the interpersonal world. We argue that (1) much of motivated interpersonal cognition depends upon the calibration of commitment and relationship threats, and that (2) commitment develops from the process of identification.

THEORETICAL FOUNDATIONS

Theoretical developments in the psychology of commitment in the 1980s were inspired by the ideas that relationship survival was an important outcome of study for social scientists, and that psychological processes were likely implicated in the survival rates. Those from a sociological tradition point out that married couples stay together more than couples who are living together (Bumpass, Martin, & Sweet, 1991), perhaps because, from a structural perspective, marriage is more difficult to end than is living together. Relationship commitment researchers have conceptualized this in terms of the external constraints on leaving (Johnson, 1991) or of barriers to ending the relationship (Lund, 1985). A psychological analysis of the "marriage effect" also considers the publicness of the act. Marriage is a public pledge that binds one to the promises and vows of the wedding ceremony (Kiesler, 1971). An internal attitude (vow) is strengthened by its public expression.

Extending the marriage effect was the finding that couples with children are more likely to stay together than those without children. Again, the research identified a descriptive feature of a relationship that implied a psychological process leading to relationship survival. The ability of a measure of psychological commitment (rather than a structural proxy for it) to predict relationship survival was most striking in the 15-year follow-up to the Boston Couples Study (Bui, Peplau, & Hill, 1996). Commitment was operationalized in terms of intent to marry and three items from the attachment subscale of Rubin's (1970) Love Scale. Participants' level of commitment, assessed while they were dating, accounted for 21% of the variance in who remained together 15 years later.

In social psychology, at least four theoretical contributions to psychological commitment in the 1980s played a role in the development of the theoretical framework we present in this chapter. First, Kelley (1983) was concerned with the overlap between love and commitment. He theorized that although there should be significant overlap between the constructs, they are nevertheless distinct (Fehr, 1988). Moreover, he believed that one way to ascertain commitment was via a stress test, similar to the strain test for a bridge. This notion has been a core element of our program of research for the past 12 years because we theorize that acute challenges to love and satisfaction provide a test of commitment.

Kelley's general formulation for commitment was to examine the mean difference between rewards and costs, relative to the variance in this difference. Thus, the volatility in the reward–cost differential is critical to commitment (Arriaga, 2001). Similar to the findings of research on subjective well-being (e.g., Diener, Sandvik, & Pavot, 1990), a person should be more committed to a relationship that is consistently above midpoint than to a relationship with lots of highs and lows because there would be less variability in the reward–cost differential in the former case than in the latter.

Brickman (1987) conceptualized commitment in nonhedonic terms. For Brickman, commitment is a rationalizing process, not a rational one. It is rooted in the values and meaning a person ascribes to a relationship. Others have conceptualized this in terms of identity (Burke & Reitzes, 1991) and self-definition (Gollwitzer & Wicklund, 1985). Like Kelley, Brickman recognized the importance of costs, or negative elements. However, instead of taking an attributional approach and seeing costs as a way to reveal commitment, Brickman, coming from a dissonance tradition, believed that costs are integrated through a Hegelian dialectical synthesis of positive and negative forces. Consistent with this idea, Murray and Holmes (1993) found that people could turn their partners' faults into virtues.

Whereas Brickman proposed a broad conceptualization of commitment to life goals in general, Michael Johnson developed (1973) and refined (1991) a framework for understanding commitment to close relationships in particular. Drawing on both sociological and psychological perspectives, Johnson first proposed a distinction between "personal commitment" and "structural commitment." Personal commitment is a satisfaction-based commitment emphasizing choice and volition, whereas structural commitment reflects external constraints on leaving a relationship. Johnson subsequently expanded on this framework by adding a third type of commitment, moral commitment, which reflects internal constraints on leaving a relationship because one values (1) continuity in general, (2) continuity in the context of romantic relationships, or, more particularly, (3) continuity in the context of the romantic relationship with a specific other.

Concurrent with the development of Johnson's theoretical framework for studying commitment to close relationships was the investment model derived from interdependence theory. Whereas Thibaut and Kelley (1959) had theorized about the roles of expectations (comparison level) and quality of alternatives (comparison level for alternatives) in interpersonal relationships, Rusbult (1980) added the idea of "investment." Other more

Using the Inclusion of Other in the Self Scale (IOS; Aron, Aron, &
Smollan, 1992) to assess identification and the six-item Assessment of Relationship Commitment (ARC), we repeatedly find correlations between
.50 and .65. Consistent with our theoretical framework, the meaning of
the relationship also correlates with identification and commitment. People
identify with relationships that are a source of meaning in their lives and,
in turn, they commit to these relationships.

Interestingly, in this line of research, we found that deliberating about
relationship goals correlates negatively and highly with identification and
commitment, suggesting that a lack of commitment to specific relationship
goals (e.g., whether to travel together to Europe for the summer) is reflected in a lack of identification and commitment to the relationship in
general. Finally, avoidance of attachment within the specific relationship
(but not avoidance in general) also correlated highly and negatively with
identification and commitment, suggesting that relationship-specific avoidance may represent a degree of disidentification in close relationships.

To examine the process of identification per se, we have drawn on
theory and research about self-determination. Ryan and Deci (2000) posit
that motivation is not simply an extrinsic–intrinsic dichotomy but instead
a continuum from external regulations for behavior to increasingly internalized regulations. Whereas an introjected regulation is characterized by
guilt, an identified regulation signifies that one considers the goal or behavior to be personally important. In an initial attempt to examine these
motives and commitment, we adapted a measure of identified and introjected regulations to the study of caregivers of those with Alzheimer's disease. The correlations between each type of regulation and moral commitment were similar, although only the correlation with identified regulation
attained statistical significance. This suggests that moral commitment, at
least with the unique sample of chronically stressed caregivers, has elements of both motivations. However, it was identified regulation that correlated with subjective well-being and benign appraisals of threatening
caregiver scenarios. Moreover, links between identification and both threat
appraisals and well-being were mediated by commitment.

One of the challenges in examining identification and close relationships is that there appear to be gender differences in identification.
Whereas women's self-construals are oriented toward their relationships
with others, men's self-construals are more individualistic (Cross & Madson, 1997). Consequently, women identify with relationships across their
social network, incorporating these into their self-concept. Men, in contrast, do not identify with such relationships by default. The process of
identification still operates for men, but it is more specific to certain relationships than to others.

An implication of this gender difference is that women, at the outset
of a relationship, would identify with the relationship and therefore should

be motivated to exhibit commitment-related cognitions and behaviors. Men should not exhibit such thoughts and actions until they have identified with, and committed to, the particular relationship. This idea may account for a disparate set of gender differences in commitment. For example, women who are moderately committed were found to devalue an attractive alternative, but generally only men high in commitment devalued the attractive alternative (Lydon, Meana, Sepinwall, Richards, & Mayman, 1999). Similarly, women in dating relationships showed relationship illusions by rating their partner more positively than the partner rated himself, but only married men showed the same type of relationship illusions (Murray, Holmes, & Griffin, 1996a, 1996b).

As a test of this idea, Gagné and Lydon (2003) examined the relationship illusions of dating couples. Two studies sought to replicate the gender differences found by Murray and her colleagues (1996a, 1996b). Moreover, the reasoning was that men would show relationship illusions if they identified with the relationship and were also committed to it. In the first study, men's commitment level moderated their illusions such that men low in commitment actually rated their partners less positively than the partners rated themselves, but men high in commitment showed the reverse.[2] In the second study, identification was assessed using the IOS. Here again, identification also moderated men's illusions. Moreover, commitment mediated the identification–illusions relation. Men who identified with the relationship, incorporating it into their sense of self, were more committed, and consequently showed greater relationship illusions.

Although identification suggests a somewhat positive and self-determined motivational basis for commitment, the notions of avoidant commitment (Frank & Brandstätter, 2002), barriers (Levinger, 1976; Lund, 1985), and structural commitment (Johnson, 1991) suggest less self-determined bases for commitment. The work of Frank and Brandstätter (2002) is particularly interesting because the authors examined approach and avoidance commitment for predicting changes in relationship satisfaction, personal well-being, and relationship survival. *Approach commitment* was based on intrinsic and identified motives and was conceptualized as having a promotion focus; approach commitment was positively associated with changes in relationship satisfaction and personal well-being. *Avoidance commitment* was based on identified and relatively less self-determined introjected motives, and it was conceptualized as having a prevention focus. This type of commitment was associated with relationship duration. As goal researchers attest, introjected motives can promote persistence, but persistence may belie important cognitive and affective effects of being externally regulated in one's behavior.

We have begun some fine-grained analyses of the motivational bases of commitment (Menzies-Toman & Lydon, 2005) in an effort to identify distinct relationship signatures of cognitive–affective units and behavior (see

Mischel & Shoda, 1999). We created measures of intrinsic, identified, and introjected motives for being in a close relationship. For example, intrinsic motivation was assessed via endorsement of the statement "I am in my relationship because my partner and I have fun together," identified motivation via the statement " . . . because my partner and I share the same attitudes and values," and introjected motivation via the statement " . . . because I would feel guilty if I broke up with my partner." In an Internet survey of approximately 500 participants, we found that both intrinsic and identified motives correlated .50 with our relationship commitment scale but introjected motives did not. However, as we and Johnson would expect, introjected motives were higher among married people than among those dating or living together. Thus, introjection is associated with externally based, structural commitment. In contrast, intrinsic motives were highest among daters. Interestingly, the level of identified motives was consistent across relationship groups. Moreover, identification was the only motivation measure with a direct link to perspective taking. That is, the ability to take the perspective of one's partner is a distinguishing feature of identification.

In sum, we propose that various bases of commitment can be organized in terms of the process of identification. Meaning captures identification with the relationship and interdependence captures identification with the specific individual other. The interplay of self and interpersonal cognitions contribute to the identification process that serves as a platform for commitment.

MOTIVATED INTERPERSONAL COGNITION

A great deal of research in social psychology has documented the motivational nature of interpersonal perception and cognition. This has received considerable attention in the area of close relationships in the past 20 years. Early work emphasized that the overall positive tone of a relationship (i.e., relationship satisfaction) could guide attributions for partner behavior (Bradbury & Fincham, 1990). This was in keeping with Holmes's (1981) idea that overarching macromotives guide relationship processes in a top-down fashion. Subsequently, Fletcher and Fincham (1991) delineated cognitive processes that might link partner A's behavior to partner B's experience and understanding of the behavior.

Critical contributions by commitment researchers specified relationship-maintaining and relationship-protecting cognitions and linked these to measures of relationship commitment (Rusbult & Buunk, 1993). Incorporating commitment into the theoretical and empirical mix highlighted the motivational underpinnings of such processes as idealization and relationship illusions. At the same time, the biased cognitions provided some explanation for why commitment might lead to relationship survival.

CALIBRATING COMMITMENT AND ADVERSITY

Our point is that, although commitment may motivate positive relationship thoughts and behaviors under normal circumstances, commitment most likely motivates responses under adverse circumstances, that is, when something is happening that threatens relationship survival. If identification is the critical latent variable driving commitment, adversity may be the critical diagnostic tool for testing commitment. Motivated interpersonal cognition should be elicited when commitment levels are calibrated appropriately with levels of adversity.

It seems that all theoretical approaches to commitment have to deal with the issue of adversity, or costs. The investment model specifies that costs should be negatively associated with satisfaction, and consequently negatively associated with commitment. As we outlined earlier in describing Brickman's ideas, those from a dissonance tradition consider costs as positively associated with commitment. As costs increase, commitment increases in order to justify and redeem the initial decision to pursue the relationship. Finally, Kelley (1983), from an attributional perspective, theorized that costs allow the actor and the observers to infer commitment with greater confidence than possible when costs are low and satisfaction is high.

Our program of research started with the Kelley perspective and used adversity as a stress test for commitment (Lydon & Zanna, 1990). In addition to correlational and longitudinal evidence of this, we found in an experimental analogue that students were more willing to attend an 8:00 A.M. experiment that was relevant to their values than one that was irrelevant to their values, but that the differences were obscured when the participant could come at any convenient time of the day. This pattern of findings is suggestive of a prevention focus (Shah & Higgins, 1997) whereby people maintain their commitment even when expectancies are low (adversity is high) because the goal has high value.

If our idea of a stress test is correct, then well-known relationship biases should be associated with commitment, especially under conditions of threat. Consider studies of relationship illusions and the "perceived superiority effect." In one study of university students, the suggestion that one's relationship was unlikely to last prompted committed participants to report more positive, relative to negative, features of their relationships and their partners compared to control and accuracy conditions (Rusbult, Van Lange, Wildschut, Yovetich, & Verette, 2000). We found that simply prompting people to deliberate about a relationship goal (Gagné & Lydon, 2001) produced the same sort of effect. Highly committed participants responded to deliberation by further exaggerating the superiority of their partners compared to controls, whereas those low in commitment did not. It should be noted that everyone (all 100 participants) believed that their partners were better than the average dating partner of their peers. The threat of deliberating about a "yet to be resolved" relationship goal heightened this effect for those committed to the relationship. These findings underscore the motivational quality of the processes studied. Because people are committed to their relationships, they are prepared to defend them. Threats necessitate such defenses.

Of course, adversity is on as much of a continuum as commitment. This led us to theorize that relationship maintenance involves a delicate calibration between adversity and commitment. Obviously, if adversity exceeds commitment, then the adversity should overwhelm the relationship and lead to maladaptive relationship behaviors and the ultimate demise of the relationship. Less obvious, we reasoned that if commitment exceeds adversity, then there should not be an activation of relationship maintenance responses because there is not sufficient threat. This is consistent with the ideas of energy mobilization (Wright & Brehm, 1989) and optimal functioning (Csikszentmihalyi & Csikszentmihalyi, 1988). For example, in the workplace, if the level of challenge is lower than one's skill level, then those skills are unlikely to be elicited.

With student populations, one of the most salient threats is the availability of an attractive alternative relationship partner. All major theories of relationship commitment specify the availability of attractive alternatives as a key variable associated with commitment (Johnson, 1991; Levinger, 1976; Rusbult, 1991), with the idea being that the availability of alternatives should undermine commitment. However, Kelley (1983) understood that people act on their environments, and he theorized that one should respond to attractive alternatives by dismissing either their availability or their attractiveness.

Kelley's theorizing led to a set of studies on the devaluation of alternatives, or the tendency to rate attractive alternative relationship partners as less attractive. For example, Johnson and Rusbult (1989) obtained a negative linear relationship between participants' commitment level and their ratings of a highly attractive alternative. Those who were more committed to their relationships rated the attractive target as less attractive. This effect was not obtained for the targets who were rated low or moderate in attractiveness.

Because of the negative linear relation obtained, the assumption in the literature was that the more committed someone is to his or her relationship, the greater the devaluation. Lydon et al. (1999) theorized that the commitment–devaluation relation was more complex and belied a broader issue about when people defend their relationships. For Lydon and his colleagues, the "devaluation effect" was a great context in which to test the idea of calibration. In reexamining the original devaluation effect, they sought to prove that potentially important differences between dating and marriage were being overlooked. They theorized that as a group, those highly committed to their dating relationships may be best cast as moderately committed when compared to married people, who report similar high levels of commitment on a commitment scale. Using the same logic, those married but low on a commitment scale were conceptualized as moderately committed. The framework, then, was to cross a commitment measure (low–high) with an individual's marital status (married–unmarried) to create three levels of commitment.

Given the calibration idea, the original paradigm was thought to have created a moderate level of threat. In theory, then, those who are highly committed should not be threatened and therefore should not devalue when simply presented with the file of an attractive, available "participant." However, if the level of threat could be increased, then highly committed married participants should devalue the appeal of the alternative and moderately committed participants should cease devaluation. This theory was tested by creating a paradigm to supposedly test the validity of computer matching compared to when people decide for themselves. Participants completed surveys and had their pictures taken, and then returned a couple of weeks later to review the file of someone else in the study. The file folder always included the same biography and the same picture. Threat was experimentally manipulated by leading half of the participants to believe that the attractive and romantically available person had selected them. In other words, participants were now reviewing and rating an attractive person who was attracted to them (high threat). Consistent with the hypothesis, the only participants to devalue the target, compared to baseline ratings by single participants, were those moderately committed who were in the moderate threat condition and those highly committed in the high threat condition.

Subsequent research (Lydon, Fitzsimons, & Naidoo, 2003) created a low threat condition by having participants rate how they believed a friend would rate the target. Single and low commitment participants rated the attractive available relationship partner as equally attractive under low and moderate threat conditions. However, committed daters rated the target as less attractive in the moderate condition. In other words, it was okay to say that one's friend (even a friend in a dating relationship) would rate the person as highly attractive, but it was not okay for participants themselves to say that they found the person to be attractive. Note too that these effects were obtained for strong evaluative and threatening statements about the romantic appeal of the partner, not simply the physical attractiveness of the partner. It is less threatening to say that someone is attractive than to connect the dots and say explicitly that the person would be an appealing dating partner.

Of course, as Kelley mentioned, another way to deal with the threat of an attractive alternative is to simply avoid the alternative. We examined a generalized tendency to ward off attractive alternatives by using a virtual reality paradigm (Burton, Lydon, & Bell, 2000). Participants were presented with four images to manipulate in virtual reality, including a picture of a model of their preferred sex. The original finding was that those in relationships (dating and married) avoided the attractive target, whereas single participants did not, and that measures of duty and obligation predicted the degree of avoidance (Bell & Lydon, 1997). In subsequent research we found that reminding people, particularly women, of their relationship attitudes (commitment, attachment, enthusiasm toward the relationship) is critical to eliciting avoidance. Again, gender makes a difference in a certain way, suggesting that when calibrating adversity and commitment, one would be advised to consider the potential of gender in the process. Women in some relationship adversity situations may be more equipped with relationship-maintaining tools than men.

PERCEPTUAL AND COGNITIVE MEDIATORS

So what are some of the commitment-motivated perceptual, cognitive, and behavioral tools available and utilized in response to relationship adversities? Early research first sought to identify behaviors that would help explain why commitment leads to relationship survival. For example, accommodation refers to the willingness to tolerate a partner's transgression by either engaging the issue constructively (voice) or loyally enduring it (loyalty) rather than by exhibiting more negative responses of exit or neglect. In 1991, Rusbult, Verette, Whitney, Slovik, and Lipkus found commitment to be associated with accommodation. Recently, in her dissertation research, Kimberly Burton found that by simply making salient one's relationship, a woman will increase her willingness to accommodate. Those who reported their relationship attitudes prior to an assessment of accommodation reported greater willingness to accommodate their partners' transgressions than those who reported their relationship attitudes after the assessment of accommodation. The Burton paradigm has been used to show the same effect on attributions for a partner's negative behavior. Originally, this process was thought to be driven by relationship satisfaction, in that studies showed that individuals who were happy in their relationships made more benign attributions for their partner's bad behavior than those who were unhappy in their relationships (Bradbury & Fincham, 1990). However, early studies on attributions in relationships did not examine relational identity or commitment. In our research, all that was necessary to activate women's relational identities was to ask them a few factual questions about their relationships. Subsequently, when they completed the Relationship Attributions Measure (Fincham & Bradbury, 1992), they reported more benevolent attributions for their partners' negative behaviors than did those in the control condition (Burton & Lydon,

2004). Additional research suggests that this effect is tied to relational identities. Women with highly relational (interdependent) self-construals were influenced by the relationship activation manipulation, whereas those low in relational interdependence were not. It seems that the more a relationship is tied to one's self-concept and identity, the more likely it is that the person will engage in benevolent attributions.

Whereas attributions involve the interpretation of a partner's bad behavior, our research suggests an even more immediate, proximal relationship defense (Menzies-Toman & Lydon, in press). We had participants write a few sentences about a transgression committed by their romantic partner. The instructions were to simply give the facts. Participants' level of commitment was assessed prior to the writing of the paragraphs. Participants rated the severity of the transgressions and later, blind to these ratings and participants' commitment levels, research assistants made their own ratings of the severity of the transgressions. Results revealed that there were no differences in the objective ratings of transgression severity as a function of commitment level. Those highly committed wrote about transgressions as severe as those relatively low in commitment. However, commitment level predicted the discrepancy between objective ratings and subjective ratings such that highly committed participants perceived the transgression as less severe.

Across these various studies, a picture emerges of a number of lines of defense in response to a partner transgression. There is some evidence to suggest that more than one of these tools may be used in response to the relationship adversity (Finkel, Rusbult, Kumashiro, & Hannon, 2002). However, our research suggests that the selection of specific tools and the number of tools used may again be a matter of calibration. We found that the objective level of severity of a transgression interacted with the commitment-perceptual dampening effect. For transgressions particularly high in objective severity, even those committed to the relationship could not deny the severity. However, those committed were, at that point, more prepared to accommodate the transgression than their less-committed counterparts. Thus, when the more immediate perceptual line of defense failed in the face of transgressions that were objectively high in severity, committed individuals were able to utilize a second line of defense to dampen the potential harm to the relationship.

Despite the limits of perceptual bias in response to partner transgressions, one should not underestimate the power of commitment-motivated appraisals across a range of relationship adversities. Our first foray into the appraisal process was with our sample of individuals in long-distance dating relationships. In that study, those most committed to their relationship increased their appraisals of investments over time. This was also found in another longitudinal study of dating relationships (Agnew, Van Lange, Rusbult, & Langston, 1998). When relationship costs are seen as investments, they may appear to be less negative and instead be thought of as worthwhile and simply part of the price to pay for obtaining something of value. In the long-distance dating study, while those who were committed to their relationships increased their appraisals of investment, they simultaneously increased their appraisals of meaning. By ascribing more meaning to the relationship, they increased its value, thereby making the incurring of costs a more worthwhile investment.

Relatedly, it appears that commitment is associated with benign appraisals of stressors. In the study of family members caring for a loved one diagnosed with Alzheimer's disease, those high in moral commitment appraised difficult prototypical caregiving scenarios as challenges more than as threats (Pierce, Lydon, & Yang, 2001). Moreover, those high in moral commitment exhibited greater persistence in the caregiving role. Thus, the appraisal of stressors as challenges rather than threats may have helped sustain these caregivers.[3]

In both the long-distance dating study and the caregivers study, committed individuals were faced with naturally occurring relationship adversities. In the laboratory, as mentioned above, one way to operationalize relationship adversity is with the presence of an attractive alternative relationship partner. Interestingly, in this context, we have also found evidence of commitment motivating a way of thinking in addition to more evaluative or behavioral responses to the relationship threat. The paradigm to create threat involved participants in dating relationships having 5-minute interactions in the waiting room with an ostensible other research participant, who happened to be attractive, single, and of the opposite sex. In the control condition, the confederate was unavailable.

In one of our studies using this paradigm, we found evidence for a type of relational thinking elicited by relational threats (Burton, Lydon, & Bauer, 2003). Relationship commitment was assessed approximately 10 days prior to the lab session as part of a general social survey. At the lab session, after the time with the confederate, participants completed some questionnaires and then were presented with a picture of a park scene with two people in the distance who might be walking along together. Participants' written descriptions of the photograph were later independently coded for relational thinking. A significant interaction between gender and threat condition was obtained. For women, commitment level correlated with relational thinking in the high threat condition but not in the low threat condition, whereas for men, commitment level did not correlate with relational thinking in either condition. These results are consistent with the notion of cognitive interdependence, suggesting that commitment may motivate at least women to reaffirm the "we-ness" of their relationship when threatened.

The motivation to quell the threat of an attractive alternative is so great that it can even at times, for some people, trump the fundamental attribution error. Participants received positive feedback from an attractive single confederate and were lead to believe that the person provided the feedback freely or was constrained by the experimenter to provide positive feedback. Previous research showed that people ignore constraint information about positive feedback and infer that the judgment reflects the confederate's true feelings. Khan, Gagné, Lydon, and To (2004) found that people committed to their dating relationships defended against this positive feedback in one of two ways. Dating individuals low in self-esteem discounted the positive feedback, whereas single people low in self-esteem did not. However, dating individuals high in self-esteem, who did not discount the feedback, subsequently devalued the alternative. That is, people in dating relationships sought to reduce the threat of receiving positive feedback from an attractive single person, but depending on their level of self-esteem they utilized different strategies to accomplish their relationship maintenance goal. These results underscore the fact that, unlike the typical closed situation in an experiment with only one relationship maintenance response available, in the real world people may avail themselves of one of a variety of strategies from the relationship cognition toolbox depending upon the exigencies of the current situation interacting with chronic personal and interpersonal tendencies.

EXPLICIT AND IMPLICIT PROCESSES

Almost all commitment research relies on either self-report scales or relationship status to operationalize commitment. In theory, motivational constructs should conform to social cognitive principles, and therefore commitment should vary in its chronic accessibility and its contextual activation. Yet, on the face of it, commitment appears to be a highly controlled process. It is a matter of inhibiting hedonic self-interest. Thus, commitment may motivate behaviors to respond to explicit threats but may be less effective in response to implicit threats. And yet it would seem that when people are tired or caught unaware they are most vulnerable and most in need of relationship protective strategies. It would seem important, then, that commitment develop to the point at which it could operate implicitly for some people, in at least some situations. As important as this may be both for theoretical and applied reasons, it has been a challenge to researchers to demonstrate whether and when commitment operates implicitly.

We found some evidence for this in our first study of avoiding attractive alternatives in virtual reality. As reported earlier, people in relationships pushed the attractive model away. However, in a second phase of the study, participants also explored four rooms that flashed images in random places along the back wall of each room. Two of the rooms included flashing images of the attractive model. After exploring the four rooms, the participants were presented with a balloon on a table. Their task was to lift the balloon from the table and carry it into any one of the four rooms. In contrast to their behavior minutes earlier of pushing the image of the attractive model away, those in relationships actually carried the balloon to one of the rooms with the model rather than to either of the two control rooms.

It may be that commitment is more effective in responding to explicit conscious threats and less so in responding to implicit threats. Alternatively, it may be that commitment is subject to ego-depletion effects (Baumeister, Bratslavsky, Muraven, & Tice, 1998). After exerting relationship regulatory strength by pushing the image away, participants may have become more vulnerable to the stealth effects of the implicit presentation of the attractive models.

The ability to defend the relationship when ego-depleted may depend upon one's implicit commitment and not just on explicit commitment. In an initial investigation of this theory (Burton, Lydon, & Patall, 2003), we manipulated ego depletion following a procedure used by Baumeister and colleagues (1998; see also Finkel & Campbell, 2001) whereby participants in romantic relationships suppress their emotional reactions to funny and sad films while those in the control condition express their emotional reactions to these films. Prior to this task, an effort was made to assess implicit relationship commitment and satisfaction. Participants answered a series of 12 trivia questions (e.g., "What is your favorite ice cream?" "Name a province in Canada that begins with the letter *A*"). The 11th question asked participants the name of their romantic partner. This was designed to activate participants' mental representations of their romantic relationship prior to a lexical decision task. Participants were exposed to a series of 48 words and nonword letter strings on a computer screen and were instructed to respond as quickly as possible as to whether the letter string was a word or a nonword. Among the words were eight words associated with commitment (e.g., *loyalty*) and eight words associated with satisfaction (e.g., *happy*). Response latencies to these words (controlling for response times to neutral words) were used as measures of implicit commitment and satisfaction to predict accommodation.

The measure of implicit satisfaction predicted accommodation under ego depletion and it did so independent of a premeasure of relationship satisfaction. Unfortunately, the measure of implicit commitment did not predict accommodation. The preliminary results for implicit satisfaction are open to some alternative interpretations. Although we tried to activate a mental representation of the romantic relationship by asking the name of the romantic partner, we do not know if we were successful. If we were not, then our measure of relationship satisfaction may merely have been a measure of implicit mood or self-esteem.

The alternative explanation for the satisfaction measure, along with the null findings for commitment, point to one of the difficulties in assessing implicit commitment. Response latencies to commitment words are not meaningful if not assessed in the context of the romantic relationship. Even then, the way the relationship is brought to mind may matter. Consider a study in which we had participants report on a transgression committed by their partner. The severity of the transgressions was coded and results revealed that they correlated with subsequent response latencies to commitment words. But what does the response latency measure represent? It may be that one's own implicit commitment influenced the elicitation of transgressions. Alternatively, the response latencies may be less a measure of one's own commitment and instead a measure of perceived partner commitment. The person who can only think of a rather trivial transgression by the partner might then more quickly and easily think of commitment than the person who recalled a serious transgression by the partner.

To address this issue, we conducted another study in which we primed either "I," "he," or "she" (opposite sex to heterosexual research participants), or "it." These primes were presented in conjunction with a lexical decision task including commitment words. We also manipulated whether the lexical decision task was performed before or after recalling and describing a transgression, although appraisals of transgressions always were done last. The finding was that when the lexical decision task was first, the accessibility of commitment words when paired with "I" predicted objective ratings (made by trained coders) of the severity of the subsequent transgression reported. When primed with "he," "she" or "it," reaction times to commitment words were not associated with objective ratings of the severity of the transgressions. Essentially, the chronic accessibility of one's own commitment predicted the objective severity of the transgression recalled. However, when the lexical decision task came second, reaction times in the "I" condition predicted biased appraisals. That is, the extent to which thinking of a transgression activated one's own commitment led to dampened appraisals of the severity of the transgression (own ratings, controlling for objective ratings). In addition to these basic findings, this research is exciting in the potential it offers for research on commitment accessibility and activation.

Another promising approach has recently been taken by Etcheverry and Le (2003). They presented participants with sentence stems from a commitment scale, leaving off the final word—for example, the statement "Imagining myself with my partner in the distant future is . . . ," Followed by a pause and the appearance of either the word "hard" or the word "easy." The statement would appear twice—once paired with "hard" and the other with "easy." Fourteen sentence stems with two alternatives each created a measure of commitment accessibility based on 28 response latencies. The 28 statements were interspersed with 30 additional filler statements.

Etcheverry and Le found that this measure of commitment accessibility interacted with self-reported commitment in predicting relationship survival 7 months later. The main effect for self-reported commitment was qualified by accessibility such that highly committed participants were more likely to be together 7 months later if commitment was highly accessible. An issue to consider here is whether one is trying to assess implicit commitment or accessibility. Although the two terms are often used interchangeably, an implication of an implicit measure is that it is outside of conscious awareness.

In addition to our efforts to subtly cue an individual's relationship commitment prior to a lexical decision task, we have had recent success studying commitment to an academic goal (Burton & Lydon, 2004). We were interested in the motivational bases of commitment. So we had a group of students in a psychology class complete a lexical decision task with the course number flashed on the screen for 20 milliseconds, followed by a mask. Included were words representing intrinsic, identified, and introjected motives for the goal of mastering the course material. Response time latencies to identified words correlated with grades on the final exam 6 weeks later, after controlling for grades on the earlier in-class exams.

In addition to measuring implicit commitment or commitment accessibility, most recently we have been examining commitment activation. When is commitment brought to mind? Although one might try using a lexical decision task for this, it would seem less than ideal as one word ("commitment") could prime other words on subsequent trials. Instead, we have utilized a word-fragment completion procedure (Menzies-Toman & Lydon, 2003).

The idea of the study was to create a relationship threat to see if it activated commitment. The procedure involved students visualizing themselves having an interaction with an attractive-looking person of the opposite sex at a cafe. At the end of the interaction, the other person asks the participant for his or her phone number. We refer to this as the "unambiguous threat condition." A second ambiguous threat condition also included the other person making a passing mention of his girlfriend or her boyfriend. Still, the person asked for the phone number. The control condition involved an interaction with a person of the same sex. After completing the visualization, participants received a "distractor task" of completing word fragments. Six word fragments could be completed as a commitment word or an alternative word (e.g., "lo_ _ l" as "local" or "loyal").

There were no differences between the two threat conditions. However, women completed more commitment word fragments in the threat conditions than in the control condition. Men were not influenced by the threat manipulation. This is consistent with earlier results we obtained for accommodation after an interaction with an attractive confederate who was presented as single versus married. Men, when the availability of alternatives was made salient, decreased their willingness to accommodate. However, women responded to the same manipulation by increasing their accommodation. We suspect that the effect for women is due, at least in part, to the activation of commitment.

Another way to look at this is to conceptualize the threat–commitment sequence as an "if–then" contingency. Women, for various reasons, may have a chronic "if–then" contingency that "*if* an attractive guy approaches, *then* I should defend the relationship." Gollwitzer and Schaal (1998) claim that such contingencies can be formed by a single act of mental will—what they refer to as "implementation intentions." Whereas women may have habitual patterns of commitment responses to attractive alternatives (Aarts & Dijksterhuis, 2000) in theory, men should be able to respond similarly if they form implementation intentions.

We tested this idea using a guided visualization of participants being on their own for the weekend. On Friday evening, friends at dinner tease the participant about being "single" for the weekend. One friend remarks that his girlfriend is bringing her roommate to join them later in the evening when they go to the pub ("You know—the cute one that likes you"). At the end of the guided visualization, the participant is at the pub and the girl approaches. The participant is prompted with the statement "When the girl approaches, I will _____ to protect my relationship."

Of course, even with the cover story about vividness and mental simulations, and the participant randomly selecting one of seven scenarios (all of which, of course, are the same scenario in the implementation intention condition), it would seem rather obvious to have a female confederate appear and interact with the research participant. Instead, we tested avoidance by presenting objects on a computer screen to be manipulated, including images of attractive male and female models. As predicted, men kept the image of the attractive model further away in the implementation intention condition than in the control condition, suggesting that the chronic if–then response of women might be formed and activated by a situational cue.

COUPLES AND DEVELOPMENTAL TRAJECTORIES

A more complete *social* cognitive approach to relationship commitment is one that considers both members of the dyad. It is not clear that much is gained from knowing his commitment as well as her commitment (Attridge, Berscheid, & Simpson, 1995). However, this may be different when a distinction is made between the person who leaves a relationship versus the person who is left. Commitment appears to predict relationship survival better when the criterion is stay versus leave and those who were left by their partner are excluded (the idea being, of course, that one's own commitment may not effectively constrain one's partner). Moreover, given some of the gender differences described above, it would seem important to examine commitment and its motivational bases for both members of a couple.

But all that aside, the important reason, from an interpersonal cognition perspective, to study couples is that not only are people committed to varying extents, but that they also vary in their perceptions of their partner's commitment. Our first investigation of this issue involved a sample of 100 dating couples in which at least one member of the couple was graduating from university that term, and the couple was facing the prospect of being apart the following year. Participants completed our six-item commitment scale (ARC) both for themselves and then also in terms of what they thought their partner's commitment was. Having both sets of scores allowed us to look not only at the similarity in commitment within the dyad but also at the extent to which one's commitment was projected onto perceptions of partner commitment controlling for that partner's actual commitment. This is referred to as the "bias path." The path from partner actual commitment to one's perception of partner commitment represents the "accuracy path" (Kenny & Acitelli, 2001). Structural equation modeling revealed evidence of both bias and accuracy.

Given both bias and accuracy in perceptions of partner commitment, one next step would be to extend the paths out to other relationship variables and relationship survival. Consider, for example, a biased perception that the partner is highly committed to the relationship because one is projecting one's own high level of commitment. On the one hand, this may foster misplaced trust in the partner and leave one vulnerable to unforeseen disappointment. Yet it is possible that the biased perception will fuel one's own caring and supportive behaviors that may eventually increase the partner's actual commitment.

The other and related direction we would like to see for future research is the charting of the developmental trajectories of relationship commitment. This research would incorporate many of the issues discussed above, examining how perceptions and cognitions over time influence commitment, the role of adversity in the development of commitment, and the effects of gender differences in the rate at which commitment develops. We theorize that situations imbued with social meaning will precipitate changes in the level of commitment in a nonlinear fashion. Early on in a relationship, a relatively mundane event such as agreeing to attend a movie that stars an actor that one hates would signal some commitment. Later in the relationship, social gatherings with the dating partner's friends or, more so, family, would likely take commitment to another level. Resolving significant conflicts in a relationship also should alter the level of commitment. We find particularly interesting the "travel test," when two people are together all day and night for some number of days.

In positing a nonlinear course to the development of commitment, we are envisioning something akin to a step function, whereby commitment level jumps to a higher level following the successful resolution of socially meaningful events. Returning to the issue of couples, such a developmental framework also leads to interesting questions and hypotheses about events that are construed in different ways by the members of the dyad.

EXPANDING THE CALIBRATION MODEL

The original formulation of the calibration hypothesis focused on the interplay between levels of commitment and levels of threat. However, as we summarize in Figure 6.1, numerous components are in play when studying commitment to close relationships. First, the process of identification likely implicates issues of meaning, interdependence, and gender. On the other side of the equation is an array of motivated responses to defuse or dampen relationship threats. Moreover, the motivation to defend and protect the relationship can operate at an implicit as well as an explicit level and particular contexts likely increase its activation.

First, in specifying more precisely the mechanisms at work in calibrating commitment and adversity with motivated cognition tools, we might

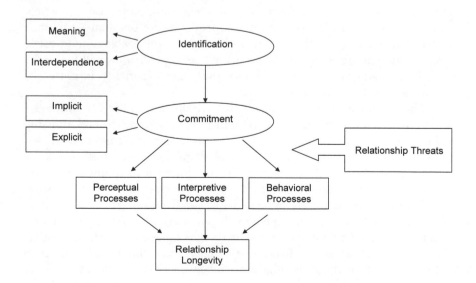

FIGURE 6.1. An expanded model of commitment calibration.

do well to delineate among the types of relationship threats, for they may elicit different relationship protective responses. Second, we might begin to consider the conclusional needs that likely influence the tool selected and used. For example, in one situation or at one time in the relationship, the need may be to regulate one's emotions, another time it may be to actively work to improve the relationship, and a third time it may be to simply try to persist. We theorize that different motivational bases for maintaining the relationship, such as intrinsically based enlightened self-interest, identification, or introjection, will underlie the different patterns of responses to relationship threats, providing distinct relationship signatures. Third, and finally, the issue of implicit commitment points to new directions concerning implicit threats and implicit relationship protective responses. What are the implications of threats posed out of awareness such as subliminally priming a room with an attractive alternative? Moreover, how do individuals develop a repertoire of effective relationship regulation strategies that can be employed in efficient and effortless ways that are seamlessly integrated into one's routine social interactions?

SUMMARY AND CONCLUSION

People who are dedicated to their relationships are devoted to their partners and have relationships that last. But the simple commitment to relationship survival relation belies the mediating pathways of perception, cognition, and behavior. Theory and research on commitment has mutually informed both the areas of social cognition and of interpersonal relationships. To social cognition research, commitment provides a resounding "Yes" to the question of whether cognitive and perceptual biases are "hot." To interpersonal relationships research, commitment illuminates how and why relationship properties lead to outcomes such as relationship longevity by emphasizing the cognitive pathways.

The challenge now is to examine interpersonal cognition in general, and commitment in particular, of both members of a dyad, and to study this over time. Then we will more thoroughly understand when and why people leave relationships and begin to understand why, despite their own commitment, they were left.

NOTES

1. Interdependence can also operate cognitively (Agnew et al., 1998) as individuals think in terms of a unit or identity relation. This conceptualization of interdependence is very much in line with theoretical formulations of identification.
2. Relationship satisfaction did not moderate men's illusions.

3. Similarly, in a study of trainees as fighter pilots, commitment assessed with the hardiness scale predicted greater challenge appraisals relative to threat appraisals (Florian, Mikulincer, & Taubman, 1995).

REFERENCES

Aarts, H., & Dijksterhuis, A. (2000). Habits as knowledge structures: Automaticity in goal-directed behavior. *Journal of Personality and Social Psychology, 78*, 53–63.

Agnew, C. R., Van Lange, P. A., Rusbult, C. E., & Langston, C. A. (1998). Cognitive interdependence: Commitment and the mental representation of close relationships. *Journal of Personality and Social Psychology, 74*, 939–954.

Aron, A., Aron, E. N., & Smollan, D. (1992). Inclusion of Other in the Self Scale and the structure of interpersonal closeness. *Journal of Personality and Social Psychology 63*, 596–612.

Arriaga, X. B. (2001). The ups and downs of dating: Fluctuations in satisfaction in newly formed romantic relationships. *Journal of Personality and Social Psychology, 80*, 754–765.

Attridge, M., Berscheid, E., & Simpson, J. A. (1995). Predicting relationship stability from both partners versus one. *Journal of Personality and Social Psychology, 69*, 254–268.

Baumeister, R., Bratslavsky, E., Muraven, M., & Tice, D. (1998). Ego depletion: Is the self a limited resource? *Journal of Personality and Social Psychology, 74*, 1252–1265.

Baumeister, R. F., & Leary, M. R. (1995). The need to belong: Desire for interpersonal attachments as a fundamental human motivation. *Psychological Bulletin, 117*, 497–529.

Becker, H. S. (1960). Notes on the concept of commitment. *American Journal of Sociology, 66* 32–42.

Bell, C., & Lydon, J. (1997, June). *Avoiding attractive alternatives in virtual reality.* Paper presented at the annual meeting of the Canadian Psychological Association, Toronto, Ontario.

Berscheid, E., Snyder, M., & Omoto, A. M. (1989). The Relationship Closeness Inventory: Assessing the closeness of interpersonal relationships. *Journal of Personality and Social Psychology, 57*, 792–807.

Borden, V. M. H., & Levinger, G. (1991). Interpersonal transformations in intimate relationships. In W. H. Jones & D. W. Perlman (Eds.), *Advances in personal relationships: A research annual* (Vol. 2, pp. 35–56). London: Jessica Kingsley.

Bowlby, J. (1969–1980). *Attachment and loss* (Vols. 1–3). London: Hogarth Press.

Bradbury, T. N., & Fincham, F. D. (1990). Attributions in marriage: Review and critique. *Psychological Bulletin, 107*, 3–33.

Brickman, P. (1987). Commitment. In C. B. Wortman & R. Sorrentino (Eds.), *Commitment, conflict, and caring* (pp. 1–18). Englewood Cliffs, NJ: Prentice-Hall.

Bui, K.-V. T., Peplau, L. A., & Hill, C. T. (1996). Testing the Rusbult model of relationship commitment and stability in a 15-year study of heterosexual couples. *Personality and Social Psychology Bulletin, 22*, 1244–1257.

Bumpass, L. L., Martin, T. C., & Sweet, J. A. (1991). The impact of family background and early marital factors on marital disruption. *Journal of Family Issues, 12,* 22–42.

Burke, P. J., & Reitzes, D. C. (1991). An identity theory approach to commitment. *Social Psychology Quarterly, 54,* 239–251.

Burton, K., & Lydon, J. (2004a, January). *Priming relationship identification to increase relationship supportive behavior.* In L. A. Neff (Chair), Support in close relationships: when are intimates most likely to engage in supportive behaviors? Symposium conducted at the 5th annual meeting of the Society for Personality and Social Psychology, Austin, TX.

Burton, K., & Lydon, J. (2004b). *The differential effects of intrinsic and identified motives on well-being and performance: A social cognitive approach to self-determination theory.* Unpublished manuscript, McGill University.

Burton, K. D., Lydon, J. E., & Bauer, M. (2003, August). *Commitment and the implicit activation of relational thinking under threat.* Poster session presented at the annual meeting of the American Psychological Association, Toronto, Ontario, Canada.

Burton, K., Lydon, J., & Bell, C. (2000, July). *Priming the avoidance of attractive alternatives.* Paper presented at the annual meeting of the Canadian Psychological Association, Ottawa, Ontario.

Burton, K., Lydon, J., & Patall, E. (2003, February). *Implicit relationship satisfaction and the prediction of accommodation.* Poster session presented at the 4th annual meeting of the Society for Personality and Social Psychology, Los Angeles, CA.

Cross, S. E., & Madson, L. (1997). Models of the self: Self-construals and gender. *Psychological Bulletin, 122,* 5–37.

Csikszentmihalyi, M., & Csikszentmihalyi, I. S. (1988). *Optimal experience: Psychological studies of flow in consciousness.* New York: Cambridge University Press.

Deci, E. L., & Ryan, R. M. (1991). A motivational approach to self: Integration in personality. In R. A. Dienstbier (Ed.), *Nebraska Symposium on Motivation: Vol. 38. Perspectives on motivation* (pp. 237–288). Lincoln: University of Nebraska Press.

Diener, E., Sandvik, E., & Pavot, W. G. (1990). Happiness is the frequency, not intensity, of positive versus negative affect. In F. Strack, M. Argyle, & N. Schwarz (Eds.), *The social psychology of subjective well-being* (pp. 119–139). Elmsford, NY: Pergamon Press.

Etcheverry, P. E., & Le, B. (2003, February). *Accessibility of commitment and the prediction of relationship continuance.* Poster session presented at the annual meeting of the Society for Personality and Social Psychology, Los Angeles, CA.

Fehr, B. (1988). Prototype analysis of the concepts of love and commitment. *Journal of Personality and Social Psychology, 55,* 557–579.

Fincham, F. D., & Bradbury, T. N. (1992). Assessing attributions in marriage: The Relationship Attribution Measure. *Journal of Personality and Social Psychology, 62,* 457–468.

Finkel, E. J., & Campbell, W. K. (2001). Self-control and accommodation in close relationships: An interdependence analysis. *Journal of Personality and Social Psychology, 81,* 263–277.

Finkel, E. J., Rusbult, C. E., Kumashiro, M., & Hannon, P. A. (2002). Dealing with betrayal in close relationships: Does commitment prmote forgiveness? *Journal of Personality and Social Psychology, 82,* 956–974.

Fletcher, G. J. O., & Fincham, F. D. (1991). Attribution processes in close relationships. In G. J. O. Fletcher & F. D. Fincham (Eds.), *Cognition in close relationships* (pp. 7–35). Hillsdale, NJ: Erlbaum.

Florian, V., Mikulincer, M., & Taubman, O. (1995). Does hardiness contribute to mental health during a stressful real-life situation?: The roles of appraisal and coping. *Journal of Personality and Social Psychology, 68,* 687–695.

Frank, E., & Brandstätter, V. (2002). Approach versus avoidance: Different types of commitment in intimate relationships. *Journal of Personality and Social Psychology, 82,* 208–221.

Gagné, F. M., & Lydon, J. E. (2001). Mind-set and close relationships: When bias leads to (in)accurate predictions. *Journal of Personality and Social Psychology, 81,* 85–96.

Gagné, F. M., & Lydon, J. E. (2003). Identification and the commitment shift: Accounting for gender differences in relationship illusions. *Personality and Social Psychology Bulletin, 29,* 907–919.

Gollwitzer, P. M., & Kirchhof, O. (1998). The willful pursuit of identity. In J. Heckhausen & C. S. Dweck (Eds.), *Motivation and self-regulation across the life span* (pp. 389–423). Cambridge, UK: Cambridge University Press.

Gollwitzer, P. M., & Schaal, B. (1998). Metacognition in action: The importance of implementation intentions. *Personality and Social Psychology Review, 2,* 124–136.

Gollwitzer, P. M., & Wicklund, R. A. (1985). Self-symbolizing and the neglect of others' perspectives. *Journal of Personality and Social Psychology, 48,* 702–715.

Holmes, J. G. (1981). The exchange process in close relationships: Microbehavior and macromotives. In M. J. Lerner & S. C. Lerner (Eds.), *The justice motive in social behavior* (pp. 261–284). New York: Plenum Press.

Johnson, D. J., & Rusbult, C. E. (1989). Resisting temptation: Devaluation of alternative partners as a means of maintaining commitment in close relationships. *Journal of Personality and Social Psychology, 57,* 967–980.

Johnson, M. P. (1973). Commitment: A conceptual structure and empirical application. *Sociological Quarterly, 14,* 395–406.

Johnson, M. P. (1991). Commitment to personal relationships. In W. H. Jones & D. W. Perlman (Eds.), *Advances in personal relationships* (Vol. 3, pp. 117–143). London: Jessica Kingsley.

Kelley, H. H. (1983). Love and commitment. In H. H. Kelley, E. Berscheid, A. Christensen, J. H. Harvey, T. L. Huston, G. Levinger, et al. (Eds.), *Close relationships* (pp. 265–314). New York: Freeman.

Kenny, D., & Acitelli, L. K. (2001). Accuracy and bias in the perception of the partner in a close relationship. *Journal of Personality and Social Psychology, 80,* 439–448.

Khan, A., Gagné, F., Lydon, J., & To, M. (2004). *When flattery gets you nowhere: Discounting positive feedback as a relationship maintenance strategy?* Unpublished manuscript.

Kiesler, C. (1971). *The psychology of commitment: Experiments linking behaviour to belief.* New York: Academic Press.

Kunda, Z. (1990). The case for motivated reasoning. *Psychological Bulletin, 108,* 480–498.

Levinger, G. (1976). A social psychological perspective on marital dissolution. *Journal of Social Issues, 32*, 21–27.

Lund, M. (1985). The development of investment and commitment scales for predicting continuity of personal relationships. *Journal of Social and Personal Relationships, 2*, 3–23.

Lydon, J. E., Dunkel-Schetter, C., Cohan, C. L., & Pierce, T. (1996). Pregnancy decision making as a significant life event: A commitment approach. *Journal of Personality and Social Psychology, 71*, 141–151.

Lydon, J. E., Fitzsimons, G. M., & Naidoo, L. (2003). Devaluation versus enhancement of attractive alternatives: A critical test using the calibration paradigm. *Personality and Social Psychology Bulletin, 29*, 349–359.

Lydon, J. E., & Gagné, F. M. (2004). *The Assessment of Relationship Commitment (ARC): Four studies validating a 6-item measure.* Unpublished manuscript, McGill University.

Lydon, J. E., Meana, M., Sepinwall, D., Richards, N., & Mayman, S. (1999). The commitment calibration hypothesis: When do people devalue attractive alternatives? *Personality and Social Psychology Bulletin, 25*, 152–161.

Lydon, J. E., Pierce, T., & O'Regan, S. (1997). Coping with moral commitment to long distance dating relationships. *Journal of Personality and Social Psychology, 73*, 104–113.

Lydon, J. E., & Zanna, M. P. (1990). Commitment in the face of adversity: A value-affirmation approach. *Journal of Personality and Social Psychology, 58*, 1040–1047.

McAdams, D. (2001). The psychology of life stories. *Review of General Psychology, 5*, 100–122.

Menzies-Toman, D. A., & Lydon, J. E. (2003, February). *Relationships under threat: Gender differences in the contextual activation of commitment accessibility.* Poster session presented at the 4th annual meeting of the Society for Personality and Social Psychology, Los Angeles, CA.

Menzies-Toman, D. A., & Lydon, J. E. (2005, January). *Beyond commitment: Self-determination theory and relationship maintenance processes.* Poster session presented at the 6th annual meeting of the Society for Personality and Social Psychology, New Orleans, LA.

Menzies-Toman, D. A., & Lydon, J. E. (in press). Commitment motivated benign appraisals of partner transgressions: Do they facilitate accommodation? *Journal of Social and Personal Relationships, 22.*

Mischel, W., & Shoda, Y. (1999). Integrating dispositions and processing dynamics within a unified theory of personality: The cognitive–affective personality system. In L. A. Pervin & J. P. Oliver (Eds.), *Handbook of personality: Theory and research* (2nd ed., pp. 197–218). New York: Guilford Press.

Murray, S. L., & Holmes, J. G. (1993). Seeing virtues in faults: Negativity and the transformation of interpersonal narratives in close relationships. *Journal of Personality and Social Psychology, 65*, 707–722.

Murray, S. L., Holmes, J. G., & Griffin, D. W. (1996a). The benefits of positive illusions: Idealization and the construction of satisfaction in close relationships. *Journal of Personality and Social Psychology, 70*, 79–98.

Murray, S. L., Holmes, J. G., & Griffin, D. W. (1996b). The self-fulfilling nature of positive illusions in romantic relationships: Love is not blind, but prescient. *Journal of Personality and Social Psychology, 71,* 1155–1180.

Pierce, T., Lydon, J. E., & Yang, S. (2001). Enthusiasm and moral commitment: What sustains family caregivers of those with dementia? *Basic and Applied Social Psychology, 23,* 29–41.

Rokeach, M. (1979). Some unresolved issues in theories of beliefs, attitudes, and values. *Nebraska Symposium on Motivation, 27,* 261–304.

Rubin, Z. (1970). Measurement of romantic love. *Journal of Personality and Social Psychology, 16,* 265–273.

Rusbult, C. E. (1980). Commitment and satisfaction in romantic associations: A test of the investment model. *Journal of Experimental Social Psychology, 16,* 172–186.

Rusbult, C. E. (1983). A longitudinal test of the investment model: The development (and deterioration) of satisfaction and commitment in heterosexual involvements. *Journal of Personality and Social Psychology, 45,* 101–117.

Rusbult, C. E., & Buunk, B. P. (1993). Commitment processes in close relationships: An interdependence analysis. *Journal of Social & Personal Relationships, 10,* 175–204.

Rusbult, C. E., Van Lange, P. A. M., Wildschut, T., Yovetich, N. A., & Verette, J. (2000). Perceived superiority in close relationships: Why it exists and persists. *Journal of Personality and Social Psychology, 79,* 521–545.

Rusbult, C. E., Verette, J., Whitney, G. A., Slovik, L. F., & Lipkus, I. (1991). Accommodation processes in close relationships: Theory and preliminary empirical evidence. *Journal of Personality and Social Psychology, 60,* 53–78.

Ryan, R. M., & Deci, E. L. (2000). The darker and brighter sides of human existence: Basic psychological needs as a unifying concept. *Psychological Inquiry, 11,* 319–338.

Shah, J., & Higgins, E. T. (1997). Expectancy * value effects: Regulatory focus as determinant of magnitude and direction. *Journal of Personality and Social Psychology, 3,* 447–458.

Sorrentino, R. M., & Higgins, E. T. (Eds.). (1986–1990). *Handbook of motivation and cognition: Foundations of social behavior* (Vols. 1–2). New York: Guilford Press.

Thibaut, J. W., & Kelley, H. H. (1959). *The social psychology of groups.* New York: Wiley.

Wright, R. A., & Brehm, J. W. (1989). Energization and goal attractiveness. In L. A. Pervin (Ed.), *Goal concepts in personality and social psychology* (pp. 169–210). Hillsdale, NJ: Erlbaum.

7

A Relationship-Specific Sense of Felt Security

How Perceived Regard Regulates Relationship-Enhancement Processes

SANDRA L. MURRAY *and* JAYE DERRICK

> Had I said that, had I done this,
> So might I gain, so might I miss.
> Might she have loved me? Just as well
> She might have hated, who can tell!
> —ROBERT BROWNING,
> "The Last Ride Together"

However sarcastic the tone, Browning's words capture an inferential goal common to most romantic pursuits: discerning the quality of another's caring. In fact, petals are plucked off daisies, and innocuous events, such as a glance, a frown, or a smile, are imbued with meaning in the hopes of concluding that another truly cares. Such (motivated) attentiveness to the evidence is not all that surprising given that the need to belong is thought to be a fundamental human motivation, one as basic as the need to drink or eat (Baumeister & Leary, 1995). Finding evidence of a desirable, sought-after, and beloved intimate's love and acceptance thus has the potential to soothe belongingness needs and to affirm one's own worthiness of love.

Simultaneously, though, risking love and closeness also leaves people vulnerable to the pain of rejection and the threat to self-esteem it represents (Leary, Tambor, Terdal, & Downs, 1995). In fact, rather than abating after an initial, successful romantic overture, the psychological costs of rejection likely only increase with greater interdependence and closeness (Braiker & Kelley, 1979). After all, as (temporarily) crushing as it might be to have a request for a first date rejected or to have a dating relationship end after a few months, such threats likely pale in comparison to believing that one's spouse is disinterested in providing needed support, too selfish to make personal sacrifices for the relationship, or too attracted to the physical attributes of available opposite-sex others.

In this chapter, we examine how people balance the need to risk closeness, and see the best in one's partner and relationship, against the need to protect themselves from the possibility of rejection. In so doing, we hope to integrate early research illustrating the benefits of positive illusions and motivated cognition (see Murray, 1999, for a review) with a more recent focus on dependence regulation (Murray, Holmes, & Griffin, 2000; Murray, Holmes, Griffin, Bellavia, & Rose, 2001; Murray, Bellavia, Rose, & Griffin, 2003). Our central thesis is that finding a stable, relationship-specific sense of felt security in a partner's regard and love acts as a psychological switch that allows people to put self-protection aside, and take the risk of loving, idealizing, and becoming attached to an imperfect partner (Murray, Holmes, & Griffin, 2000; Murray et al., 2001; Murray, Bellavia, Rose, & Griffin, 2003).

Accordingly, we begin our chapter by describing how much of people's self-esteem is at stake in romantic attachments, particularly in situations where the threat of rejection is salient. We then describe the many common situations in relationship life that highlight the potential risks of dependence, and thus necessitate the kinds of benevolent, motivated transformations that can put relationship-promotion and self-protection motives into conflict. Next we outline the data supporting our central thesis by describing how feeling positively regarded by one's partner regulates how this tension is resolved in daily life. We conclude by describing the self-fulfilling effects of finding (or failing to find) this relationship-specific sense of felt security.

THE SELF-ESTEEM STAKES

Self-esteem is in large part relational in nature (Andersen & Chen, 2002; Baldwin, 1992; Leary & Baumeister, 2000). Specifically, Leary and his colleagues believe that self-esteem acts as a "sociometer" that gauges the risks of interpersonal rejection (Leary, Cottrell, & Misha, 2001; Leary, Haupt, Strausser, & Chokel, 1998; Leary et al., 1995). On a situation-to-situation basis, this sociometer is thought to function such that signs of another's waning approval diminish self-esteem, and thus activate the need to seek approval and interpersonal connections. For instance, the general need to enhance feelings of inclusion even sensitizes people with low self-esteem to signs of a stranger's approval or disapproval (Nezlek, Kowalski, Leary, Blevins, & Holgate, 1997; Rudich & Vallacher, 1999).

Further underscoring the interpersonal basis of self-esteem, attachment theorists believe that infants develop chronic models of the self as being worthy of love and care in the context of early interactions with consistently available and responsive caregivers (Bowlby, 1982; Hazan & Shaver, 1994). Similarly, symbolic interactionists have characterized the self as a "looking-glass," one that mirrors the actual and imagined reactions of others (e.g., Cooley, 1902; Mead, 1934; Shrauger & Schoeneman, 1979). For instance, across causal acquaintanceships, close friendships, parent–child relationships, and romantic relationships, people's views of themselves closely mirror the image of themselves they perceive in the eyes of others (Felson, 1989; Kenny, 1994; McNulty & Swann, 1994; Murray, Holmes, & Griffin, 2000). In fact, people's sense of themselves is so sensitive to interpersonal ties that simply being exposed to a novel person who happens to resemble a significant other within one's life shifts the content of the working self-concept to resemble the sense of self that is experienced in the presence of this significant other (Hinkley & Andersen, 1996). Moreover, even disapproving audiences that are activated outside of consciousness have the potential to undermine self-esteem (Baldwin, Carrell, & Lopez, 1990).

The self-esteem gains of eliciting acceptance, and the self-esteem costs of eliciting disinterest or disapproval, are likely magnified in close romantic relationships. For instance, dating and married intimates who believe their hoped-for selves are understood and nurtured by their partner report less discrepancy between their actual and ideal selves as time passes (Drigotas, Rusbult, Wieselquist, & Whitton, 1999; Ruvolo & Brennan, 1997). The opposite is true for people who feel less affirmed. Similarly, dating intimates who believe their partner sees them more positively on specific interpersonal qualities see themselves more positively on those same traits over time (Murray, Holmes, & Griffin, 2000). Dating intimates also incorporate their partner's perceived strengths in their self-concepts as time passes (Aron, Paris, & Aron, 1995).

THE RELATIONSHIP-PROMOTION WINDFALL

Just as romantic life is replete with situations, such as an affectionate hug or a comforting remark, that can function to affirm and bolster self-esteem, it is also filled with situations that highlight the risks of rejection, and the potential practical and self-esteem costs of depending on another's (fallible) goodwill. After all, couples are interdependent at many different levels—from negotiating preferences to see an action flick as opposed to a romantic comedy, to merging one partner's relaxed, laissez-fair personality style with the other's more controlled style, to finding a comfortable balance between closeness and autonomy within the relationship (e.g., Braiker & Kelley, 1979; Kelley, 1979; Holmes, 2002). Given such diversity and breadth of interdependence, discovering negative features of the partner's personality, significant conflicts, and the necessity of compromise and sacrifice is inevitable.

As a consequence, people may often find themselves in situations where they need to make a choice (whether deliberative or not) between self-protection and relationship promotion. In the language of interdependence theory (Rusbult & Buunk, 1993), people implicitly decide between acting to protect their own interests as opposed to the relationship's interests (i.e., "given" versus "effective" matrix considerations). For instance, in the face of Sally's unsolicited criticisms of his movie or leisure preferences, Harry may be caught between the desire to defend himself by lashing out at Sally in turn, and the desire to protect the relationship, by making a charitable attribution for her critical remark. In the event of conflict between Sally's need to spend an evening working and Harry's need for companionship at an important social gathering, Sally may also need to decide whether to risk rejection by asking Harry to sacrifice some of his needs to meet her own. When feeling uncertain of his professional aptitudes, Harry may need to decide whether to take the chance of disclosing such self-doubts in the hope of eliciting her comfort and support. In situations where Harry has transgressed and broken a promise, Sally must decide whether to risk letting her outcomes depend on Harry's actions again in the future.

As these situations illustrate, the safe, self-protective choice is most often the choice that minimizes dependence on the other's goodwill. In the last scenario, for instance, deciding not to trust Harry's promises, and reducing her reliance on Harry for the satisfaction of her own goals, likely protects Sally from feeling letdown and rejected in the future. However, such a self-protective choice also compromises Sally's trust in Harry, and limits Harry's future opportunities to demonstrate his trustworthiness, putting the well-being of the relationship at greater risk. Accordingly, in the face of such dilemmas, people in satisfying relationships typically put protecting the welfare of the relationship ahead of self-protection. That is, they make generous leaps of faith, and put the best possible (behavioral and cognitive) spin on the evidence available.

For instance, people in satisfying marriages generously attribute their partner's transgressions to transient features of the situation (Bradbury & Fincham, 1990). They also inhibit self-protective inclinations to respond in kind to a partner's misdeeds, and instead respond constructively (Rusbult, Verette, Whitney, Slovik, & Lipkus, 1991). People in satisfied, committed relationships also sacrifice their own self-interest to meet the needs of their partner (Van Lange et al., 1997). They are also more willing to respond to their partners' needs as they arise rather than adhering to a safer, tit-for-tat, strategy in the provision and receipt of benefits (Grote & Clark, 2001). People in committed dating relationships even minimize or benevolently misconstrue their partner's possible attraction to others rather than being hypersensitive to any cue that might suggest rejection is possible (Simpson, Ickes, & Blackstone, 1995).

Perhaps as a consequence of such situated generosity, dating and married intimates in satisfying relationships see strengths or virtues in their partner that they do not see in others (Rusbult, Van Lange, Wildschut, Yovetich, & Verette, 2000), and that are also not apparent to their friends (Murray, Holmes, Dolderman, & Griffin, 2000) or even to their partner (Murray, Holmes, & Griffin, 1996a; Neff & Karney, 2002). People in satisfying dating relationships even organize their beliefs about their partner's qualities in ways that link faults to compensatory thoughts about greater virtues (Murray & Holmes, 1999). Through these types of cognitive and behavioral accommodation processes, satisfied intimates keep their partner's imperfections from compromising their faith in their partner's basic responsiveness to their needs and minimize the potential for cycles of negativity to develop (Gottman, 1994).

In our initial investigation of such motivated cognitive processes, we asked both members of dating and married couples to describe themselves, their partner, and their ideal partner on a series of interpersonally oriented attributes (Murray et al., 1996a). We then defined *illusions* as the qualities that people see in their partner that their partner does not see in himself or herself. In other words, we defined illusions as a residual term: Harry's perception of Sally, controlling for Sally's perception of herself. In a longitudinal follow-up, we collected these measures of positive illusions and measures of relationship well-being three times over the course of a year in a sample of established dating couples (Murray, Holmes, & Griffin, 1996b).

Although people's perceptions of their partner in part reflected the "reality" of their partner's self-image, people's hopes for an ideal partner also colored their perceptions. To the extent that Sally's ideal partner was warm and generous, for instance, she projected such traits onto Harry, seeing him more positively than he saw himself on these dimensions. Such benevolently filtered perceptions were critical for relationship well-being. Dating and married intimates both reported greater satisfaction in their relationships when they saw their partner more generously than their partner saw him- or herself. In fact, people were also happier in their relationships when their partner put the best possible spin on the available evidence and idealized them. Over the longer term, such benevolently biased perceptions also had positive, self-fulfilling effects. People ultimately reported relatively greater satisfaction, less conflict, and fewer doubts about their dating partner the more they idealized their partner, and the more their partner idealized them initially. As time passed, people in stable dating relationships even shifted their definitions of an ideal partner to match the qualities they perceived in their own partner, illustrating the flexible, adaptive nature of motivated construal processes.

Thus, to be happy in the face of the normal risks and vicissitudes of romantic life, people need to risk framing their behavioral options and construing their partner's traits and motives in the best possible light. Although such motivated transformations are critical for maintaining a sense of trust in the partner and satisfaction in the relationship (Holmes & Rempel, 1989; Murray, 1999), enhancing the value of the partner and relationship in this way also magnifies the self-threat posed by the prospect of rejection, and thus heightens the stakes of risking dependence. After all, feeling rejected by a valued, cherished other who approximates one's ideal partner presumably poses a much greater threat to self-esteem than being rejected by someone of only passing interest.

A RESOLUTION?: FINDING FELT SECURITY IN THE PARTNER'S ACCEPTANCE

How do people balance the tension between the need to make generous leaps of faith and the desire to protect themselves against feeling unduly vulnerable? Attachment and interdependence theories are based on the implicit assumption that people regulate closeness (and thus dependence) with a sense of felt security, not letting themselves risk vulnerability and feel fully in love and committed until they are confident of their partner's reciprocated affections and commitment (Berscheid & Fei, 1977; Bowlby, 1982; Holmes & Rempel, 1989; Kelley, 1983). Accordingly, we reasoned that similar psychological constraints or brakes may also regulate relationship-enhancement processes (Murray, Holmes, & Griffin, 2000; Murray, Bellavia, Rose, & Griffin, 2003).

Specifically, people should only allow themselves to risk giving a partner the cognitive and behavioral "benefit of the doubt," and putting a positive spin on the available evidence when they believe their partner's acceptance and love is secure (Murray, Holmes, & Griffin, 2000; Murray et al., 2001). After all, people are not likely to feel as vulnerable in forgiving a partner's transgressions if they expect this partner to be equally forgiving of their own foibles. To find this sense of security in a partner's acceptance, people likely need to believe that their partner sees qualities in them worth valuing (Leary & Baumeister, 2000). For instance, dating and married intimates report feeling more accepted and loved by their partner when they believe their partner sees them more positively on specific interpersonal qualities (Murray et al., 2001). In other words, Sally is not likely to believe that Harry will always love her if she has trouble pinpointing qualities in herself that he values, especially ones he could not easily find in another (Tooby & Cosmides, 1996).

In our first investigation of dependence regulation processes in dating and marital relationships, we asked both members of the couple to describe how they believed their partner saw them on a series of interpersonally oriented attributes, our measure of perceived regard (Murray, Holmes, & Griffin, 2000). For instance, Sally would be asked to describe Harry's perceptions of her status on traits such as warm, responsive, critical, and kind. We also asked participants to describe how they saw their partner on the same traits. As we expected, dating and married intimates both found more to value in their partner's traits, the more positively they believed their partner saw them on these same traits (Murray, Holmes, & Griffin, 2000). A parallel dependence regulation effect emerged when we substituted perceptions of the partner's love as the index of perceived regard (Murray et al., 2001). Thus, finding a sense of felt security in a partner's love and acceptance may act as a psychological switch that allows people to feel safe seeing a partner's qualities in the most generous light possible. On the other side of the coin, people who feel less valued and loved by their partner find less to value in that same partner. Distancing oneself from the relationship in this way likely functions as a self-protective defense for people who believe that their partner is not all that committed to the relationship (because tying oneself to a relationship in which rejection seems likely is too risky a psychological proposition).

If establishing a sense of confidence in a partner's acceptance is a fundamental relationship goal, its motivating influence in shaping perception and behavior should be evident throughout a relationship's development. Consistent with this logic, the perception of another's attraction to the self is a more potent force in triggering attraction and love at relationship inception than considerations of this person's qualities per se (Aron, Dutton, Aron, & Iverson, 1989; Hazan & Diamond, 2000). As new relationships develop, moreover, people actively monitor their partner's behaviors for signs of selflessness, and thus reason to trust in their partner's willingness to respond to their needs (Fraley & Shaver, 2000; Holmes & Rempel, 1989; Wieselquist, Rusbult, Foster, & Agnew, 1999). Even in stable marriages, people still seek their spouse's admiration and approval, reporting that they want their spouse to see them much more positively than they see themselves (Murray, Holmes, & Griffin, 2000). In specific situations, self-threats also activate the attachment system, and thus the need to seek another's literal or symbolic comfort (Collins & Feeney, 2000). In fact, priming failure-related thoughts automatically activates thoughts of seeking proximity to others (Mikulincer, Birnbaum, Woddis, & Nachmias, 2000; Mikulincer, Gillath, & Shaver, 2002).

Despite people's general needs for belongingness, and the specific goal of establishing a sense of felt security in a partner's regard, people troubled by dispositional insecurities, such as low self-esteem, have difficulty finding evidence of a partner's acceptance in even the most accommodating behavioral realities. In both dating and marital relationships, people with low

self-esteem underestimate how positively their partner sees them on specific traits (Murray, Holmes, & Griffin, 2000) and even underestimate how
much their partner loves them (Murray et al., 2001). People who are more
sensitive to rejection or more preoccupied in attachment style (and thus
lower in self-esteem) also underestimate their dating partner's relationship
satisfaction and commitment (Downey & Feldman, 1996; Tucker & Anders, 1999). Thus, people who chronically feel less positively regarded by
their partner lack the level of confidence in a partner's acceptance and caring that they need to satisfy felt security goals. Consequently, the goal of
satisfying felt security needs becomes chronically accessible (Fraley &
Shaver, 2000). In contrast, people with higher self-esteem and less dispositional anxiety about rejection more accurately perceive how positively
their partner regards them, and thus felt security goals are likely to be
largely satiated.

    We believe a conceptual focus on relationship-specific expectations of
acceptance might help explain why certain dispositional vulnerabilities,
such as low self-esteem (e.g., Murray, Holmes, MacDonald, & Ellsworth,
1998), chronic rejection sensitivity (Downey, Freitas, Michaelis, & Khouri,
1998), and insecure attachment styles (e.g., Collins & Feeney, 2000;
Simpson, Rholes, & Nelligan, 1992; Trobst, 2000) can be so problematic
in both dating and marital relationships. That is, more negative general
models of self may go hand in hand with diminished satisfaction because
such self-doubts typically interfere with people's ability to form (explicit or
implicit) representations of specific others that foster optimistic inferences
about a specific partner's positive regard and caring. Consistent with this
hypothesis, perceptions of a partner's regard mediates the link between
self-esteem and satisfaction in both dating and marital relationships
(Murray, Holmes, & Griffin, 2000). Moreover, if the vulnerability imposed
by general models rests in the specific representations they foster, even people who are normally troubled by dispositional vulnerabilities may respond adaptively to threat if they believe their partner sees qualities in
them that merit attention, nurturance, and care. Illustrating this logic,
women who are anxious–ambivalent in attachment style, yet nonetheless
believe that their partners will be responsive and caring during the transition to parenthood, remain satisfied in their marriages during this stressful
time. The opposite is true for anxious–ambivalent women without this relationship-specific sense of being valued (Rholes, Simpson, Campbell, &
Grich, 2001).

REGULATING THE RISK OF REJECTION IN DAY-TO-DAY MARRIED LIFE

What are the consequences of more or less chronically activated relationship-
specific felt security goals for how people interpret and respond to situa-

tions that highlight the risks of dependence? Recently, we have argued that chronic perceptions of a partner's regard for the self govern the operation of a *relationship-specific sociometer,* one that gauges the risks of a partner's rejection on a daily basis, and then structures affective, cognitive, and behavioral responses to felt rejection in situ (Murray, Bellavia, Rose, & Griffin, 2003; Murray, Griffin, Rose, & Bellavia, 2003). Figure 7.1 presents the conceptual model underlying our thinking. Specifically, feeling more or less positively regarded by a partner may determine how readily rejection concerns are activated in any given situation (i.e., Path A, the activation threshold of this sociometer), whether feeling rejected undermines self-esteem (i.e., Path B, the calibration function of this sociometer), and how people respond mentally and behaviorally to the experience of feeling rejected (i.e., Path C, the behavioral consequences of this sociometer).

In developing this model, we reasoned that studying couples in the midst of negotiating specific situations, such as conflicts, might provide an ideal way of examining these dynamics. Consistent with such logic, recent theorizing within social psychology suggests that a person's motives, personality, and general expectations can best be revealed within specific diagnostic situations (Holmes, 2002; Mischel & Shoda, 1995). Put another way, the differences between people who feel more or less chronically regarded by their partner may emerge most clearly in situations where the threat of rejection is salient. Such differences may be less obvious in more accepting or neutral circumstances. Accordingly, we decided to conduct a diary study so that we might sample a wide range of situations within the daily lives of married couples.

We asked both members of 154 married couples from the Buffalo

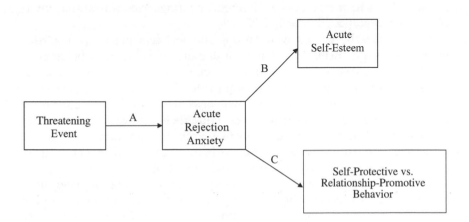

FIGURE 7.1. The situational regulation of felt security.

community to each complete a paper-and-pencil diary for 21 days (Murray, Bellavia, Rose, & Griffin, 2003; Murray, Griffin, Rose, & Bellavia, 2003). Both members of the couple attended a 1.5-hour session at our laboratory where they completed a package of background measures, and also received instructions for completing the diary each day. Each diary asked participants to check which self- or relationship-relevant events had occurred that day (e.g., "had a minor disagreement," "partner criticized me," "I insulted my partner," "I told my partner I loved him/her"), and to complete *state* items tapping self-esteem that day (e.g., "good about myself"), how rejected/accepted they felt by their partner that day (e.g., "rejected or hurt by my partner," "worried about disappointing my partner"), evaluations of the partner that focused on perceptions of the partner's responsiveness (e.g., "my partner is selfish," "my partner is taking me for granted"), and how close they felt to their partner that day (e.g., "in love with my partner," "happy in my relationship").

Reading the Tea Leaves: Appraisal Sensitivity

What types of acceptance- or rejection-related inferences should people who feel more or less positively regarded draw from specific events (Path A in Figure 7.1)? As we reasoned earlier, people who chronically feel less positively regarded by their partner (i.e., lows) lack the level of confidence in a partner's acceptance and caring they need to satisfy felt security goals. Accordingly, the chronic activation of this goal (whether conscious or not) should sensitize lows to information relevant to the satisfaction of this goal (e.g., Bargh & Ferguson, 2000; Gardner, Pickett, & Brewer, 2000; Holmes & Rempel, 1989; Vorauer & Ross, 1996). In this way, the need to find signs of a specific partner's positive regard and acceptance should oversensitize lows to the perceived "if–then" contingencies warranting interpersonal acceptance (Baldwin, 1992).

Consequently, people who chronically feel less positively regarded may more readily detect rejection in mundane events such as being criticized at work, seeing a spouse in a bad mood, or experiencing a marital conflict. Ironically, though, in scanning the available behavioral data, lows may actually hope to soothe their own insecurities by finding conclusive evidence that their partner really does value them. However, they are not likely to be all that even-handed in this search. Instead, they may process information in risk-averse ways, too ready to perceive and generalize from signs of rejection and too hesitant to trust signs of acceptance.

We expected this asymmetry to emerge because feelings of uncertainty and consequent concerns about making incorrect inferences often result in people processing information in a cautious or risk-averse fashion (Holmes & Rempel, 1989; Taylor, 1991). That is, people may become more hesitant to believe what they hope to be true as the costs of being wrong in this inference increase. Even though detecting signs of rejection might hurt in the short term, such sensitivity may better protect intimates who feel less positively regarded by their partner against the greater hurt of inferring acceptance, risking attachment, and then later reaching the all more hurtful conclusion that they were never really accepted after all. In this way, the combination of relatively negative chronic expectations and risk aversion may prime people who are looking for signs of acceptance to overinterpret signs of rejection as they monitor both their own and their partner's behavior.

Imagine, for instance, that Sally gets criticized at work for failing to complete a project on time. To the extent that she feels unsure of Harry's regard, Sally may be reluctant to disclose this personal failing for fear he might be angry with or disappointed in her. Consistent with this logic, Baldwin and Sinclair (1996) argue that people low in self-esteem—and thus people who generally doubt the acceptance of others—automatically associate failure with interpersonal rejection. In dating relationships, people with low self-esteem also react to experimentally induced doubts about their intelligence with greater concerns about their partner's likely rejection (Murray et al., 1998). As a consequence, people who chronically feel less valued may be overly sensitized to their own failures, seeing such failings as a sign that a partner's rejection is likely to be forthcoming.

Now imagine that Sally comes home to find Harry in a generally irritable mood, grumbling about the lack of food in the fridge. Rather than brushing this off, Sally may worry that such grumbling signifies broader displeasure with her or the relationship. Consistent with this logic, Holmes and Rempel (1989) argue that uncertainty about a partner's trustworthiness sensitizes married intimates to the motivational implications of their behaviors. Accordingly, people who feel less positively regarded by their spouse should scrutinize their partner's daily relationship behaviors for hints of negative behaviors that might suggest rejection is imminent.

Supporting this hypothesis, people with lower self-esteem (and thus less confidence in their partner's regard) overinterpret their dating partner's (hypothetical) negative moods, seeing them as symptomatic of a partner's ill feelings toward the self (Bellavia & Murray, 2003). They also react to experimentally induced signs of a partner's irritation by anticipating rejection (Murray, Rose, Bellavia, Holmes, & Kusche, 2002). Similarly, dating intimates high on attachment-related anxiety interpret a partner's hypothetical (Collins, 1996) and actual misdeeds in suspicious ways that are likely to exacerbate hurt feelings (Simpson, Rholes, & Phillips, 1996). People who chronically anticipate interpersonal rejection also attribute negative intent to a new romantic partner's hypothetical negative behaviors (Downey & Feldman, 1996).

On the other side of the coin, confident expectations that a partner sees positive qualities in the self may inoculate highs against all but the most threatening situations. For people who feel more positively regarded, felt security goals are likely to be largely satiated (and thus quiescent). Rather than looking for signs of a partner's approval, such people may instead approach their relationships with an eye toward confirming and maintaining benevolent expectations about a partner's caring. When people chronically feel positively regarded, their own failings and their partner's negative behaviors may be more easily discounted, and consequently may hurt less. Consistent with this hypothesis, people who generally anticipate interpersonal acceptance—that is, people high in self-esteem—actually compensate for experimentally induced doubts about their own intelligence or considerateness by exaggerating how much their partner accepts and loves them (Murray et al., 1998).

To examine our hypotheses about "appraisal sensitivity," we first operationalized the chronic activation of felt security goals, our between-persons variable, as people's perceptions of their partner's regard for them on specific interpersonal qualities, such as warm, critical, responsive, and demanding. (We had asked people to describe how they believed their partner saw them on these traits.) Thus, the activation of felt security goals refers to the perception that the partner sees relatively few positive qualities in oneself. Conversely, the satiation of felt security goals refers to the perception that the partner sees many positive qualities in oneself.[1]

We then identified three types of threatening events (our within-person independent variables): the incidence of conflict on a given day (e.g., "we had a minor disagreement," "we had a serious argument"), the number of negative partner behaviors perceived on any given day (e.g., "partner was irritated or angry with me," "partner criticized or complained about me," "partner insulted me," and how negative a mood or psychological state the partner was actually in each day (e.g., the partner's responses to items such as "anxious," "sad/depressed," "unsure of myself"). We also identified a category of positive events by summing the number of positive partner behaviors perceived each day (e.g., "partner told me he/she loves me," "partner praised me," "partner was physically affectionate").

We next identified three measures of rejection anxiety (our within-person dependent variables): perceptions of the partner's rejection (e.g., "rejected or hurt by my partner," "partner doesn't understand me," "partner wasn't there for me"), anxiety about the partner's acceptance (e.g., "worried about disappointing partner," "unsure whether partner is happy in our relationship," "partner is bored with me"), and comfort in the partner's acceptance (e.g., "partner loves me," "partner accepts me as I am," "partner sees the best in me").

As diary data is nested in nature (day is nested within person, and person is nested within couple), we employed a multilevel modeling program to analyze the data. Specifically, our appraisal sensitivity hypotheses postulate cross-level interactions: within-person effects, such as the link between perceptions of conflict on one day, and feelings of rejection the next, are moderated by a between-persons effect, feeling more or less positively regarded by one's spouse. Accordingly, we conducted a series of multilevel models predicting one day's feelings of rejection (or acceptance) from the *prior* day's feelings of rejection (or acceptance), the *prior* day's triggering event, chronic perceptions of the partner's regard, and the cross-level prior day's triggering event by chronic perceptions of the partner's regard interaction. (More detailed descriptions of our analytic procedures are available in Murray, Bellavia, Rose, & Griffin, 2003, and Murray, Griffin, Rose, & Bellavia, 2003.)

These analyses yielded significant cross-level interactions consistent with our appraisal sensitivity hypotheses (Murray, Bellavia, Rose, & Griffin, 2003). Generally, married intimates who felt less positively regarded, and thus were presumably trying to gauge the likelihood of acceptance in any specific context, read rejected-related meaning into negative, but not positive, situations. That is, lows felt more rejected on days after their partner had been in a worse-than-average mood (as compared to low-threat days). In contrast, people who chronically felt more positively regarded actually felt more accepted and loved by their partner (and less rejected) on days after they had reported higher than average levels of conflict or negative partner behaviors (compared to low-threat days). Thus, chronic perceptions of a partner's regard set the activation threshold of relationship-specific sociometers at high or low levels, leading people to interpret specific situations in ways that reinforce chronic feelings of being more or less positively regarded.

Although we believe these results illustrate the consequences of felt security goal activation on appraisal processes, at least three alternate explanations are possible. The first alternative is that people who feel less positively regarded may read more rejection into reasonably mundane signs of negativity because such events chronically recur in their relationships. For people who feel more valued, however, occasional signs of negativity may be more easily discounted because they rarely occur. To examine this possibility, we conducted a set of control analyses where we separately controlled for the mean levels of conflict, the mean levels of negative partner behaviors, and the mean level of negative partner mood. In these control analyses, people who felt less positively regarded were still more troubled by greater lingering concerns about rejection than highs on the days after they had detected a greater than average number of potential trouble signs in their marriages.

The second alternative is that people who feel less positively regarded may actually possess partners who value them less, and really do behave in ways that warrant greater concerns about rejection. This possibility seems unlikely. First, further analyses revealed that people who felt less positively regarded read more into a partner's perceived negative behaviors than highs when we controlled for that aspect of their perceptions that was grounded in their partner's actual, or at least, self-reported behavior that day. Second, when we controlled for the partner's actual appraisal of the intimate, and thus the kernel of truth in these reflected appraisals, people who felt less positively regarded still read more into negative situations.

The third alternative is that the apparent effects of relationship-specific needs for a partner's acceptance might actually reflect the effects of general approval motivations. That is, perceptions of a partner's regard might moderate these dynamics because perceived regard is a proxy for a more general mental model, such as global self-esteem. To evaluate this possibility, we included global self-esteem as a control variable in our analyses, and we still found the expected effects. Therefore, perceptions of a partner's regard, a relationship-specific representation, confer a resilience or vulnerability not contained in more general representations.

The Self-Esteem Stakes: Self-Esteem Sensitivity

Unfortunately for lows, the rejections they too readily perceive should also sting or hurt more (Path B in Figure 7.1). That is, people who feel less positively regarded by their partner should internalize experiences of rejection, feeling worse about themselves in the face of their partner's perceived or actual rejection (because acute feelings of rejection present a greater proportional loss to an already impoverished self-esteem resource). To the extent that Sally is unsure of Harry's affections, for instance, her feelings of self-esteem should be highly contingent on recent experiences with feeling accepted or rejected within the relationship. Consistent with this "self-esteem sensitivity" hypothesis, Leary and Baumeister (2000) argued that chronic low self-esteem, and thus general expectations of rejection, renders being rejected in any specific situation all the more painful. For instance, low, but not high, self-esteem people feel worse about themselves in the face of strangers' rejection (Nezlek et al., 1997). Similarly, low, but not high, self-esteem dating intimates respond to induced fears of their partner's rejection with diminished state self-esteem (Murray et al., 2002, Experiment 3).

For people who chronically feel more positively regarded, however, the contingencies surrounding interpersonal acceptance may not be all that salient (e.g., Baldwin & Sinclair, 1996). Instead, people who chronically feel more valued may think and behave in ways that suggest they are relatively immune to such contingencies (at least in the context of the relatively mundane events of daily relationship life). Consistent with this logic, Leary and Baumeister (2000) suggest that some of the self-esteem protective (or self-deceptive) tactics of high self-esteem people, such as derogating the source of criticism, may reflect a kind of cognitive, and perhaps automatic, override of the sociometer. As a result, on those occasions when highs do perceive signs of a partner's perceived or actual rejection, resilient expectations of acceptance should lessen the sting of this potential threat to self-esteem, leaving their feelings of self-worth much less sensitive to situated aberrations in their perceptions of their spouse's acceptance.

To examine these self-esteem sensitivity hypotheses, we again operationalized the activation of felt security goals, our between-persons variable, as people's perceptions of their partner's regard for them on specific interpersonal qualities. In these analyses, the daily measures of felt rejection, anxiety about acceptance, and felt acceptance then became our within-person independent variables. We then created a measure of state self-esteem each day, our within-person dependent variable, by averaging responses to items tapping self-evaluative emotions (e.g., "good about myself," "unsure of myself," "unlikable," "lonely"). Next, we conducted multilevel models predicting today's self-esteem from the prior day's self-esteem, the prior day's rejection anxieties, chronic perceptions of the partner's regard, and the cross-level prior day's rejection anxieties by chronic perceived regard interaction.

These analyses yielded a significant cross-level interaction consistent with our self-esteem sensitivity hypothesis (Murray, Griffin, Rose, & Bellavia, 2003). That is, chronic perceptions of a partner's regard predicted how much concerns about a partner's rejection deflated self-esteem. People who felt less positively regarded reported feeling worse about themselves on days after they experienced more anxiety about their partner's acceptance (as compared to low-anxiety days). In contrast, for people high on perceived regard, one day's anxieties about acceptance did not turn into the next day's self-doubts. Thus, operating at a relationship-specific felt security deficit sensitized lows to the contingencies of acceptance, leaving their feelings about themselves much more vulnerable to situationally heightened anxieties about their partner's acceptance.

We interpreted these effects as evidence of the greater self-esteem costs of perceiving rejection when people are operating at a felt security deficit, and thus actually seeking greater reason to trust in the partner's acceptance. Alternate explanations for these results are again possible, however. The most obvious one is that signs of a partner's impending disaffection might hurt the self-esteem of lows more because their partner is behaving in an objectively worse fashion, and not because chronically activated felt security concerns sensitize them to perceived rejections. To examine this possibility, we conducted a number of additional analyses where we controlled for the partner's self-reported negative (and positive) behavior each day, and analyses that controlled for the partner's actual appraisal of the participant on the interpersonal qualities measure. In all of these analyses, people who felt less positively regarded still felt significantly worse about themselves on days after they reported greater than average levels of anxiety about their partner's acceptance (relative to low-anxiety days).

The second possibility is that feeling rejected threatens the self-esteem of lows more than that of highs because lows are operating at a general rather than a relationship-specific inclusion deficit. That is, the moderating effects of perceived regard might be masking the moderating effects of global self-esteem. Accordingly, we included global self-esteem as a control variable in the analyses described above, and we still found significant moderating effects of perceived regard.

Maintaining Safety from Harm: Behavioral Regulation

The findings thus far suggest that people who chronically feel less positively regarded are not only more likely than highs to perceive rejection in the aftermath of routine relationship threats, but they are also more likely to internalize such (incorrectly) perceived rebuffs. How might the greater self-esteem threat posed by rejection affect the capacity of lows to put the needed positive mental and behavioral spin on things when they are feeling acutely rejected and self-protective motivations are likely heightened (Path C in Figure 7.1)?

For instance, in making a charitable attribution for Sally's snippy comments about his capacity to dress himself, Harry protects a belief in Sally's generally more sanguine disposition, but leaves his self-esteem again vulnerable to future criticisms if his faith in Sally proves to be unfounded. In specific situations, then, the tendency to read rejection and hurt into daily events may make it difficult for intimates who chronically feel less positively regarded by their partner to respond constructively to difficulties. Instead, they might react to the self-esteem sting of rejections with anger, and with the defensive step of actively distancing from the source of the hurt: the partner or the relationship. Devaluing the partner, lashing out behaviorally, or reducing feelings of closeness likely all function to lessen the acute threat to self-esteem posed by feeling rejected (Murray et al., 1998). After all, one need not believe the message if the messenger can be discredited. Accordingly, intimates who chronically feel less positively regarded may settle for the sense of safety that comes from avoiding situations that put themselves at risk for further harm, thus opting for self-protection over relationship promotion.

Consistent with this logic, people typically react to acute rejection experiences by strangers by aggressing against those who ostracized them, suggesting that people's most immediate impulse is to return hurts in a tit-for-tat fashion (Twenge, Baumeister, Tice, & Stucke, 2001). In romantic relationships, people who are dispositionally prone to questioning another's acceptance also seem to react in this self-protective (perhaps self-vindicating) way. Low self-esteem people respond to induced anxieties about rejection by derogating their partner's traits (Murray et al., 1998; Murray et al., 2002). More anxiously attached women also display greater anger toward their partner in situations in which their partner may not have been as responsive as they hoped (Rholes, Simpson, & Orina, 1999). Women chronically high on rejection sensitivity also respond to a potential dating partner's disinterest by evaluating that partner more negatively (Ayduk, Downey, Testa, Yen, & Shoda, 1999). They are also more likely to initiate conflicts on days after they felt more rejected by their partner; indeed, simply priming rejection-related words activates hostility-related thoughts for these women (Ayduk et al., 1999).[2]

In contrast, for people who chronically feel more positively regarded, resilient expectations of acceptance seem to lessen the self-esteem sting of rejection in ways that might allow them to put protecting the relationship ahead of defending against a perceived blow to the self. As a result, people who feel more positively regarded may more readily compensate for signs of difficulty by drawing closer, emphasizing the strengths of their partner and relationship. In a sense, highs may find a sense of safety in their relationships through the kinds of cognitive and behavioral transformations that diminish the threat and enhance the value of the relationship. Consistent with the idea that felt acceptance fosters generosity, unconsciously primed thoughts of security and acceptance diminish people's normal tendencies to derogate outgroup members (Mikulincer & Shaver, 2001) and increase people's desire to seek support from others in dealing with a personal crisis (Pierce & Lydon, 1998). Similarly, consciously activated feelings of being unconditionally accepted reduce people's tendency to disparage others in response to a threat to the self (Schimel, Arndt, Pyszczynski, & Greenberg, 2001).

To explore our hypotheses about behavioral regulation, we again operationalized the activation of felt security goals, our between-persons variable, as people's perceptions of their partner's regard for them. In these analyses, the daily measures of felt rejection, anxiety about acceptance, and felt acceptance again served as our within-person independent variables. We then created two different categories of within-person dependent variables, one tapping self-protective responses to felt rejection, and the other tapping relationship-promotive responses. Specifically, the level of negative, cold, and distancing behaviors directed at the partner each day served as our measure of distancing or self-protection (e.g., "criticized or complained about my partner," "ignored my partner," "snapped or yelled at my partner"), and the level of closeness expressed toward the partner each day served as our measure of relationship promotion (e.g., "in love with my partner," "happy in my relationship"). We then conducted multilevel models predicting today's behavioral response from that same behavior on the prior day, the prior day's rejection anxieties, chronic perceptions of the partner's regard, and the cross-level prior day's rejection anxieties by chronic perceived regard interaction.

These analyses yielded significant cross-level interactions consistent with our hypotheses about behavioral regulation (Murray, Bellavia, Rose, & Griffin, 2003). As we expected, unfulfilled needs for a partner's approval predisposed people to respond to acute feelings of rejection and vulnerability by self-protectively distancing themselves from their partner. Specifically, people who felt less positively regarded reacted to feelings of hurt and anxiety about acceptance on one day by treating their partner in more cold, critical, and rejecting ways the next day (relative to low-vulnerability days). Thus, people who felt less accepted reacted to the acute pain of rejection by giving their partners less power to hurt them in the future—a self-protective reaction. Resilient expectations of acceptance, however, allowed people who felt more positively regarded to put protecting the relationship ahead of defending against a perceived slight or hurt to the self. These people actually drew relatively closer to their partner on days after they felt most vulnerable rather than responding to hurt with hurtful actions in a tit-for-tat exchange of negative behaviors.

These findings suggest that feeling more or less positively regarded by one's partner does regulate how people resolve the possible tension between self-protection and relationship-promotion motives on a day-to-day basis, but alternative explanations are again possible. Perhaps the most obvious alternative is that people who feel less positively regarded may respond to feeling acutely rejected and vulnerable with hurtful action because they are defending themselves against a battery of real criticisms and complaints (not because they are overly sensitized to rejection). However, we still found the interactions described above in analyses where we controlled for the partner's mean level of self-confessed rejecting behavior, suggesting that the actions that lows take in response to acute vulnerability are largely unwarranted by their partner's actual behavior. A second possibility is that people who feel less positively regarded may respond to situated hurts by distancing themselves because they are involved in less satisfying relationships marked by habitual patterns of reciprocated negativity (e.g., Gottman, 1994). To explore this possibility, we controlled for satisfaction in the analyses described above, and we still found the expected effects. The third possibility is that the moderating effects of perceived regard really reflect the moderating influence of a more general representation: global self-esteem. Again, though, the control analyses revealed consistent moderating effects of perceived regard when we controlled for global self-esteem. Thus, relationship-specific expectations of acceptance play a role in governing how people respond to situated experiences of rejection that is not already captured by more general models.

THE SELF-FULFILLING EFFECTS OF FELT SECURITY REGULATION

Since the experience of slights and hurts at the hands of a romantic partner is inevitable, the challenge in maintaining a satisfying relationship rests in preventing such situated threats from triggering the defensive devaluation of the partner (and the delivery of reciprocal slights). Confident expectations of acceptance seem to dull the self-esteem sting of rejection in ways that allow people to see an (occasionally) hurtful partner in the best possible light. For people who feel less positively regarded, however, the slightest offense is likely to be seen as a sign of impending rejection, motivating them to reject and devalue their partner, and thus to distance themselves from the sting of any further perceived slights. In this way, the desire to protect themselves against hurt could ultimately and ironically lead people who are trying to find signs of acceptance to undermine the attachment bonds they presumably want to preserve.

In fact, in the diary study, the *partners* of people who felt less positively regarded (correctly) believed that they were the target of more hurtful and rejecting behaviors on days after lows had felt most vulnerable (Murray, Bellavia, Rose, & Griffin, 2003). Even though they were not annoyed or upset initially, the partners of lows were also more likely to see lows as being selfish and demanding on days after lows had felt most hurt and vulnerable. Further illustrating the potential for such self-fulfilling effects, women who chronically anticipate rejection behave more negatively toward their dating partner during conflicts, and elicit more rejecting behavior in that specific instance (Downey et al., 1998). Moreover, on days after rejection-sensitive women feel acutely rejected by their dating partner, their partner reports greater dissatisfaction (Downey et al., 1998). Consequently, repeated experiences with a partner who seems to read too much into relatively mundane problems, and then lashes out in return, may set the stage for cycles of reciprocated negative affect and behavior that hallmark marital distress (Gottman, 1994).

The Cognitive and Behavior Signature of Relationship Resilience

The fact that such self-fulfilling effects emerged over the short term led us to wonder how people's habitual means of regulating the risk of rejection might affect how the relationship unfolds over the longer term. For instance, if Sally is likely to internalize rejections, feeling worse about herself in the face of Harry's imagined rebuffs, will that affect how her marriage fares over time? Will it affect her more general beliefs about her own worthiness of love and the level of acceptance she anticipates from others? In turn, if Sally's habitual response to feeling hurt, and having her esteem threatened, is to criticize Harry in return, or to start a fight about an unrelated matter, will that eventually erode both her and Harry's satisfaction? Alternately, if Harry is able to respond to feeling rejected by actually drawing closer to Sally rather than pushing her away, will that affect Sally's capacity to sustain her trust in Harry?

Our most current research stems from such possibilities. Consider again the paths illustrated in Figure 7.1. Each of these paths can be thought of as a person-specific affective, cognitive, or behavioral response profile—a within-person pattern of covariation that is evident by following a person across situations and days. For instance, the magnitude and direction of the slope linking one day's rejection anxiety to the next day's self-esteem for any individual person in the diary study taps the level of that person's habitual self-esteem sensitivity to rejection. Similarly, the magnitude and direction of the slope linking one day's rejection anxiety to the next day's cold rejecting behavior to the partner taps that person's habitual tendency to respond to feeling rejected by self-protectively behaving badly. Alternately, such a slope might reflect another person's more relationship-promotive tendency to respond to rejection anxiety by drawing closer to a partner, and expressing need for love and support.

We believe that the microprocess of felt security regulation we observed in the diary study underlies a much broader cycle of relationship development and change. Through repeated exposure to similar situations, the residues of specific, daily experiences may eventually be represented as cognitive, affective, and behavioral signatures—"if–then" associations that are highly accessible in memory, and automatically activated in threatening situations (Baldwin, 1992; Bargh & Ferguson, 2000). A relationship's ultimate fate may thus rest in the nature of the relational schemas that people develop in their interactions with their partner. Over time, these individualized, relationship-specific patterns of thinking and relating may then shape more general expectations about one's own worthiness of love and the benevolence of others.

In our most recent research, we have been exploring these possibilities. As a first, exploratory study, we collected 1-year follow-up data from the married couples involved in our diary study (see Murray, Griffin, Rose, & Bellavia, 2003, for further details). We then operationalized one type of self-esteem sensitivity signature (Path B in Figure 7.1) as the size of the within-person slope linking yesterday's anxiety about acceptance to today's diminished self-esteem (derived from multilevel analyses). We also operationalized one type of self-protective behavioral regulation signature as the within-person slope linking yesterday's felt rejection to today's negative behavior toward the partner (again derived from a multilevel model). Next we related these within-person slopes to changes in satisfaction over time.

These analyses revealed promising support for the idea that the ultimate fate of relationships may rest in part in how people regulate the tension between self-protection and relationship-promotion motives on a day-to-day basis. First, reacting to perceived rejections with diminished self-esteem predicted declines in marital satisfaction (Murray, Bellavia, Rose, & Griffin, 2003). When people reacted to one day's anxieties about their partner's rejection by reporting diminished self-esteem the next day, their partner reported significantly greater declines in satisfaction over the year. Second, when women's strategic response to feeling rejected was to behave badly, their husband reported greater declines in satisfaction. The more women reacted to one day's felt rejection by behaving in a more negative and rejecting way toward their husband on subsequent days, the greater the decline in their husband's satisfaction over the year. Impressively, these effects emerged in analyses that controlled for the mean levels of the self-related affect, or behavior in question, suggesting that the ultimate fate of people's relationships really may rest in the mental and behavioral associations they form to specific situations (see Mischel & Shoda, 1995, and Holmes, 2002, for similar reasoning). Accordingly, in our next major project, we will continue to explore these types of dynamics in newlywed couples.

CONCLUSION

On the brighter side, marital relationships offer a unique opportunity for the protection and enhancement of self-esteem (see Aron, Aron, Tudor, & Nelson, 1991; Drigotas et al., 1999). On the darker side, the prospect of the loss of spousal admiration also poses a substantial threat to self-esteem (Baumeister & Leary, 1995). Given such stakes, it is not all that surprising that people only allow themselves to make the leap of faith that relationship promotion entails when they trust in their partner's ongoing positive regard and acceptance. For people who find this sense of trust, a partner's perceived love and support provides sufficient safety to risk being generous in one's attributions, and accommodating, and self-sacrificing in one's behavior. For people who lack this sense of trust, however, signs of a partner's day-to-day irritation or annoyance more readily undermine the more precarious sense of self-esteem that made confidence in a partner's acceptance difficult to achieve in the first place. Rather than eliciting the partner's comfort and approval, however, such oversensitivity to rejection only seems to lead to self-protective reactions that are likely to alienate the partner over time, creating the very reality that intimates who feel less positively regarded are motivated to avoid.

ACKNOWLEDGMENT

The preparation of this chapter was supported by Grant No. SBR 9817282 from the National Science Foundation and by Grant No. MH 60105-02 from the National Institute of Mental Health.

NOTES

1. In drawing these parallels, we are not trying to argue that feeling understood by a partner is unimportant to felt acceptance. In fact, Reis and Shaver's (1988) process model of intimacy is based on the assumption that perceptions of a partner's caring depend on the per-

ception of being understood. Similarly, Swann, Hixon, and De La Ronde (1992) reported that low self-esteem people report greater intimacy in their marriage when their partner sees them as negatively as they see themselves. From our perspective, however, people need to be able to pinpoint particular reasons why their partner is likely to love and value them before they are likely to seek a partner's understanding or validation of their more negative qualities.

2. The idea that lows react to acute feelings of rejection by finding fault in their partner and engaging in overtly rejecting behaviors may seem inconsistent with a basic tenet of the sociometer model—namely, that feelings of rejection are thought to function as an alarm system that activates compensatory processes and approach behaviors aimed at securing acceptance (Heatherton & Vohs, 2000; Leary, Tambor, Terdal, & Downs, 1995; Vohs & Heatherton, 2001; Williams, Cheung, & Choi, 2001; Williams & Sommer, 1997). In routine social interactions, though, people need not seek acceptance from someone who appears to be rejecting. Instead, they may readily alleviate feelings of rejection by approaching novel others. In romantic relationships, however, people may not have this luxury, as they are often caught in the position of feeling hurt by the very person whose acceptance they most need. It is for this reason that we believe that a sense of acceptance needs to be secured in romantic relationships *before* intimates are likely to be willing to respond to acute feelings of hurt and vulnerability by behaving constructively, drawing closer, and thus approaching the source of that hurt.

REFERENCES

Andersen, S. M., & Chen, S. (2002). The relational self: An interpersonal social-cognitive theory. *Psychological Review, 109*, 619–645.

Aron, A., Aron, E. N., Tudor, M., & Nelson, G. (1991). Close relationships as including other in the self. *Journal of Personality and Social Psychology, 60*, 241–253.

Aron, A., Dutton, D. G., Aron, E. N., & Iverson, A. (1989). Experiences of falling in love. *Journal of Social and Personal Relationships, 6*, 243–257.

Aron, A., Paris, M., & Aron, E. N. (1995). Falling in love: Prospective studies of self-concept change. *Journal of Personality and Social Psychology, 69*, 1102–1112.

Ayduk, O., Downey, G., Testa, A., Yen, Y., & Shoda, Y. (1999). Does rejection elicit hostility in rejection sensitive women? *Social Cognition, 17*, 245–271.

Baldwin, M. W. (1992). Relational schemas and the processing of social information. *Psychological Bulletin, 112*, 461–484.

Baldwin, M. W., Carrell, S. E., & Lopez, D. F. (1990). Priming relationship schemas: My advisor and the pope are watching me from the back of my mind. *Journal of Experimental Social Psychology, 26*, 435–454.

Baldwin, M. W., & Sinclair, L. (1996). Self-esteem and "if . . . then" contingencies of interpersonal acceptance. *Journal of Personality and Social Psychology, 71*, 1130–1141.

Bargh, J. A., & Ferguson, M. J. (2000). Beyond behaviorism: On the automaticity of higher mental processes. *Psychological Bulletin, 126*, 925–945.

Baumeister, R. F., & Leary, M. R. (1995). The need to belong: Desire for interpersonal attachments as a fundamental human motivation. *Psychological Bulletin, 117*, 497–529.

Bellavia, G., & Murray, S. L. (2003). Did I do that?: Self-esteem related differences in reactions to romantic partners' moods. *Personal Relationships, 10*, 77–96.

Berscheid, E., & Fei, J. (1977). Romantic love and sexual jealousy. In G. Clanton & L. G. Smith (Eds.), *Jealousy* (pp. 101–109). Englewood Cliffs, NJ: Prentice-Hall.

Bowlby, J. (1982). *Attachment and loss: Vol. 1. Attachment.* London: Hogarth Press.

Bradbury, T. N., & Fincham, F. D. (1990). Attributions in marriage: Review and critique. *Psychological Bulletin, 107,* 3–23.

Braiker, H. B., & Kelley, H. H. (1979). Conflict in the development of close relationships. In R. L. Burgess & T. L. Huston (Eds.), *Social exchange in developing relationships* (pp. 135–168). New York: Academic Press.

Collins, N. L. (1996). Working models of attachment: Implications for explanation, emotion and behavior. *Journal of Personality and Social Psychology, 71,* 810–832.

Collins, N. L., & Feeney, B. C. (2000). A safe haven: An attachment theory perspective on support seeking and caregiving in intimate relationships. *Journal of Personality and Social Psychology, 78,* 1053–1073.

Cooley, C. H. (1902). *Human nature and the social order.* New York: Schocken Books.

Downey, G., & Feldman, S. I. (1996). Implications of rejection sensitivity for intimate relationships. *Journal of Personality and Social Psychology, 70,* 1327–1343.

Downey, G., Freitas, A. L., Michaelis, B., & Khouri, H. (1998). The self-fulfilling prophecy in close relationships: Rejection sensitivity and rejection by romantic partners. *Journal of Personality and Social Psychology, 75,* 545–560.

Drigotas, S. M., Rusbult, C. M., Wieselquist, J., & Whitton, S. W. (1999). Close partner as sculptor of the ideal self: Behavioral affirmation and the Michelangelo phenomenon. *Journal of Personality and Social Psychology, 77,* 293–323.

Felson, R. B. (1989). Parents and the reflected appraisal process: A longitudinal analysis. *Journal of Personality and Social Psychology, 56,* 965–971.

Fraley, R. C., & Shaver, P. R. (2000). Adult romantic attachment: Theoretical developments, emerging controversies, and unanswered questions. *Review of General Psychology, 4,* 132–154.

Gardner, W., Pickett, C. L., & Brewer, M. B. (2000). Social exclusion and selective memory: How the need to belong influences memory for social events. *Personality and Social Psychology Bulletin, 26,* 486–496.

Gottman, J. M. (1994). *What predicts divorce?: The relationship between marital processes and marital outcomes.* Hillsdale, NJ: Erlbaum.

Grote, N. K., & Clark, M. S. (2001). Perceiving unfairness in the family: Cause or consequence of marital distress? *Journal of Personality and Social Psychology, 80,* 281–293.

Hazan, C., & Diamond, L. M. (2000). The place of attachment in human mating. *Review of General Psychology, 4,* 186–204.

Hazan, C., & Shaver, P. R. (1994). Attachment as an organizational framework for research on close relationships. *Psychological Inquiry, 5,* 1–22.

Heatherton, T. F., & Vohs, K. D. (2000). Interpersonal evaluations following threats to self: Role of self-esteem. *Journal of Personality and Social Psychology, 78,* 725–736.

Hinkley, K., & Andersen, S. M. (1996). The working self-concept in transference: Significant-other activation and self-change. *Journal of Personality and Social Psychology, 71,* 1279–1295.

Holmes, J. G. (2002). Interpersonal expectations as the building blocks of social cognition: An interdependence theory perspective. *Personal Relationship, 9,* 1–26.

Holmes, J. G., & Rempel, J. K. (1989). Trust in close relationships. In C. Hendrick (Ed.), *Review of personality and social psychology: Close relationships* (Vol. 10, pp. 187–219). Newbury Park, CA: Sage.

Kelley, H. H. (1979). *Personal relationship: Their structures and processes.* Hillsdale, NJ: Erlbaum.

Kelley, H. H. (1983). Love and commitment. In H. H. Kelley, E. Berscheid, A. Christensen, J. H. Harvey, T. L. Huston, G. Levinger, E. McClintock, L. A. Peplau, & D. R. Peterson (Eds.), *Close relationships* (pp. 265–314). New York: Freeman.

Kenny, D. A. (1994). *Interpersonal perception: A social relations analysis.* New York: Guilford Press.

Leary, M. R., & Baumeister, R. F. (2000). The nature and function of self-esteem: Sociometer theory. In M. P. Zanna (Ed.), *Advances in experimental social psychology* (Vol. 32, pp. 2–51). San Diego, CA: Academic Press.

Leary, M. R., Cottrell, C. A., & Misha, P. (2001). Deconfounding the effects of dominance and social acceptance on self-esteem. *Journal of Personality and Social Psychology, 81,* 898–909.

Leary, M. R., Haupt, A. L., Strausser, K. S., & Chokel, J. T. (1998). Calibrating the sociometer: The relationship between interpersonal appraisals and state self-esteem. *Journal of Personality and Social Psychology, 74,* 1290–1299.

Leary, M. R., Tambor, E. S., Terdal, S. K., & Downs, D. L. (1995). Self-esteem as an interpersonal monitor: The sociometer hypothesis. *Journal of Personality and Social Psychology, 68,* 518–530.

McNulty, S. E., & Swann, W. B. (1994). Identity negotiation in roommate relationships: The self as architect and consequence of social reality. *Journal of Personality and Social Psychology, 67,* 1012–1023.

Mead, G. H. (1934). *Mind, self and society.* Chicago: University of Chicago Press.

Mikulincer, M., Birnbaum, G., Woddis, D., & Nachmias, O. (2000). Stress and accessibility of proximity-related thoughts: Exploring the normative and intra-individual components of attachment theory. *Journal of Personality and Social Psychology, 78,* 509–523.

Mikulincer, M., Gillath, O., & Shaver, P. R. (2002). Activation of the attachment system in adulthood: Threat-related primes increase the accessibility of mental representations of attachment figures. *Journal of Personality and Social Psychology, 83,* 881–895.

Mikulincer, M., & Shaver, P. R. (2001). Attachment theory and intergroup bias: Evidence that priming the secure base schema attenuates negative reactions to outgroups. *Journal of Personality and Social Psychology, 81,* 97–115.

Mischel, W., & Shoda, Y. (1995). A cognitive–affective system theory of personality: Reconceptualizing situations, dispositions, dynamics, and invariance in personality structure. *Psychological Review, 102,* 246–268.

Murray, S. L. (1999). The quest for conviction: Motivated cognition in romantic relationships. *Psychological Inquiry, 10,* 23–34.

Murray, S. L., Bellavia, G., Rose, P., & Griffin, D. (2003). Once hurt, twice hurtful: How perceived regard regulates daily marital interaction. *Journal of Personality and Social Psychology, 84,* 126–147.

Murray, S. L., Griffin, D. W., Rose, P., & Bellavia, G. (2003). Calibrating the sociometer: The relational contingencies of self-esteem. *Journal of Personality and Social Psychology, 85*, 63–84.

Murray, S. L., & Holmes, J. G. (1999). The (mental) ties that bind: Cognitive structures that predict relationship resilience. *Journal of Personality and Social Psychology, 77*, 1228–1244.

Murray, S. L., Holmes, J. G., Dolderman, D., & Griffin, D. W. (2000). What the motivated mind sees: Comparing friends' perspectives to married partners' views of each other. *Journal of Experimental Social Psychology, 36*, 600–620.

Murray, S. L., Holmes, J. G., & Griffin, D. (1996a). The benefits of positive illusions: Idealization and the construction of satisfaction in close relationships. *Journal of Personality and Social Psychology, 70*, 79–98.

Murray, S. L., Holmes, J. G., & Griffin, D. (1996ab). The self-fulfilling nature of positive illusions in romantic relationship: Love is not blind, but prescient. *Journal of Personality and Social Psychology, 71*, 1155–1180.

Murray, S. L., Holmes, J. G., & Griffin, D. W. (2000). Self-esteem and the quest for felt security: How perceived regard regulates attachment processes. *Journal of Personality and Social Psychology, 78*, 478–498.

Murray, S. L., Holmes, J. G., Griffin, D. W., Bellavia, G., & Rose, P. (2001). The mismeasure of love: How self-doubt contaminates relationship beliefs. *Personality and Social Psychology Bulletin, 27*, 423–436.

Murray, S. L., Holmes, J. G., MacDonald, G., & Ellsworth, P. (1998). Through the looking glass darkly?: When self-doubts turn into relationship insecurities. *Journal of Personality and Social Psychology, 75*, 1459–1480.

Murray, S. L., Rose, P., Bellavia, G., Holmes, J., & Kusche, A. (2002). When rejection stings: How self-esteem constrains relationship-enhancement processes. *Journal of Personality and Social Psychology, 83*, 556–573.

Neff, L. A., & Karney, B. R. (2002). Judgments of a relationship partner: Specific accuracy but global enhancement. *Journal of Personality, 70*, 1079–1112.

Nezlek, J. B., Kowalski, R. M., Leary, M. R., Blevins, T., & Holgate, S. (1997). Personality moderators of reactions to interpersonal rejection: Depression and trait self-esteem. *Personality and Social Psychology Bulletin, 23*, 1235–1244.

Pierce, T., & Lydon, J. (1998). Priming relational schemas: Effects of contextually activated and chronically accessible interpersonal expectations on responses to a stressful event. *Journal of Personality and Social Psychology, 75*, 1441–1448.

Reis, H. T., & Shaver, P. (1988). Intimacy as an interpersonal process. In S. W. Duck (Ed.), *Handbook of personal relationships* (pp. 367–389). London: Wiley.

Rholes, S. W., Simpson, J. A., Campbell, L., & Grich, J. (2001). Adult attachment and the transition to parenthood. *Journal of Personality and Social Psychology, 81*, 421–435.

Rholes, S. W., Simpson, J. A., & Orina, M. M. (1999). Attachment and anger in an anxiety-provoking situation. *Journal of Personality and Social Psychology, 76*, 940–957.

Rudich, E. A., & Vallacher, R. R. (1999). To belong or to self-enhance?: Motivational bases for choosing interaction partners. *Personality and Social Psychology Bulletin, 25*, 1387–1404.

Rusbult, C. E., & Buunk, B. P. (1993). Commitment processes in close relationships:

An interdependence analysis. *Journal of Social and Personal Relationships, 10,* 175–204.

Rusbult, C. E., Van Lange, P. A. M., Wildschut, T., Yovetich, N. A., & Verette, J. (2000). Perceived superiority in close relationships: Why it exists and persists. *Journal of Personality and Social Psychology, 79,* 521–545.

Rusbult, C. E., Verette, J., Whitney, G. A., Slovik, L. F., & Lipkus, I. (1991). Accommodation processes in close relationships: Theory and preliminary research evidence. *Journal of Personality and Social Psychology, 60,* 53–78.

Ruvolo, A., & Brennan, C. J. (1997). What's love got to do with it?: Close relationships and perceived growth. *Personality and Social Psychology Bulletin, 23,* 814–823.

Schimel, J., Arndt, J., Pyszczynski, T., & Greenberg, J. (2001). Being accepted for who we are: Evidence that social validation of the intrinsic self reduces general defensiveness. *Journal of Personality and Social Psychology, 80,* 35–52.

Shrauger, J. S., & Schoeneman, T. J. (1979). Symbolic interactionist view of the self-concept: Through the looking glass darkly. *Psychological Bulletin, 86,* 549–573.

Simpson, J. A., Ickes, W., & Blackstone, T. (1995). When the head protects the heart: Empathic accuracy in dating relationships. *Journal of Personality and Social Psychology, 69,* 629–641.

Simpson, J. A., Rholes, W. S., & Nelligan, J. S. (1992). Support seeking and support giving within couples in an anxiety-provoking situation: The role of attachment styles. *Journal of Personality and Social Psychology, 62,* 434–446.

Simpson, J. A., Rholes, W. S., & Phillips, D. (1996). Conflict in close relationship: An attachment perspective. *Journal of Personality and Social Psychology, 71,* 899–914.

Swann, W. B., Hixon, J. G., & De La Ronde, C. (1992). Embracing the bitter "truth": Negative self-concepts and marital commitment. *Psychological Science, 3,* 118–121.

Taylor, S. E. (1991). Asymmetrical effects of positive and negative events: The mobilization-minimization hypothesis. *Psychological Bulletin, 110,* 67–85.

Tooby, J., & Cosmides, L. (1996). Friendship and the banker's paradox: Other pathways to the evolution of adaptations for altruism. *Proceedings of the British Academy, 88,* 119–143.

Trobst, K. K. (2000). An interpersonal conceptualization and quantification of social support transactions. *Personality and Social Psychology Bulletin, 26,* 971–986.

Tucker, J. S., & Anders, S. L. (1999). Attachment style, interpersonal perception accuracy, and relationship satisfaction in dating couples. *Personality and Social Psychology Bulletin, 25,* 403–412.

Twenge, J. M., Baumeister, R. F., Tice, D. M., & Stucke, T. S. (2001). If you can't join them, beat them: Effects of social exclusion on aggressive behavior. *Journal of Personality and Social Psychology, 81,* 1058–1069.

Van Lange, P. A. M., Rusbult, C. E., Drigotas, S. M., Arriaga, X. B., Witcher, B. S., & Cox, C. L. (1997). Willingness to sacrifice in close relationships. *Journal of Personality and Social Psychology, 72,* 1373–1395.

Vohs, K. D., & Heatherton, T. F. (2001). Self-esteem and threats to self: Implications for self-construals and interpersonal perceptions. *Journal of Personality and Social Psychology, 81,* 1103–1118.

Vorauer, J. D., & Ross, M. (1996). The pursuit of knowledge in close relationships: An informational goals analysis. In G. J. O. Fletcher & J. Fitness (Eds.), *Knowledge structures in close relationships: A social psychological approach* (pp. 369–396). Mahwah, NJ: Erlbaum.

Wieselquist, J., Rusbult, C. E., Foster, C. A., & Agnew, C. R. (1999). Commitment, pro-relationship behavior, and trust in close relationships. *Journal of Personality and Social Psychology, 77,* 942–966.

Williams, K. D., Cheung, C. K. T., & Choi, W. (2001). Cyberostracism: Effects of being ignored over the Internet. *Journal of Personality and Social Psychology, 79,* 748–762.

Williams, K. D., & Sommer, K. L. (1997). Social ostracism by coworkers: Does rejection lead to loafing or compensation? *Personality and Social Psychology Bulletin, 23,* 693–706.

8

The Role of Prototypes
in Interpersonal Cognition

BEVERLEY FEHR

In one of the most famous palimony cases in U.S. law, Michelle Triola sued Lee Marvin for a portion of the rather substantial financial gains he had accumulated during the 6 years of their cohabitation. Triola argued that although they were not legally married, their relationship took the "form of a marriage." In her role as wife, she had sacrificed her own career to stay at home and manage their household and now expected compensation. Not surprisingly, Lee Marvin (who had initiated the breakup) argued that their relationship did not constitute a marriage. When Triola's lawyer asked him whether he had ever loved Michelle Triola "even a little bit," Marvin replied that he had not felt the kind of love that entailed "deep regard for the other person, truthfulness, loyalty, fidelity, and a tremendous sense of selflessness toward the other person." (Ultimately, the courts were more concerned with the technicalities of whether there had been an agreement about how assets would be divided in the event of termination than with the parties' conflicting definitions of their relationship.)

This case illustrates a fundamental premise of research and theorizing on interpersonal cognition, namely, that people form concepts to represent their interpersonal experiences and, once formed, these concepts influence perception and behavior. Based on a history of her interactions with Lee Marvin, Michelle Triola formed a cognitive representation of their relationship as a marital one. She then behaved in accordance with her concept of marriage, which apparently included the belief that wives should make sacrifices for their husbands. The corollary was that there should be monetary compensation for these sacrifices should the relationship dissolve. Lee Marvin claimed to have formed quite a different representation of their relationship, one that failed to meet the requirements for "real love," let alone marriage.

The *Triola v. Marvin* case speaks to the central issue to be addressed in this chapter, namely, "How does interpersonal cognition work?" Interpersonal cognition scholars assume that people form concepts to represent their interpersonal experiences and that these concepts influence the interpretation of relationship events and guide behavioral responses. But exactly how is this information represented? Do people develop clear-cut categories to represent different kinds of interpersonal situations or patterns? Does this information take the form of types (e.g., classifying relationships into particular categories, like Michelle Triola did) or is it stored as feature lists (as in Lee Marvin's definition of love)? Are some kinds of information more likely to become part of stored relational knowledge than others? Are there different kinds of interpersonal knowledge (e.g., knowledge based on one's experiences in a given relationship vs. the knowledge that is transmitted by one's culture)? How is all of this knowledge organized in cognitive representation? And, finally, when and how is this interpersonal knowledge applied to a specific situation?

The purpose of this chapter is to provide at least some preliminary answers to these questions by drawing on social-cognitive research on knowledge structures. More specifically, I focus on knowledge of concepts that are relevant to people's interpersonal experiences and relationships (e.g., emotion, love, commitment, intimacy, anger). The topics to be discussed include the content and organization of interpersonal knowledge structures, measurement issues, the relation between experts' and lay conceptions of relational knowledge, and the cognitive processing and behavioral implications of interpersonal knowledge. These topics are examined within the framework of *prototype theory*, a cognitive theory that has made substantial contributions to the study of interpersonal cognition.

THE ANATOMY OF A CONCEPT: A PROTOTYPE PERSPECTIVE

When social scientists begin to explore any new area, their first step is to define the concept of interest. It is assumed that this task entails the identification of individually necessary and jointly sufficient criterial attributes. However, in many domains, including that of interpersonal cognition, such attempts have met with repeated failure. Nevertheless, the belief has persisted that with sufficient insight, debate, and perhaps empirical examination, the "true" definition of social-scientific concepts can be found. In other words, definitions exist in the same way that fossils exist—the challenge is to discover and unearth them. And, as in any archeological excavation, one has to expect misses and false positives along the way. All of this changed, however, when Eleanor Rosch (1973a, 1973b) published her highly influential critique of the classical view of concepts. Rosch argued that many natural language concepts cannot be defined in the classical sense (i.e., defined in terms of necessary and sufficient criterial features). Rather, such concepts are organized around their clearest cases, or best examples, which Rosch referred to as *prototypes*. Further, she argued that members of a category can be ordered in terms of their degree of resemblance to the prototypical cases, with members shading gradually into nonmembers. Boundaries between categories therefore are blurry and ill-defined, rather than precise and clear-cut, as the classical view would have it.

Rosch (see Mervis & Rosch, 1981, for a review) substantiated her claims with numerous empirical articles demonstrating that natural language concepts such as "fruit," "vegetable," and "furniture" are structured as prototypes, such that some instances of these concepts are considered more prototypical than others. Moreover, this internal structure affects the cognitive processing of categories. For example, in a reaction time study, she showed that the category membership of prototypical instances is confirmed more quickly than that of nonprototypical instances (e.g., "robin" is verified as a kind of bird more quickly than is "chicken"; Rosch, 1973b). As will be seen, Rosch's theorizing and research would eventually revolutionize the way that many social scientists think about and study concepts, particularly those relevant to interpersonal cognition.

THE EVOLUTION OF PROTOTYPE ANALYSES

Prototype analyses initially followed the precedent set by Rosch and focused on analyses of types of concepts (i.e., members of categories). This was followed by analyses of the features or attributes of concepts. Most recently, prototype analyses have been extended to more complex knowledge structures, namely, patterns of relating.

Analyses of Types

Although Rosch's research focused on natural object categories, her ideas about the cognitive representation of natural language concepts appealed to social psychologists. Jim Russell and I (Fehr & Russell, 1984) noted the many attempts, dating back to the early Greek philosophers, to find a commonly accepted definition of *emotion*. The many failures prompted Duffy (1934, 1941) and others after her to suggest that the concept be abandoned altogether. The fact that emotion had eluded definition, yet was clearly a meaningful concept in ordinary usage, made it a promising candi-

date for a prototype analysis. We undertook such an analysis by first conducting a study in which participants were asked to list types of emotion
(Fehr & Russell, 1984, Study 1). Consistent with a prototype conceptualization, there was variability in the instances that came to mind: some
kinds of emotion (e.g., happiness, anger, sadness) were listed frequently,
and others less so (e.g., respect, awe). Still others seemed to lie at the fuzzy
boundary between emotion and related concepts (e.g., tiredness, hyperac-
tive). The critical test, however, was whether these types of emotion could
be meaningfully calibrated in terms of prototypicality. We asked a new
group of participants to rate a subset of the emotion terms generated in the
first study in terms of goodness-of-example (Fehr & Russell, 1984, Study
3). Some types of emotion were, in fact, rated as better examples of the
concept of emotion than others. Moreover, prototypical instances were
verified as types of emotion more quickly than were nonprototypical instances (Fehr, Russell, & Ward, 1982). Prototypical instances also were
more easily substituted for the word *emotion* in sentences than were
nonprototypical instances (e.g., "He could not speak a word for he was so
overcome with <u>emotion</u>" sounded natural when the word *emotion* was replaced with *anger* but not when replaced with *respect*; Fehr & Russell,
1984, Study 4). To give a final example, prototypical instances also had a
greater number of features in common (known as "family resemblance")
than did nonprototypical instances (Fehr & Russell, 1984, Studies 6 and
7). Importantly, all of these indices of internal structure showed evidence
of convergence. Based on these findings, it was concluded that the concept
of emotion is, indeed, amenable to a prototype conceptualization.

Other researchers followed suit and conducted prototype analyses of
emotion (e.g., Conway & Bekerian, 1987; Mascolo, 1988; Shaver, Schwartz,
Kirson, & O'Connor, 1987; Tiller & Harris, 1984). In each of these investigations, it was concluded that the concept of emotion is better understood from a prototypical, than from a classical, perspective.

Subsequently, researchers began to conduct prototype analyses of specific emotions. Russell and I (Fehr & Russell, 1991) targeted the concept of
love. In a series of studies, we demonstrated that some types of love were
reliably rated as more prototypical than others. For example, maternal
love and friendship love were considered prototypical; romantic love and
sexual love were considered nonprototypical. In addition, various measures of internal structure (e.g., reaction time, family resemblance) were
highly intercorrelated, thereby confirming a prototype conceptualization.
Next, we undertook a prototype analysis of types of anger (Russell & Fehr,
1994) and found that types such as rage and fury were central to the concept whereas humiliation and indignation were peripheral. Again, this internal structure was corroborated using a variety of methods. Prototype
analyses also were extended to other interpersonal constructs that were not
specifically emotions (e.g., types of commitment; Fehr, 1999). Once again,

it was concluded that the target construct lent itself to a prototypical, more than to a classical, conceptualization.

Analyses of Features

The next development was to conduct prototype analyses of the features of concepts, based on the assumption that the internal structure that had been found for types of concepts might also extend to features.[1] In an initial investigation, I (Fehr, 1988, Study 1) asked participants to list features of the concepts of love and commitment. Another group of participants subsequently rated these features in terms of prototypicality (Fehr, 1988, Study 2). They found it meaningful to do so. Moreover, prototypicality ratings were correlated with other measures of internal structure. For example, prototypical features of love (e.g., trust, caring) were more salient in memory than were nonprototypical features (e.g., passion, think about the other all the time; Fehr, 1988, Study 3). Importantly, this internal structure also affected the kinds of judgments that people made about close relationships. In a scenario study, it was found that as the level of love or commitment increased in a relationship, prototypical features of these concepts were rated as increasingly applicable to the relationship. In contrast, the applicability of nonprototypical features did not vary as systematically with the level of love or commitment (Fehr, 1988, Study 5). Further, violations of prototypical features were rated as more damaging to a relationship than violations of nonprototypical features. For example, when told that Chris and Pat have a loving, committed relationship, participants regarded a betrayal of trust as much more devastating than a decline in sexual attraction (Fehr, 1988, Study 6).

Other researchers subsequently conducted prototype analyses of the features of a wide variety of concepts. Examples relevant to interpersonal cognition include analyses of the features of jealousy (Sharpsteen, 1993); romantic love (Button & Collier, 1991; Regan, Kocan, & Whitlock, 1998); love, liking, and being in love (Lamm & Weismann, 1997; Luby & Aron, 1990; see also Buss's [1988] prototype analysis of the behaviors of love); relationship quality (Hassebrauck, 1997; Hassebrauck & Fehr, 2002); respect (Frei & Shaver, 2002); compassionate love (Fehr & Sprecher, 2003); forgiveness (Kearns & Fincham, 2004); closeness (Mashek et al., 2004); and, finally, the prototype of missing a romantic partner (Le et al., 2004).

Analyses of Patterns of Relating

The most recent development in the evolution of prototype analyses has been the application of this approach to more complex knowledge structures, namely, patterns of relating (Fehr, 2004a). This research represents an integration of prototype and interpersonal script approaches and is discussed later (see section "Integrating Prototype Theory with Other Social Cognitive Models," below). As will be seen, there is evidence that patterns of relating pertaining to intimacy (e.g., "If I want to talk, my friend will listen") also show evidence of prototype structure.

THE MANY USES OF A PROTOTYPE ANALYSIS

As already discussed, Rosch (1973a, 1973b) developed prototype theory as an alternative to the classical view of concepts. And, indeed, this was the spirit in which the early emotion studies were conducted. It is perhaps ironic that the original impetus for developing the theory is no longer the primary motivation for undertaking a prototype analysis. Perhaps this only speaks to the widespread usefulness and applicability of the prototype approach. At any rate, it seems safe to say that Rosch probably never anticipated the many uses to which prototype analyses have been put.

Mapping Out the Content and Structure of Concepts

Prototype analyses frequently are conducted to answer the "What is it?" question. In other words, a prototype analysis is undertaken to flesh out the content and structure of a particular concept. Many of the first social-psychological studies on the types and features of emotion and emotion-related concepts were conducted for this reason. Recently, there has been a resurgence of studies of this sort. Examples include prototype analyses of respect (Frei & Shaver, 2002), relationship quality (Hassebrauck, 1997; Hassebrauck & Fehr, 2002), compassionate love (Fehr & Sprecher, 2003), forgiveness (Kearns & Fincham, 2004), missing a romantic partner (Le et al., 2004), and the prototypes of wanting more closeness and wanting less closeness in a relationship (Mashek et al., 2004).

The advantage of a prototype analysis is that it provides a theory-driven method for delineating the content of a given domain (at least in terms of lay conceptions). Moreover, prototypicality ratings (and other indices of internal structure) provide valuable information about the structure of that knowledge. However, in conducting such analyses, it is important that researchers not lose sight of the fact that a prototype analysis only tells us how ordinary people think about a particular concept. It does not dictate how experts should define their concepts. Some have argued that experts must base their theories and definitions on lay conceptions (e.g., Prager, 2000), but this was not the position taken by Rosch (see Fehr & Russell, 1984, and Russell, 1991b, for further discussion of this point). Certainly, lay conceptions may be used as a starting point for the development of a theory. Lay conceptions also can be the subject of experts' explanations (i.e., developing a theory of why laypeople hold a particular conception). However, the point remains that a prototype analysis is a descriptive, not a prescriptive, analysis. It tells us how something is done, not how it *must* be done.

Mapping Out Similarities and Differences between Related Concepts

Prototype analyses also have been used to delineate the similarities and differences between related concepts. For example, I (Fehr, 1988) used this approach to elucidate the similarities and differences between the concepts of *love* and *commitment*. The literature was of little use in this regard because experts disagree on the extent to which love and commitment are related, ranging from the view that they are identical concepts to the view that they are completely independent (these perspectives are discussed in greater detail later). In an attempt to clarify this issue, I asked participants to list the features of love and commitment (Fehr, 1988, Study 1). I then assessed the extent of feature overlap, whether unique features were listed for each concept, and so on. The feature lists, along with prototypicality ratings, provided a basis for identifying areas of commonality as well as the features unique to each concept, as represented in the layperson's lexicon. For example, features such as caring, devotion, and trust were generated for both love and commitment and were rated as central to both concepts. Features such as gazing at the other, excitement, and energy were listed only for love; features such as obligation, hard work, and faithfulness were listed only for commitment.

Button and Collier (1991) conducted a similar analysis to highlight commonalities and differences between the concepts of *love* and *romantic love*. Luby and Aron (1990) used this approach to map out the similarities and differences between the concepts of *love*, *liking*, and *in love* (see Lamm & Weismann, 1997, for a similar analysis). More recently, Walker and Hennig (2004) used prototype methodology to identify the similarities and differences between the concepts of *just*, *brave*, and *caring* (in the context of mapping out the prototype of a moral person). Mashek and colleagues (2004) are conducting a program of research examining whether features describing the experience of wanting more closeness are qualitatively different from the features of the experience of wanting less closeness, or whether those prototypes have the same content, but the features are simply oppositely valenced. Thus, prototype analyses have proven to be useful in delineating the similarities and differences between related concepts, with the caveat that these analyses are limited to lay people's conceptions.

Cross-Cultural Comparisons

Prototype analyses also have been used to compare conceptions of emotion across cultures. The ultimate goal of this research is to establish whether emotion concepts are universal or culturally specific (see Russell, 1991a, for a discussion of the various views on this issue). The initial investigations, at least in the realm of interpersonal constructs, involved comparisons between rather similar cultures. For example, Button and Collier (1991) examined whether the prototype of love I had derived from participants' responses on the West Coast of Canada (Fehr, 1988) would replicate on the East Coast of Canada, with both university student and community participants. Luby and Aron (1990) explored whether American participants living on the West Coast of the United States would generate a similar prototype of love. The extent of consensus across these data sets (summarized by Fehr, 1993) was remarkable, given that participants in these studies provided open-ended data that were subjected to the particular coding schemes devised by each set of investigators. Five features of love were listed frequently and received the highest prototypicality ratings in each of these data sets: trust, caring, honesty, friendship, and respect.

As part of a research program on the prototype of relationship quality (Hassebrauck, 1997), Manfred Hassebrauck and I (Hassebrauck & Fehr, 2002) compared the factorial structure of features of relationship quality (and their correlations with various relationship-relevant constructs) in German and Canadian samples. Even though the prototype measures (and other scales) were completed in different languages, the findings were highly similar across samples.

Attempts to examine the universality of emotion concepts have been conducted in more diverse cultures. These include prototype analyses of emotion terms in Palau, Micronesia (Smith & Tkel-Sbal, 1995); Turkey (Türk Smith & Smith, 1995); and Indonesia (Shaver, Murdaya, & Fraley, 2001). It is questionable whether such analyses can inform conclusions about the universality of emotion because scholars disagree on how much deviation should be permitted between cultures before one can conclude that the categorization of emotion is or is not culturally specific. Nevertheless, these cultural analyses are useful because they tell us how people in a given location conceptualize emotion.

Using Prototype Analyses to Evaluate Competing Theories

Prototype analyses also are useful in examining which experts' theories most closely resemble lay conceptions. This is not to say that experts' theories must mirror lay conceptions (as discussed earlier). However, when there are a number of competing views or theories in a given domain, it can be useful to analyze which theory most closely models the way that ordinary people think.[2] For example, Parrott and Smith (1991) explored which of five theories of embarrassment most closely mapped onto lay conceptions. To give another example, there are various competing views on the relation between love and commitment (see Fehr, 1988). Some theorists have argued that these concepts are synonymous: to "love" a person means that one is "committed" to him or her. In contrast, others have argued that these concepts are completely independent. Another view is that love is a component of commitment. The converse also has been proposed, namely, that commitment is a component of love. Kelley (1983) conceptualized love and commitment as largely overlapping, but partially independent, categories. In a prototype analysis of love and commitment, I (Fehr, 1988) found that people list many of the same features for both concepts (nearly one-third of the features listed for love were also listed for commitment; half of the features listed for commitment also were listed for love). However, each concept also possessed unique features. Based on these and other findings, I concluded that laypeople's view of the relation between love and commitment most closely conformed to Kelley's (1983) model.

Finally, the most controversial issue in the friendship literature is whether women's same-sex friendships are more intimate than men's same-sex friendships (see Fehr, 1996). The dominant view is that women's friendships are more intimate because women are more likely to engage in behaviors that create intimacy, namely, personal self-disclosure. Others have argued that women's and men's friendships are equally intimate, but that the sexes follow different routes to intimacy: women achieve intimacy via self-disclosure, while men achieve intimacy by doing activities together. Still others have suggested that women become intimate *only* through self-disclosure, whereas men become intimate through self-disclosure or activities. By conducting a prototype analysis, I (Fehr, 2004a) was able to show that both women and men list patterns of relating involving self-disclosure (e.g., "If I want to talk, my friend will listen") as producing intimacy in a friendship—more so than patterns involving activities (e.g., "If I want to have fun, my friend will go out with me"). Second, although women assign significantly higher prototypicality ratings to self-disclosure patterns than do men (i.e., rate such patterns as more likely to produce intimacy), within-gender analyses reveal that both women and men rate self-disclosure patterns significantly higher than activity patterns. Thus, the sexes agree that intimacy is achieved via self-disclosure.

This example highlights the merit of bringing a prototype analysis to bear on competing theories. The controversy over whose friendships are more intimate stems from the failure to agree on a definition of *intimacy*. Theorists who define intimacy in terms of personal self-disclosure necessarily conclude that women's friendships are more intimate than men's. However, theorists in another camp have taken exception to this definition, arguing that it is female-biased. These scholars maintain that intimacy also can be defined in terms of shared activities; on this definition, men's friendships are just as intimate as women's. As long as these different theorists are unable to agree on a definition of intimacy, they will continue to draw different conclusions over whose friendships are more intimate. A prototype analysis can inform such a debate because this approach does not pre-suppose a particular definition of intimacy. Instead, lay conceptions be-come the metric for comparing different views. And in this case, it turns out that lay conceptions of intimacy are more closely aligned with the self-disclosure theorists than with the shared activities theorists.

Prototype-Based Measurement

Personality psychologists were the first to recognize the usefulness of pro-totype analyses in constructing measurement instruments (e.g., Broughton, 1984; Broughton, Trapnell, & Boyes, 1991; Buss & Craik, 1980, 1981; Cantor, Smith, de Sales French, & Mezzich, 1980; John, Pals, & Westen-burg, 1998). Klohnen and John's (1998) prototype-based assessment of working models of attachment is perhaps most relevant to interpersonal cognition. In this research program, experts were asked to rate the extent to which various interpersonal descriptors applied to each attachment style. Subsequent studies showed that participants exemplifying different attachment styles rated themselves as most similar to the prototype (the characteristics rated most highly by the experts) of their particular style.

Social psychologists also have recognized the potential of prototype analyses to inform measurement. (Here I focus strictly on the creation of measurement instruments; the findings obtained using those instruments are discussed later.) This research has proceeded along several lines. One approach has been to assess the extent of agreement with feature lists of concepts (derived from prototype studies). For example, I (Fehr, 1994) constructed a scale to assess laypeople's conceptions of love by presenting participants with the feature lists of 15 different kinds of love (taken from Fehr & Russell, 1991). In the scale, participants are asked to rate how sim-ilar the view of love portrayed in each feature list is to their own view. The scale can be scored in terms of the individual types of love (e.g., the extent of agreement with the romantic love prototype) or ratings can be aggre-gated to assess the two major kinds of love most often investigated by social psychologists: companionate love and passionate love. A compan-ionate love score is created by summing ratings of the feature lists (proto-types) of friendship love, familial love, maternal love, and so on. A pas-sionate love score is created by summing ratings of the feature lists depicting passionate love, romantic love, infatuation, sexual love, and the like. Psychometric analyses suggest that this is a valid, reliable instrument for measuring lay conceptions of love. This measure has been used to ex-amine gender and personality differences in conceptions of love (Fehr & Broughton, 2001). Most recently, this scale was used to assess dating cou-ples' conceptions of love and the implications of similarities in those con-ceptions for relationship outcomes (Fehr & Broughton, 2004).

Conceptions of commitment have been measured in an analogous manner. For example, I (Fehr, 1994, Study 8) presented dating couples with feature lists (prototypes) of different kinds of commitment and asked them to rate how similar the view of commitment depicted in each feature list was to their own view. I then compared whether couples who conceptualized commitment in terms of its prototypical cases (i.e., summing ratings of commitment to a romantic partner, family, friends, etc.) fared better in their dating relationship than those who did not.

There are other approaches to prototype-based measurement. For example, Aron and Westbay (1996) factor-analyzed the 68 features of the concept of love I had identified earlier (Fehr, 1988). Three factors were extracted and were labeled Intimacy, Passion, and Commitment. Scales to measure these constructs were developed by averaging the prototypicality ratings of the features that loaded on each of these factors.

The most recent development has been the construction of distance-from-the-prototype measures (Boris, 2002; Hassebrauck & Aron, 2001). Hassebrauck and Aron (2001) asked participants to rate the extent to which the features of relationship quality (delineated by Hassebrauck, 1997) were present in their romantic relationship. They then calculated the distance between the participants' ratings of their relationship and the prototype of relationship quality itself (i.e., by subtracting a participant's rating of each feature from the maximum score, squaring that difference, and summing the squared difference scores).

In conclusion, prototype theory has inspired a number of approaches to measurement. One advantage of prototype-based instruments is the reliance on laypeople's understanding of the target concept. This increases the probability that the researcher and the participant are attributing the same meaning to a given concept. This seems particularly important when assessing the kinds of relationship-relevant concepts that are studied by interpersonal cognition researchers. It is, after all, the lives of ordinary people that interpersonal scholars are seeking to understand and explain.

IMPLICATIONS OF PROTOTYPES FOR INTERPERSONAL BEHAVIOR

I have a vivid memory of my dissertation proposal defense. I was trying to persuade my committee that a prototype analysis of the concepts of love and commitment would be a worthwhile pursuit. Following my presentation, my advisor, Dan Perlman, asked a question: "What about behavior?" I explained that a prototype analysis was intended to answer questions about the content and structure of laypeople's knowledge, and, although this knowledge was surely relevant to behavior, that was not the focus of my dissertation. Nevertheless, I conducted two studies to show that the prototype structure of love and commitment had implications for the kinds of judgments that people make about the dynamics of relationships (Fehr,

1988, Studies 5 and 6). However, these studies did not directly address behavior. Indeed, most prototype research is still limited to examinations of what is "in the head." Surprisingly little attention has been paid to the relationship implications of this kind of knowledge. There are a few exceptions. Aron and Westbay (1996, Study 5) administered their Intimacy, Passion, and Commitment scales along with Sternberg's (1988) Intimacy, Passion, and Commitment scales completed with reference to a romantic partner. Overall, there was little relation between conceptions of love assessed in this way and reports of intimacy, passion, and commitment in an actual relationship (possibly because of psychometric inadequacies in the Sternberg measure; see Whitely, 1993).

I explored the implications of prototypes of commitment in the context of dating relationships (Fehr, 1999, Study 8). I found that people who conceptualized commitment in terms of its most prototypical instances (e.g., commitment to spouse, romantic partner, friend) reported greater satisfaction, love, liking, and commitment (including intentions to remain in the relationship) than those who held a less prototypic conception. In another investigation, Hassebrauck and I (2002) showed that agreement with the prototypical features of relationship quality was associated with greater marital satisfaction, relationship importance, attachment to a relationship, and the like (Hassebrauck & Fehr, 2002, Study 4). There is also evidence that the more closely people judge their relationship as approximating the prototype of relationship quality, the greater their satisfaction with the relationship (Hassebrauck & Aron, 2001).

Although most of this research has focused on romantic relationships, these effects extend to friendships. In a recent investigation, I found that people are satisfied in friendships to the extent that the friendship embodies patterns of relating that are prototypical of intimacy, although this applies more strongly to female, than to male, same-sex friendships (Fehr, 2004b).

To my knowledge, actual behavior has been examined in only one study. Ross Broughton and I (Fehr & Broughton, 2004) assessed the extent to which dating partners conceptualized love in terms of its prototypical (e.g., friendship love, familial love) versus nonprototypical cases (e.g., sexual love, infatuation). As predicted, those who held a prototypical conception of love reported greater relationship satisfaction, love, and liking than those who held a nonprototypical conception. Importantly, those who held a prototypical conception of love also were less likely to end their relationship (our behavioral measure) over the course of the study. Interestingly, we also found that similarity in terms of a prototypical conception (i.e., both partners conceptualized love in terms of its prototypes) was more predictive of positive relationship outcomes than similarity in terms of a nonprototypical conception.

In a trenchant analysis of the literature on relationship knowledge structures, Reis and Knee (1996) declared that "relationship cognition can provide critical clues to understanding relationship behavior in its fullest possible light" (p. 177; Berscheid, 1994, made a similar point). The studies discussed in this section confirm that relationship knowledge structures are indeed relevant to people's thoughts, feelings, and behavior in relationships. However, these studies have just scratched the surface. An important direction for future research will be to elucidate the role of prototypes in shaping a variety of interpersonal behaviors—not just decisions about whether to terminate or remain in a relationship.

INTEGRATING PROTOTYPE THEORY WITH OTHER SOCIAL-COGNITIVE MODELS

If we are to fully understand interpersonal cognition, it will be necessary to establish links between various models. As discussed next, bridges have been built, or at least their construction attempted, between prototype theory and three social-cognitive theories: cognitive appraisal dimensions, script theory, and relational schema models. Given that these developments are still in their infancy, it is unlikely that a "grand theory" of interpersonal cognition will emerge in the near future. However, the preliminary links that have been forged suggest that such ventures are likely to be fruitful.

Cognitive Appraisal Dimensions

Fitness and Fletcher (1993) attempted to integrate prototype theory with cognitive appraisal models in an analysis of love, hate, anger, and jealousy in the context of marriage. In their first study, participants were asked to describe episodes of these emotions as experienced in their marriage. Features lists were then extracted from these accounts. Participants also were asked to rate the emotion-eliciting events in terms of cognitive appraisal dimensions such as perceived control, self and partner responsibility, amount of effort required to deal with the events, and their unexpectedness, to name a few. The researchers found, for example, that anger events were perceived as more predictable and controllable than hate or jealousy events; the cause of love was appraised as global, rather than situationally specific, and so on. In a follow-up study, Fitness and Fletcher (1993, Study 3) sought to determine which kind of information—prototype or cognitive appraisal—would be most useful in discriminating between emotions. Participants were presented with scenarios depicting emotion events as well as prototype information (i.e., a subset of the features listed for that emotion in Study 1), cognitive appraisal information (based on the Study 1 findings), or both. The results indicated that prototype and cognitive appraisal information, individually, increased the likelihood of emotion identification (relative to a control condition in which only the emotion event scenarios were presented). However, the highest rates of correct identification occurred when participants were provided with both kinds of information.

This research illustrates that prototype analyses can be usefully integrated with cognitive appraisal approaches. One reason that these approaches can be wed is that cognitive appraisals are widely regarded as one of the elements of emotion scripts. Indeed, respondents in Fitness and Fletcher's feature-listing study spontaneously reported various appraisal-like cognitions (see Shaver et al., 1987, for similar results). However, laypeople may not necessarily generate the kinds of appraisal dimensions that Fitness and Fletcher (1993) found were most useful in discriminating between emotions (e.g., whether the emotion-eliciting event was unexpected; whether the cause was situationally specific versus global). This is an issue that would be worth exploring in future research. There are a number of additional promising avenues. For example, it seems important to examine how different appraisal patterns shape the way in which the rest of the emotion script unfolds. It may well be that emotion experience follows different tracks (Ableson, 1981), depending on how the eliciting event is appraised.

Script Theory

In our inaugural prototype analysis of emotion concepts, we (Fehr & Russell, 1984) suggested that to know the meaning of a word such as *fear* is to know a script in which events unfold in a particular sequence (Abelson, 1981). The script contains prototypical antecedents, physiological reactions, facial expressions, behaviors, and so on. "The notion of script can thus be seen to extend to episodes the notion of prototype" (Fehr & Russell, 1984, p. 482). Nevertheless, there have been few attempts to integrate prototype and script analyses of concepts. Granted, as already mentioned, several researchers have generated feature lists for specific emotions, usually based on people's accounts of emotion experience (e.g., Fitness, 2000; Fitness & Fletcher, 1993; Shaver et al., 1987). However, these feature lists remain largely "standalone" accounts of emotion experience, isolated from prototype analyses of the internal structure of these concepts. Mark Baldwin and I (Fehr & Baldwin, 1996) took some preliminary steps to integrate script and prototype approaches to emotion, focusing on anger. We began by asking participants to describe, in detail, an anger experience. Next, they rated the experience in terms of prototypicality and intensity. Finally, they received a list of anger terms (taken from Russell & Fehr, 1994) and were asked to rate how well each described their feelings at the time. In analyzing the data, the first question we asked was how closely ratings of the anger terms (applied to actual anger experiences) would correspond with prototypicality ratings of these terms obtained by Russell and Fehr (1994). These correlations turned out to be substantial (in the .60 range). Interestingly, the anger terms that received the highest proto-typicality ratings (in Russell and Fehr's research) also received the highest ratings in our study of actual experiences (e.g., frustration, irritation, an-noyance, hostility). In additional analyses, we explored how ratings of the anger terms varied as a function of the instigating event. We found, for ex-ample, that participants who were angered by a betrayal event (e.g., a woman who discovered that the man she was dating was actually married) reported that they felt hurt, jealous, and depressed—but not annoyed. Those whose anger was triggered by harassment experienced feelings of aggravation, annoyance and arousal—but they did not feel hurt. Thus, the different instigators were associated with different shadings of anger. These data still need to be mined further to establish additional links between the prototype of anger and anger scripts. For example, it may be that certain physiological responses are associated with prototypical instances of anger and other–perhaps milder—reactions are associated with nonprototypical instances (e.g., heart racing may be associated with rage but not with an-noyance). One challenge in future research will be to determine the kinds of methodological and statistical analyses that are best suited for data of this sort.

Relational Schemas/Interpersonal Scripts

Several theorists have proposed that interpersonal expectations are the product of patterns of relating (e.g., Bowlby, 1969; Sullivan, 1953). For ex-ample, in developmental psychology, Bretherton (1990) developed a model of relationship expectations in which interactional schemas that are experi-ence-near form the basis of more abstract, higher order expectations. To be more specific, a child might learn patterns of relating such as "If I fall down, Mommy will comfort me" or "If I am sick, Mommy will take care of me." These patterns of relating contribute to the higher order expecta-tion of being cared for, which in turn contributes to the global expectation of being loved.

In 1992, Baldwin published a groundbreaking paper in which he pre-sented a model of relational schemas, drawing on Bretherton's (1990) hier-archical model of interpersonal expectancies as well as on classic psycho-logical theories including interpersonal theory, interdependence theory, and object-relations theory. Baldwin (1992) proposed that relational knowl-edge is stored in cognitive representation in the form of relational schemas. Relational schemas consist of three components: a self-schema (the cogni-tive representation of self), an other schema (the cognitive representation of the relational partner), and an interpersonal script representing the in-teraction between self and other. These self–other interactions are stored in an if–then contingency format (e.g., "If I sulk, my partner will withdraw"). This model, particularly the interpersonal script component, has inspired empirical investigations in a variety of domains (see Baldwin, Chapter 2, this volume). To give one example, Baldwin and I, along with our students (Fehr, Baldwin, Patterson, Collins, & Benditt, 1999), explored interpersonal scripts in the context of anger interactions. We found that self-responses to anger were contingent on expected partner reactions. For example, participants anticipated that if they responded destructively when angered (e.g., with indirect aggression), their partner would respond in kind. A constructive response on the part of self was expected to elicit a prosocial response from the partner. Thus, self-responses did not occur in a vacuum, but rather were shaped by the reaction that was anticipated from the partner.

Recently, I (Fehr, in 2004a, 2004b) sought to integrate the notion of interpersonal scripts with prototype theory. I suggested that prototype theory could be profitably incorporated into relational schema/interpersonal script models by specifying the structure of relational knowledge (interpersonal script models address the content of relational knowledge, not its structure). More specifically, I hypothesized that interaction patterns might be structured as prototypes such that some patterns of relating would be regarded as more likely to contribute to a particular expectation than others. In testing this prediction, I focused on intimacy expectations in same-sex friendships. I began by asking a university student and a community sample to generate patterns of relating that might contribute to an expectation of intimacy in a friendship (Fehr, 2004a, Studies 1 and 2). First, and perhaps most important, I found that people are able to report on this rather complex kind of relational knowledge. Both samples generated a rich and multifaceted set of interaction patterns. In a subsequent study, participants were asked to rate these interaction patterns in terms of prototypicality. They appeared to have little difficulty doing so (Fehr, 2004a, Study 3). As can be seen in Table 8.1, interaction patterns such as "If I want to talk, my friend will listen" were considered highly likely to contribute to an expectation of intimacy in a friendship, whereas patterns such as "If I am bored, my friend will spend time with me" were seen as less likely to do so. This internal structure was confirmed in a number of studies using a variety of measures. For example, in a reaction time study, prototypical interaction patterns were verified as indicative of intimacy more quickly than were nonprototypical patterns (Fehr, 2004a, Study 4). Prototypical patterns of relating also were seen as more likely to characterize close established friendships than either developing or deteriorating ones; the applicability of nonprototypical patterns did not mirror the stage of friendship as closely (Fehr, 2004a, Study 5), and so on. Overall, these studies demonstrated that more complex knowledge structures such as patterns of relating also appear to be organized as prototypes. These encour-

TABLE 8.1. Prototypicality of Intimacy Interaction Patterns

Ten highest prototypicality ratings

If I need to talk, my friend will listen.

If I am in trouble, my friend will help me.

If I need my friend, she or he will be there for me.

If someone was insulting me or saying negative things behind my back, my friend would stick up for me.

If I need food, clothing, or a place to stay, my friend will provide it.

No matter who I am or what I do, my friend will accept me.

If we have a fight or argument, we will work it out.

Even if it feels as though no one cares, I know my friend does.

Ten lowest prototypicality ratings

If I need practical help (e.g., moving, a ride, studying), my friend will provide it.

If I'm joking or laughing, my friend will laugh with me.

If I need a favor, my friend will do it.

If I am sick, my friend will take care of me.

If I am happy, my friend will be happy with me.

If I am bored, my friend will spend time with me.

If I need to borrow something, my friend will lend it.

If I just want to do nothing, my friend will be fine with that.

If I need money, my friend will lend it to me.

If I am sad, my friend is sad, too.

Note. Participants rated 48 patterns of relating; the full set of interaction patterns can be seen in Fehr (2004a). Adapted from Fehr (2004a, pp. 270–271). Copyright 2004 by the American Psychological Association. Adapted by permission.

aging findings suggest that prototype theory can be meaningfully incorporated into models that specify the content of interpersonal cognition by offering predictions about the structure of that knowledge.

These findings also underscore the contribution of prototype theory to our understanding of the "nuts and bolts" of interpersonal cognition. A prototype analysis reveals the content of knowledge in cognitive representation (in this case, knowledge of the kinds of patterns of relating that people regard as contributing to an expectation of intimacy in a friendship). Prototype theory also specifies that not all knowledge is equal: categories are organized around key exemplars, with other category members varying in their degree of resemblance to these prototypical cases. When a concept is activated, it is the key exemplars that are most likely to come to mind. This structure also influences the speed with which category-relevant information is processed. For example, in the intimacy interactions research, patterns of relating central to intimacy (e.g., "If I talk, my friend will listen") were verified as contributing to intimacy more quickly than peripheral patterns (e.g., "If I want to have fun, my friend will go out with me"). One implication is that people will be more likely to infer (and make the inference more quickly) that a friendship is intimate when their real-world interactions with a friend are characterized by prototypical, rather than nonprototypical, patterns. Moreover, when assessing whether they are satisfied with a friendship, people are likely to monitor the extent to which the friendship embodies prototypical patterns of relating. Thus, prototype theory has much to contribute to the question of how interpersonal cognition works by providing a detailed account of the cognitive representation and processing of interpersonal knowledge.

PROTOTYPE THEORY: UNRESOLVED ISSUES

As has been seen, prototype theory has had a major impact on interpersonal cognition research. In addition to addressing questions about the content and structure of interpersonal constructs, the theory has proven useful in guiding measurement, providing a unique perspective on theoretical debates, and in forging links with other social cognitive models. In short, prototype theory is a remarkable success story. Nevertheless, there are some issues that I believe will need to be addressed in order for this theory to move forward and maximize its usefulness to scholars of interpersonal cognition.

The Enigma of the Hierarchical Organization of Concepts

Rosch's predictions about the organization of concepts at the horizontal level of categorization have received overwhelming support. Although her early studies focused on object categories, subsequent research conducted by social psychologists demonstrated that the theory had wide applicability, extending to more abstract concepts such as emotion, love, anger, and so on. Moreover, as already discussed, the internal structure that Rosch predicted and found for types of concepts extends to features of concepts and even more complex knowledge structures, such as patterns of relating. A more equivocal picture emerges, however, when the focus shifts to the other main tenet of prototype theory, namely, the vertical organization of concepts.

According to Rosch (1978a; Rosch, Mervis, Gray, Johnson, & Boyes-Braem, 1976), natural language concepts are vertically organized into superordinate-, basic-, and subordinate-level categories. The hierarchy "furniture, chair, rocking chair" illustrates the superordinate, basic, and subordinate levels, respectively. The superordinate level is the most general level of categorization. The basic level is the most commonly used in natural language and is the level that maximizes cognitive efficiency. Finer grained distinctions between concepts are made at the lower, subordinate level.

Personality and social psychologists have attempted to demonstrate that the concepts they study are organized in such a hierarchy. One approach, devised by Cantor and Mischel (1979), has been to use hierarchical cluster analysis to array concepts at different levels. For example, in their analysis of person concepts, *buddhist monk, nun,* and *hasidic jew* formed a cluster labeled "religious devotee." This cluster then joined a "social activist" cluster to form a higher order "committed person" cluster. A similar approach was taken by Horowitz, de Sales French, Lapid, and Weckler (1982) in their analysis of the depressed person and the lonely person prototypes. Shaver et al. (1987) followed suit in their analysis of the features of various emotion concepts (see Conway & Bekerian, 1987; Fehr, 1994, 1999; and Shaver et al., 2001, for other examples). Although these analyses have produced interpretable findings, this approach can be criticized on the grounds that it represents a statistical solution (a hierarchical cluster analysis, by definition, produces a hierarchy) that may or may not approximate the layperson's cognitive organization of constructs.

There is another problem. According to prototype theory, concepts can be neatly ordered at different levels of categorization. This view contrasts sharply with the theory's portrayal of the horizontal dimension of categorization—a dimension characterized by fuzziness and overlapping sets. Why would human cognition have evolved such that concepts at the horizontal level would be characterized by fuzziness and blurry boundaries, but their vertical ordering would be clear-cut and precise? Russell and I (Russell & Fehr, 1994) speculated that the fuzziness that characterizes the horizontal dimension might also apply to the vertical dimension. In a series of studies on anger, we demonstrated that laypeople do not possess neat, ready-made taxonomies. Or if they do, they are unable to produce them. In fact, participants consistently violated rules of hierarchies. For example, they regarded fury as a type of anger; they also regarded anger as a type of fury. We concluded that concepts at the vertical level of categorization possess the same sorts of properties as concepts at the horizontal level: concepts overlap with one another and the boundaries between them are blurry.

In another investigation of vertical structure, I (Fehr, 1999) asked participants to organize types of commitment into a hierarchy. I made the task as easy and straightforward as possible. For example, I provided very concrete examples (e.g., Granny Smith apple → apple → fruit). In one study (Study 6), I had participants work in groups in the event that consensus could be reached if people were able to pool their expertise. Despite these efforts, it became clear that people do not possess an agreed-upon, orderly taxonomy of commitment constructs. The hierarchies varied greatly from one group to the next, both in terms of the number of levels that were created and in the placement of concepts at those levels. For example, some participants classified commitment to family as a kind of relationship commitment; others did just the opposite. Commitment to a pet was regarded as a kind of commitment to family, relatives, a friend, a sibling, and as a kind of casual commitment.

In conclusion, so far there is little evidence that laypeople organize concepts into discrete levels varying in their degree of abstraction. Perhaps researchers have not yet devised the proper way of eliciting this information from laypeople. But the singular lack of success encountered so far makes this a rather unlikely possibility. Perhaps Rosch simply got it wrong—at least when it comes to more abstract concepts such as emotion, where genus and species distinctions are unclear.[3] If, instead, the vertical organization of emotion and other interpersonal concepts is fuzzy in the same way that the horizontal level of organization is fuzzy (as the data suggest), it would seem important to further explore this fuzziness to determine whether any kind of order can be found. The fuzziness of the horizontal dimension has not been an impediment to research because of the orderliness that is afforded by internal structure (i.e., prototypes at the core, other category members can be ordered in terms of their resemblance to these cases). Whether or not an analogous structure can be found at the vertical level remains a challenging issue for future research.

Where Do Prototypes Come from?

Another, possibly thorny, issue concerns the origins of prototypes. Rosch maintained that prototypes reflect the structure of nature rather than one's personal experience with particular exemplars. In her words, "Creatures with feathers are more likely to have wings than creatures with fur" (Rosch, 1978b, p. 28). It is the co-occurrence of such features that contribute to prototypicality effects. For example, birds with both feathers and wings, such as robins, are considered more prototypical of the concept than are birds such as penguins, with their flippers and fur-like appearance. As further support for the view that prototypes are not based on personal experience, Rosch pointed to the high levels of agreement on ratings of prototypicality (e.g., Rosch, 1973b). It is this aspect of prototype theory that is often regarded as the key difference between it and exemplar models that argue that the content and organization of concepts in cognitive representation is a product of one's own idiosyncratic experiences (see, e.g., Fehr, 1988; Reis & Knee, 1996; Russell, 1991b).

Consistent with the idea that prototypes are not the result of personal experience, researchers rarely find individual differences in prototypicality ratings. For example, social psychologists have examined age, gender, attachment style, intimacy status, sexual orientation, and other individual differences in prototypes of love and have generally come up empty-handed (see Fehr, 1993, for a review). Holliday and Chandler's (1986) prototype analysis of the concept of wisdom is another example. Based on the reasonable assumption that this concept might take on different meanings across the lifespan, they explored conceptions of wisdom among university students, middle-aged adults, and the elderly. However, their data showed that the prototype of wisdom is remarkably stable across the adult lifespan.

A different picture emerges, however, when one changes the question. In standard prototype research, participants are asked to rate the extent to which a given member is a good example of a category (e.g., "Is romantic love a good example of love?"). However, in studies focused on close relationships, the question also has been worded in terms of the participant's own conception of love (e.g., "Does the prototype of romantic love match your own view of what love is?"; see, e.g., Fehr, 1994). When asked this way, reliable individual differences are found (Fehr & Broughton, 2001). Can these apparently contradictory sets of findings be reconciled? I have suggested that they can, if one is prepared to invoke the idea that relational knowledge is categorized in multiple ways (Fehr, 1993; Fehr & Broughton, 2001). For example, there may be a general, culturally shared body of relational knowledge that is being tapped when researchers ask for prototypicality ratings of a concept. There also may exist another level of knowledge that is more heavily based on one's own personal experiences, and this may be the kind of knowledge that is accessed when participants are asked about their personal views. It does not seem particularly radical to suggest that people have different storehouses of knowledge and that the questions we ask them determine which storehouse is consulted for the answer. Indeed, Surra and Bohman's (1991) model of the cognitive processes involved in relationship development posits several different kinds of knowledge structures (see Fitness, Fletcher, & Overall, 2003, for a similar model). These include conceptions of relationship constructs (the research on prototypes of love and commitment discussed in this chapter is included in this category), generalized schemas for classes of relationships, and relationship-specific schemas for past or already-established relationships. The idea of different kinds of knowledge structures is an intriguing one that raises a number of interesting questions: When do people rely on one kind of knowledge rather than another? Do these knowledge structures vary in terms of their ability to predict behavior? What effect do these knowledge structures have on one another? Can relationship-specific structures influence more generic conceptions? Does the opposite occur? Questions along these lines have received some attention in attachment research (e.g., Pierce & Lydon, 2001) but they are relevant to many other areas of interpersonal cognition as well.

CONCLUSION

It has been assumed that with sufficient debate and empirical examination, ultimately social scientific concepts can and must be precisely defined. Rosch's bold proposal that many natural language concepts cannot be defined, but instead are structured as prototypes, has revolutionized the way that psychologists think about concepts. Prototype theory also has provided social scientists with a set of tools for mapping out concepts, at least as understood by laypeople. In addition, it has given them a theory-based method for measuring concepts as well as a metric for evaluating conflicting experts' models. Prototype theory also has proven a useful addition to other social-cognitive theories of relational knowledge.

In conclusion, the quest of interpersonal cognition scholars is to understand interpersonal behavior in its "fullest possible light." Prototype theory has made substantial contributions to this quest by illuminating how interpersonal knowledge is stored and processed. This is important because as the case of Michelle Triola and Lee Marvin vividly illustrates, the cognitive representation of interpersonal experiences plays a crucial role in understanding human motivation, emotion, and, ultimately, behavior.

ACKNOWLEDGMENTS

Preparation of this chapter was supported by a grant from the Social Sciences and Humanities Research Council of Canada. I would like to express my heartfelt appreciation to Art Aron, Ross Broughton, Julie Fitness, Debra Mashek, and Lisa Sinclair for their very helpful comments on an earlier draft of this chapter. This chapter also benefited immensely from the editorial guidance of Mark Baldwin.

NOTES

1. In the early prototype studies, participants were frequently asked to generate the features of concepts, in addition to listing types. These features were then used to calculate a family resemblance score (an index of the degree to which instances of a concept share features). These scores were taken as a measure of internal structure that would be correlated with prototypicality ratings and other indices of internal structure. Thus, the focus was on the extent to which features overlap, rather than on the specific content of the features. However, researchers began to recognize that feature lists were useful in delineating the content of categories. A number of studies were conducted in which participants were asked to list the features of concepts or, more frequently, were asked to describe emotion experiences (features were then extracted from these accounts; see, e.g., Fitness & Fletcher, 1993; Shaver et al., 1987). These feature lists became known as "the" prototype of a particular emotion. However, these investigations did not examine internal structure (i.e., the features were not rated in terms of prototypicality).

2. Aron and Westbay (1996) did not set out with the goal of determining which expert's model of love would best map onto a factor analysis of the features identified in Fehr's (1988) prototype of love. However, they found that the three factors that emerged closely resembled the intimacy, passion, and commitment components of Sternberg's (1986) triangular model of love.

3. Some (e.g., Wierzbecka, 1984) have argued that Rosch got it wrong, even for more concrete objects. The basic argument is that taxonomic categorization, in general, does not play nearly as important a role in human cognition as psychologists such as Rosch have assumed.

REFERENCES

Abelson, R. P. (1981). Psychological status of the script concept. *American Psychologist, 36*, 715–729.

Aron, A., & Westbay, L. (1996). Dimensions of the prototype of love. *Journal of Personality and Social Psychology, 70*, 535–551.

Baldwin, M. W. (1992). Relational schemas and the processing of social information. *Psychological Bulletin, 112*, 461–484.

Berscheid, E. (1994). Interpersonal relationships. *Annual Review of Psychology, 45*, 79–129.

Boris, T. S. (2002). *Prototype matching on the features of love in dating relationships.* Unpublished honors thesis, University of Winnipeg, Winnipeg, Manitoba, Canada.

Bowlby, J. (1969). *Attachment and loss: Vol. 1. Attachment.* New York: Basic Books.

Bretherton, I. (1990). Communication patterns, internal working models, and the intergenerational transmission of attachment relationships. *Infant Mental Health Journal, 11*, 237–252.

Broughton, R. (1984). A prototype strategy for construction of personality scales. *Journal of Personality and Social Psychology, 47*, 1334–1346.

Broughton, R., Trapnell, P. D., & Boyes, M. C. (1991). Classifying personality types with occupational prototypes. *Journal of Research in Personality, 25*, 302–321.

Buss, D. M. (1988). Love acts: The evolutionary biology of love. In R. J. Sternberg & M. L. Barnes (Eds), *The psychology of love* (pp. 100–118). New Haven, CT: Yale University Press.

Buss, D. M., & Craik, K. H. (1980). The frequency concept of disposition: Dominance and prototypically dominant acts. *Journal of Research in Personality, 43*, 379–392.

Buss, D. M., & Craik, K. H. (1981). The act frequency analysis of personal dispositions: Aloofness, gregariousness, dominance, and submissiveness. *Journal of Research in Personality, 49*, 174–192.

Button, C. M., & Collier, D. R. (1991, June). *A comparison of people's concepts of love and romantic love.* Paper presented at the Canadian Psychological Conference, Calgary, Alberta.

Cantor, N., & Mischel, W. (1979). Prototypes in person perception. *Advances in Experimental Social Psychology, 12*, 3–52.

Cantor, N., Smith, E. E., de Sales French, R., & Mezzich, J. (1980). Psychiatric diagnosis as prototype categorization. *Journal of Abnormal Psychology, 89*, 181–193.

Conway, M. A., & Bekerian, D. A. (1987). Situational knowledge and emotions. *Cognition and Emotion, 1*, 145–191.

Duffy, E. (1934). Emotion: An example of the need for reorientation in psychology. *Psychological Review, 41*, 184–198.

Duffy, E. (1941). An explanation of "emotional" phenomena without the use of the concept "emotion." *Journal of General Psychology, 25*, 283–293.

Fehr, B. (1988). Prototype analysis of the concepts of love and commitment. *Journal of Personality and Social Psychology, 55*, 557–579.

Fehr, B. (1993). How do I love thee . . . ?: Let me consult my prototype. In S. Duck (Ed.), *Understanding personal relationships: Vol. 1. Individuals in relationships* (pp. 87–120). Newbury Park, CA: Sage.

Fehr, B. (1994). Prototype-based assessment of laypeople's views of love. *Personal Relationships, 1,* 309–331.

Fehr, B. (1996). *Friendship processes.* Newbury Park, CA: Sage.

Fehr, B. (1999). Lay people's conceptions of commitment. *Journal of Personality and Social Psychology, 76,* 90–106.

Fehr, B. (2004a). Intimacy expectations in same-sex friendships: A prototype interaction-pattern model. *Journal of Personality and Social Psychology, 86,* 265–284.

Fehr, B. (2004b). A prototype model of intimacy interactions in same-sex friendships. In D. Mashek & A. Aron (Eds.), *Handbook of interpersonal intimacy and closeness* (pp. 9–26). New York: Oxford University Press.

Fehr, B., & Baldwin, M. (1996). Prototype and script analyses of laypeople's knowledge of anger. In G. J. O. Fletcher & J. Fitness (Eds.), *Knowledge structures and interaction in close relations: A social psychological approach* (pp. 219–245). Hillsdale, NJ: Erlbaum.

Fehr, B., Baldwin, M., Patterson, S., Collins, L., & Benditt, R. (1999). Anger in close relationships: An interpersonal script analysis. *Personality and Social Psychology Bulletin, 25,* 299–312.

Fehr, B., & Broughton, R. (2001). Gender and personality differences in conceptions of love: An interpersonal theory analysis. *Personal Relationships, 8,* 115–136.

Fehr, B., & Broughton, R. (2004). *Individual and dyadic conceptions of love: Implications for thoughts, feelings, and behavior in close relationships.* Unpublished manuscript, University of Winnipeg.

Fehr, B., & Russell, J. A. (1984). Concept of emotion viewed from a prototype perspective. *Journal of Experimental Psychology: General, 113,* 464–486.

Fehr, B., & Russell, J. A. (1991). The concept of love viewed from a prototype perspective. *Journal of Personality and Social Psychology, 60,* 425–438.

Fehr, B., Russell, J. A., & Ward, L. M. (1982). Prototypicality of emotions: A reaction time study. *Bulletin of the Psychonomic Society, 20,* 253–254.

Fehr, B., & Sprecher, S. (2003, June). *Prototype analysis of compassionate love.* Paper presented at the Compassionate Love Conference, Normal, IL.

Fitness, J. (2000). Anger in the workplace: An emotion script approach to anger episodes between workers and their superiors, co-workers and subordinates. *Journal of Organizational Behavior, 21,* 147–162.

Fitness, J., & Fletcher, G. J. O. (1993). Love, hate, anger, and jealousy in close relationships: A prototype and cognitive appraisal analysis. *Journal of Personality and Social Psychology, 65,* 942–958.

Fitness, J., Fletcher, G. J. O., & Overall, N. (2003). Interpersonal attraction and intimate relationships. In J. Cooper & M. Hogg (Eds.), *The Sage handbook of social psychology* (pp. 258–278). Newbury Park, CA: Sage.

Frei, J. R., & Shaver, P. R. (2002). Respect in close relationships: Prototype definition, self-report assessment, and initial correlations. *Personal Relationships, 9,* 121–139.

Hassebrauck, M. (1997). Cognitions of relationship quality: A prototype analysis of their structure and consequences. *Personal Relationships, 4,* 163–185.

Hassebrauck, M., & Aron, A. (2001). Prototype matching in close relationships. *Personality and Social Psychology Bulletin, 27,* 1111–1122.

Hassebrauck, M., & Fehr, B. (2002). Dimensions of relationship quality. *Personal Relationships, 9,* 253–270.

Holliday, S. G., & Chandler, M. (1986). *Wisdom: Explorations in adult competence* (Human Development Monograph No. 17). Basel, Switzerland: Carger.

Horowitz, L. M., de Sales French, R., Lapid, J. S., & Weckler, D. A. (1982). Symptoms and interpersonal problems: The prototype as an integrating concept. In J. C. Anchin & D. J. Keisler (Eds.), *Handbook of interpersonal psychotherapy* (pp. 168–190). New York: Pergamon Press.

John, O. P., Pals, J. L., & Westenberg, P. M. (1998). Personality prototypes and ego development: Conceptual similarities and relations in adult women. *Journal of Personality and Social Psychology, 74,* 1093–1108.

Kearns, J. N., & Fincham, F. D. (2004). A prototype analysis of forgiveness. *Personality and Social Psychology Bulletin, 30,* 838–855.

Kelley, H. H. (1983). Love and commitment. In H. H. Kelley, E. Berscheid, A. Christensen, J. H. Harvey, T. L. Huston, G. Levinger, E. McClintock, L. A. Peplau, & D. R. Peterson (Eds.), *Close relationships* (pp. 265–314). New York: Freeman.

Klohnen, E. C., & John, O. P. (1998). Working models of attachment: A theory-based prototype approach. In J. A. Simpson & W. S. Rholes (Eds.), *Attachment theory and close relationships* (pp. 115–140). New York: Guilford Press.

Lamm, H., & Wiesmann, U. (1997). Subjective attributes of attraction: How people characterize their liking, their love, and their being in love. *Personal Relationships, 4,* 271–284.

Le, B., Loving, T. J., Fiorentino, R., Quill, M., Porricelli, L., & Adams, S. (2004, July). *"Wish you were here": A prototype analysis of missing a romantic partner.* Paper presented at the conference of the International Association for Relationship Research, Madison, WI.

Luby, V., & Aron, A. (1990, July). *A prototype structuring of love, like, and being-in-love.* Paper presented at the Fifth International Conference on Personal Relationships, Oxford, UK.

Mascolo, M. F. (1988). A prototype analysis of the structure and content of basic level emotion concepts. *Dissertation Abstracts International, 49*(2-A), 222.

Mashek, D., Le, B., Bloom-Feshbach, A., Gardner-Mims, W., Israel, K., & Thomas, S. (2004, July). *Central descriptors of wanting more vs. wanting less closeness.* Paper presented at the conference of the International Association for Relationship Research, Madison, WI.

Mervis, C. B., & Rosch, E. (1981). Categorization of natural objects. *Annual Review of Psychology, 32,* 89–115.

Parrott, W. G., & Smith, S. F. (1991). Embarrassment: Actual vs. typical cases, classical vs. prototypical representations. *Cognition and Emotion, 5,* 467–488.

Pierce, T., & Lydon, J. E. (2001). Global and specific relational models in the experience of social interactions. *Journal of Personality and Social Psychology, 80,* 613–631.

Prager, K. J. (2000). Intimacy in personal relationships. In S. Hendrick & C. Hendrick (Eds.), *Close relationships: A sourcebook* (pp. 229–242). Thousand Oaks, CA: Sage.

Regan, P. C., Kocan, E. R., & Whitlock, T. (1998). Ain't love grand!: A prototype analysis of the concept of romantic love. *Journal of Social and Personal Relationships, 15,* 411–420.

Reis, H. T., & Knee, C. R. (1996). What we know, what we don't know, and what we need to know about relationship knowledge structures. In G. J. O. Fletcher & J.

Fitness (Eds.), *Knowledge structures in close relationships* (pp. 169–191). Mahwah, NJ: Erlbaum.

Rosch, E. H. (1973a). Natural categories. *Cognitive Psychology, 4,* 328–350.

Rosch, E. H. (1973b). On the internal structure of perceptual and semantic categories. In T. E. Moore (Ed.), *Cognitive development and the acquisition of language* (pp. 111–144). New York: Academic Press.

Rosch, E. H. (1978a). Principles of categorization. In E. H. Rosch & B. B. Lloyd (Eds.), *Cognition and categorization* (pp. 27–71). Hillsdale, NJ: Erlbaum.

Rosch, E. H. (1978b). Human categorization. In N. Warren (Ed.), *Studies in cross-cultural psychology* (Vol. 1, pp. 1–49). London: Academic Press.

Rosch, E. H., Mervis, C. B., Gray, W. D., Johnson, D. M., & Boyes-Braem, P. (1976). Basic objects in natural categories. *Cognitive Psychology, 8,* 382–439.

Russell, J. A. (1991a). Culture and the categorization of emotion. *Psychological Bulletin, 110,* 426–450.

Russell, J. A. (1991b). In defense of a prototype approach to emotion concepts. *Journal of Personality and Social Psychology, 60,* 37–47.

Russell, J. A., & Fehr, B. (1994). The varieties of anger: Fuzzy concepts in a fuzzy hierarchy. *Journal of Personality and Social Psychology, 67,* 186–205.

Sharpsteen, D. J. (1993). Romantic jealousy as an emotion concept: A prototype analysis. *Journal of Social and Personal Relationships, 10,* 69–82.

Shaver, P. R., Murdaya, U., & Fraley, R. C. (2001). Structure of the Indonesian emotion lexicon. *Asian Journal of Psychology, 4,* 201–224.

Shaver, P. R., Schwartz, J., Kirson, D., & O'Connor, C. (1987). Emotion knowledge: Further explorations of a prototype approach. *Journal of Personality and Social Psychology, 52,* 1061–1086.

Smith, K. D., & Tkel-Sbal, D. (1995). Prototype analyses of emotion terms in Palau, Micronesia. In J. A. Russell, J. Fernandez-Dols, A. S. R. Manstead, & J. C. Wellenkamp (Eds.), *Everyday conceptions of emotion* (pp. 85–102). Dordrecht, The Netherlands: Kluwer Academic.

Sternberg, R. (1988). *Construct validation of a triangular theory of love.* Unpublished manuscript (cited in Aron & Westbay, 1996).

Sullivan, H. S. (1953). *The interpersonal theory of psychiatry.* New York: Norton.

Surra, C. A., & Bohman, T. (1991). The development of close relationships: A cognitive perspective. In G. J. O. Fletcher & F. D. Fincham (Eds.), *Cognition in close relationships* (pp. 281–305). Hillsdale, NJ: Erlbaum.

Tiller, D. K., & Harris, P. L. (1984). *Prototypicality of emotion concepts: A discussion of normative data.* Unpublished manuscript, Oxford University, Oxford, UK.

Türk Smith, S., & Smith, K. D. (1995). Turkish emotion concepts: A prototype analysis. In J. A. Russell, J. Fernandez-Dols, A. S. R. Manstead, & J. C. Wellenkamp (Eds.), *Everyday conceptions of emotion* (pp. 103–119). Dordrecht, The Netherlands: Kluwer Academic.

Walker, L. J., & Hennig, K. H. (2004). Differing conceptions of moral exemplarity: Just, brave, and caring. *Journal of Personality and Social Psychology, 86,* 629–647.

Whitely, B. E. (1993). Reliability and aspects of the construct validity of Sternberg's Triangular Love Scale. *Journal of Personal and Social Relationships, 10,* 475–480.

Wierzbicka, A. (1984). *Apples* are not a "kind of fruit": The semantics of human categorization. *American Ethnology, 11,* 313–328.

9

Including Close Others in the Cognitive Structure of the Self

ARTHUR ARON, DEBRA MASHEK, TRACY McLAUGHLIN-VOLPE,
STEPHEN WRIGHT, GARY LEWANDOWSKI, *and* ELAINE N. ARON

The self as a knowledge structure separate from the knowledge structures of others has been a useful abstraction in social-cognitive research. However, such an abstraction can also mislead. In this chapter we summarize a model (and supporting research) that treats cognition regarding the self as intrinsically interconnected with, indeed as inseparable from, cognition regarding others. This view of self-related cognition as linked in its essence to cognition regarding others is not, of course, a new idea. In psychology generally it has its roots in William James (1890/1948) and in social psychology in Cooley (1902) and Mead (1934), among others.

This is, however, a radical view in the context of contemporary social cognition. On the one hand, there is a large body of research on the links of knowledge structures of self and others (for a review, see Aron, 2003). On the other hand, most other approaches in this tradition treat self and other as distinct knowledge structures that may have various relations to each other, such as the relational schema approach (e.g., Baldwin, 1992) or the working model of self-and-other approach (e.g., Collins & Read, 1994). In these approaches, one holds knowledge structures such as "If I do X, other is likely to respond Y." We do not doubt the utility of such conceptualizations. Indeed, we suspect that they coexist and have interesting relationships with the kinds of self-including-other structures that are the focus of our own approach. The point we are making here is just that the approach that is the focus of this chapter is different in fundamental ways from the more usual approaches, though we see each as having its own potential contributions to make to understanding human cognition related to the link of the self and its interpersonal world.

The first half of this chapter summarizes our basic model and supporting research. We begin with a brief overview of previous ideas about including other in the self and the genesis of our own theoretical model, followed by a somewhat more systematic statement of our position and a review of relevant research by ourselves and others to date. The second half of the chapter describes several new directions for applying this idea, including distinguishing including other in the self from familiarity and similarity; identifying neural substrates of the connection of self and other; understanding what it means to feel "too close" in an intimate relationship; implications for relationships of self-expansion motivation; group identification as including the group in the self; the effect of including outgroup members in the self on attitudes about the outgroup; and including communities in the self.

THE BASIC MODEL

The notion that in a relationship each is included in each other's self is consistent with a wide variety of social-psychological ideas about relationships. For example, Reis and Shaver (1988) identified intimacy as mainly being a process of an escalating reciprocity of self-disclosure in which each individual feels his or her innermost self validated, understood, and cared for by the other. Perhaps the most prominent idea in social psychology directly related to the present theme is the "unit relation," a fundamental concept in Heider's (1958) cognitive account of interpersonal relations. This notion is also related to Ickes, Tooke, Stinson, Baker, and Bissonnette's (1988) idea of "intersubjectivity"—which Ickes and his colleagues made vivid by citing Merleau-Ponty's (1945) description of a close relationship as a "double being" and Schutz's (1970) reference to two people "living in each other's subjective contexts of meaning" (p. 167).

Several currently active lines of theory-based social-psychological research focus on closely related themes. For example, in a series of experimental and correlational studies, Tesser (1988) has shown that a relationship partner's achievement, so long as it is not in a domain that threatens the self by creating a negative social comparison, is "reflected" by the self (i.e., the self feels pride in the achievement as if it were the self's). Another relevant line of work focuses on what is called "fraternal relative deprivation" (Runciman, 1966), in which the relative disadvantage of the group to which self belongs affects the self as if it were the self's own deprivation. Yet another example is work arising from social identity theory (Tajfel &

Turner, 1979), which posits that one's identity is structured from member-ship in social groups.

In the field of marketing, Belk (1988) has proposed a notion of owner-ship in which "we regard our possessions as part of ourselves" (p. 139), an idea that has been the subject of considerable theoretical discussion and several studies. For example, Sivadas and Machleit (1994) found that items measuring an object's "incorporation into self" (items such as "helps me achieve my identity" and "is part of who I am") form a separate factor from items assessing the object's importance or relevance to the self. Ahuvia (1993) integrated Belk's self-extension approach with our inclu-sion-of-other-in-the-self model and proposed that processes hypothesized in the domain of personal relationships also apply to relations to physical objects and experiences. In an interview study, Ahuvia showed that people sometimes describe their "love" of things in much the same way that they describe their "love" of relationship partners, that they often consider this "real love," and that they treat these "love objects" as very much a part of their identity. These ideas about including the owned object in the self are also related to the notion of relationship as each "possessing" the other (e.g., Reik, 1944).

In the relationship domain, Agnew, Van Lange, Rusbult, and Langston (1998) explicitly linked the inclusion-of-other-in-the-self model with inter-dependence, describing it as "cognitive interdependence—a mental state characterized by a pluralistic, collective representation of self-in-relationship" (p. 939). Cialdini, Brown, Lewis, Luce, and Neuberg (1997) linked the inclusion-of-other-in-the-self model to evolutionary theories of relation-ships. They suggested that interpersonal closeness as experienced as includ-ing other in the self may be how we recognize those with whom we share genes (a kind of literal, physical, self–other inclusion) in the interest of knowing with whom one should share resources to enhance collective fit-ness. Finally, although there has been no explicit work on the possible link, we think that there may be a close connection between self–other inclusion and communal relationships (e.g., Clark & Mills, 1979, 1993). That is, we see including other in the self as the foundation for spontaneously being concerned with the others' needs (since close others' needs are my needs), and thus both directly facilitating communal motivation (attention to and acting on close others' needs) and having possibly functioned historically to help create a social norm of communal orientation in close relation-ships.

The notion of relationship as an overlap of selves has been popular more generally among psychologists and sociologists, starting at least with James (1890/1948). For example, Bakan (1966) wrote about "commu-nion" in the context of his expansion on Buber's (1937) "I–Thou" rela-tionship. Jung (1925/1959) emphasized the role of relationship partners for providing or developing otherwise unavailable aspects of the psyche, so leading to greater wholeness. Maslow (1967) took it for granted that "beloved people can be incorporated into the self" (p. 103). And from a symbolic-interactionist perspective, McCall (1974) described "attachment" as "incorporation of . . . [the other's] actions and reactions . . . into the content of one's various conceptions of the self" (p. 219).

We first developed our specific model of including other in the self in the context of trying to understand attraction and satisfaction in close relationships (Aron & Aron, 1986). We began with the question of why people would enter or maintain a relationship. Our conclusion was that it would be for the same reasons they are motivated to do anything beyond basic survival, a set of exploratory-type motives we labeled "self-expansion," the desire to explore, enhance opportunities, and generally increase potential efficacy. (Indeed, "survival of the fittest" might be retermed "survival of the most expanded"; hence the success of sexual reproduction and perhaps the explanation for why social animals have done so well.)

This raised the question of how such a motivation would lead specifically to entering and maintaining relationships. Based on our familiarity with the various historical lines of thinking just noted, we concluded that by entering a relationship one gains to some extent the other's resources, perspectives, and identities. Instead of just being me, I am now both me *and* you. I not only have my resources, for example, but to some extent yours as well.

Originally, we viewed this only as a model of close relationships. Indeed, close relationships remains the main focus of our work. However, over the years, we have become increasingly convinced that to some extent this process operates even in relatively casual relationships (e.g., Cialdini et al., 1997) and in a variety of contexts in which what is included is not another person, but a group (e.g., Tropp & Wright, 2001) or a community (Mashek, Stuewig, Furukawa, & Tangney, 2004). In one set of studies, even "nature" is argued to be included in the self (Schultz, 2002). We consider some of these extensions in the second half of this chapter.

What Is Meant by Including Another Person in the Self?

The basic idea of our model (Aron & Aron, 1986; Aron, Aron, & Norman, 2001; Aron, Mashek, & Aron, 2004), as noted, is that when in a close relationship with another person one includes in the self, to some extent, the other person's resources, perspectives, and identities. (In adult close relationships, such as a friendship or a Western marriage, this inclusion is typically mutual.) The "resources" of the other that we argue are potentially included in the self include material, knowledge (conceptual, informational, procedural), and social assets that can facilitate the achievement of goals. Perceiving oneself as including another's resources in the self refers to perceiving oneself as having access to those resources. It is as if, to some extent, the other's resources are one's own. In some cases, the other's resources are quite literally also one's own, as where married partners share a bank account. In other cases, one reasonably expects the other to make his or her resources available to self, such as with most knowledge resources (e.g., "I can do this because my partner will show me how"). In still other cases, one may feel as if what the other has is one's own even when it is not in actuality. This might occur, for example, when a North American adolescent feels that a family car is his or her own even when the parents do not see it that way. From the point of view of the self at a given point in time, these various cases are largely equivalent. (These may of course have quite different implications for interactions with the close other, but such issues are beyond the scope of the present chapter.) From a cognitive perspective, we have described our model as implying shared cognitive elements of self and close others (e.g., Aron & Fraley, 1999). Similarly, referring specifically to shared traits, Smith, Coates, and Walling (1999) proposed a localist connectionist model of this principle.

Resources

The *resource aspect* of inclusion of other in the self is particularly central from a motivational point of view. This is because perceiving another's resources as one's own means that the outcomes (rewards and costs) the other receives are to some extent experienced as one's own. Thus, for example, helping other is helping self; interfering with other is interfering with self. This analysis also implies that the evaluative and affective responses to an other's acquisition and loss of resources (notably including social status) are to some extent the same as if the acquisition or loss was with regard to one's own resources.

Perspectives

The *perspective aspect* of inclusion refers to experiencing (consciously or unconsciously) the world to some extent from the other's point of view. Thus, for example, when another person is included in the self, various self-related attributional and cognitive biases should also apply with regard to one's attributions and cognitions with regard to that other person.

Identity

The *identity aspect*, as we are using the term, refers to the features that distinguish the self from other people. These features include the traits, memories, and other characteristics that locate the person in social and physical space. Thus, for example, our model implies that people may easily confuse their own traits or memories with those of a close other. Note that what distinguishes the self from others includes the self's particular relationships and group memberships. Such collective aspects of identity in a sense bind one to other people (those that are in the relationship or group). Yet, at the same time, they distinguish the self from people in general (indeed, a particular pattern of relationships and group memberships may identify an individual uniquely). Further, an extension of the identity aspect of our model (discussed in the second part of this chapter) with significant implications for intergroup relations is the hypothesis that people to some extent include close others' group memberships in the self.

The Process of Including Other in the Self

Our usage of these three aspects of other included in self (resources, perspectives, and identities) allows considerable room for overlap. Nevertheless, distinguishing among them has proven valuable heuristically for emphasizing different aspects of what we propose is included of another person in the self. Thus, in analyzing the process by which one comes to include the other in the self, we have tentatively suggested (Aron, Mashek, & Aron, 2004) that inclusion of another's perspectives and identities in the self to some extent follows from the inclusion of that other's resources. That is, the designation of a particular person's perspectives and identities are largely with reference to the particular person that is affected by a set of outcomes. For example, If I am concerned about your outcomes, I am evaluating the world as you would, and I am holding your perspectives. Similarly, if the material, knowledge, and social impact of events that happen to you are happening to me, then your place in the material and social world is my place in the material and social world, and I am holding your identities.

Thus, from a motivational point of view, the main benefit of including an other in the self would be the resources aspect. The perspectives and identities aspects may follow as a generally even more likely-to-be-unconscious side effect, a restructuring of the cognitive system. Thus, a common process might be one in which a person is motivated (generally not consciously) to seek a relationship with another person in order to have the benefit of that other person's social, knowledge, material, and other resources. As the relationship is forming, the other person makes his or her resources readily available to the self. This in turn leads to a cognitive reorganization that makes that other's resources seem as if they were one's own, and thus coming to take on the other's perspectives and identities as one's own. In the mutual case, one is motivated to make one's own resources available to the other, creating a reciprocal ongoing process strengthening the conscious and unconscious experience of including each other's resources (and thus perspectives and identities) in the self.

There are, however, other plausible scenarios that would seem to describe the process for at least some cases of including other in the self. For example, to some extent, relational status (e.g., being "best friends") may also lead, by association, to perceiving the other as included in the self. Thus, for example, Sedikides, Olsen, and Reis (1993) demonstrated that people spontaneously use who is in a relationship with whom to cluster their recall of persons. But given the great variance in degree of felt closeness among people of the same relational status with self, we would expect something like the process suggested above, that begins with including another person's resources in the self, to be most central.

Another possibility is that taking on another person's perspectives and identities as one's own are direct goals in themselves, that there is a motivation (again, not usually conscious) to include more than the other's possessions, information, social networks, and other resources. It may be as if we also desire to *be* the other ("My child I am watching perform is myself"), not to lose one's self, but to add "substance" to it.

Evidence That People Include Close Others' Resources in the Self

Having briefly summarized the background and some key principles of the model, we turn to the research support, focusing first on the resources aspect. As we have noted, a central implication of including another person's resources in the self is that the self's responses to the other's rewards and costs, opportunities and obstacles, successes and failures should be to some extent as if they were to the self's own rewards and so forth. Aron, Aron, Tudor, and Nelson (1991, Study 1 and follow-ups) examined this implication in three studies in which participants made a series of allocation decisions involving themselves and another person. As predicted, in each study participants distributed money about equally to themselves and the other when the other was their best friend, but they distributed more to themselves than to the other when the other was a mere acquaintance. Importantly, these results held up even when participants believed that the other could not know about their allocations (thus making unlikely interpretations involving expected effects of how the other would feel about their allocations). Medvene, Teal, and Slavich (2000) adopted quite a different approach to this issue. In their study of couples in romantic relationships, they found a standard *equity effect*, greatest satisfaction for those who are neither under- nor overbenefited. However, this pattern was significantly weaker for those who perceived their relationship as having high levels of interconnectedness. Medvene et al. predicted this pattern based on the idea that if the partner is part of the self, the partner's benefits are one's own, and if partners do not distinguish between own and other's outcomes, the meaning of over- or underbenefited in relation to the partner is undermined.

Another relevant line of research suggests that social comparison processes are dramatically altered to be more like self-comparisons when the other is either already close to self or closeness is created by a priming manipulation (Beach et al., 1998; MacKay, McFarland, & Buehler, 1998; McFarland, Buehler, & MacKay, 2001; O'Mahen, Beach, & Tesser, 2000). For example, Beach et al. (1998) showed that participants' affective reaction to the success of their task partner outperforming the self was less negative if the performance was in a domain believed to be important to the partner—that is, the importance to the partner was treated to some extent as importance to self. Similarly, MacKay et al. (1998) showed that false feedback about a task partner's performance affected one's own mood only when the task partner was also a close relationship partner. Employing an experimental paradigm, Gardner, Gabriel, and Hochschild (2002) showed that priming inclusion of other in the self completely undermined the negative effect of partner outperforming the self; also, the degree of celebration in the close partner's success was correlated with the degree of including other in the self. Similarly, Stapel and Koomen (2001) found that participants primed with "we" (as compared to those primed with "I" or "it") were more likely to feel positively about themselves after reading about the success of a person like themselves.

It is important to acknowledge that other models have been proposed to explain why people sometimes treat a close other's outcomes like their own. For example, interdependence theory (Kelley & Thibaut, 1978; Rusbult & Arriaga, 2000) emphasizes the notion that individuals transform gut-level self-interest into joint- or other-interest in the context of evaluating long-term benefits to self. We think that this is a likely mechanism that operates in close relationships. But we also think that there are important cases of acting for the benefit of close others that can not be fully explained in this way, but can be explained by the idea of including other in the self. Thus, for example, we believe that an interdependence analysis would have predicted a bigger difference between the other-will-know- and the other-will-not-know-of-one's-allocation-decisions conditions in the Aron et al. (1991) allocation decision studies reviewed earlier.

Another theoretical model that seems to explain cases of acting for the benefit of close others is Clark and Mills's (1993) communal norm theory. Clark and Mills propose that people spontaneously attend to the needs of close others largely because it is normatively appropriate to do so. Again, we think that it is quite likely that this mechanism operates in close relationships. But, also as before, we think that there are important cases of treating close others' outcomes like one's own that can not be fully explained in this way, but can be explained by the concept of including close others in the self. Thus, for example, the communal norm view would seem to suggest that what determines degree of caring for others' outcomes is primarily the relationship category. However, several of the studies noted above found that even within relationship categories, the impact on the other's outcomes were moderated by the degree of including other in the self. Also, Medvene et al.'s (2000) study included a standard measure of communal orientation, but individual differences on this measure did not significantly moderate the equity effect that was, as noted above, moderated by inclusion of other in the self.

Thus, we tentatively conclude that, while multiple mechanisms may drive the treating of a close other's outcomes as one's own, there are various lines of data that seem specifically consistent with at least one such mechanism being including a close other's resources in the self.

Evidence That People Include Close Others' Perspectives in the Self

As noted, we propose that to some extent individuals can take on another person's perspectives of appreciating the world. For example, when a long-term married individual attends a ballet, the individual may experience the ballet not only through the individual's own eyes, but also, as it were, through the spouse's eyes. This process also seems to apply to concern about the social impressions the other makes. For example, Schlenker and Britt (2001) demonstrated that people will systematically manage information they convey about close friends to make a better impression on others. Similarly, Konrath and Ross (2003) examined whether people would extend to close others the usual effect found for self in which past successes are recalled as more recent and past failures as more distant than they actually were. Consistent with the notion of including a close other's perspectives in the self, Konrath and Ross found the same effect as is usually found for self when participants recalled past events for romantic partners, but only when those partners were close and not when they were distant. In addition, the social comparison studies we reviewed briefly in the previous section also can be interpreted as due to shared perspectives.

As we also noted earlier, a key implication of the perspectives aspect of the model is with regard to extending to others self-related attributional biases. In this regard, several studies have found that the usual actor–observer difference in the tendency to make situational versus dispositional attributions (Jones & Nisbett, 1971) is smaller when the other is someone close to self, such as a best friend or romantic partner (Aron et al., 1991, Introduction to Study 2; Aron & Fraley, 1999; Sande, Goethals, & Radloff, 1988). The idea here is that the self is experiencing the other person's perspective as the self's own ("I know why he did it—like me, he did what was appropriate for the situation").

We also conducted a series of studies extending a paradigm developed by Lord (1980, 1987) that focuses on a self-relevant cognitive bias in recall of imaged information. In the Lord paradigm, participants are presented with a series of nouns, for each of which they are to form a vivid, elaborated image of a particular person interacting with the object the noun rep-

resents. Later, participants are given a free recall test for the nouns. As predicted from his model of self as background to experience, Lord found
fewer nouns recalled that were imaged with self as compared to nouns imaged with others, such as media personalities. In our studies (Aron et al.,
1991, Study 2 and follow-up), in addition to self and a nonclose other, participants also imaged nouns with a close other: their mother. Our results
replicated Lord's for self and nonclose other. But *also*, as predicted, we
found that nouns imaged with the *close* other, the participant's mother,
were recalled about the same as for those imaged with self. This result was
found both when the nonclose other was an entertainment personality and
in a replication in which the nonclose other was mother's best friend. Thus,
just as our perspective as self serves as a background to experience, our
perspective with regard to close others—but not with regard to nonclose
others—also seems to serve as a background to experience.

Evidence That People Include Close Others' Identities in the Self

A consistent finding in a long-standing line of research on the "self-
reference effect" is an advantage in terms of memory and response time
for self-relevant versus other-relevant processing. For example, in a meta-
analysis of 126 articles and book chapters on just the memory aspect of the
self-reference effect, Symons and Johnson (1997) found consistently better
memory for words studied in relation to self than for words studied in relation to other persons. However, they also found that there were significantly smaller self-reference minus other-reference differences when the
other was someone close to self. Thus, being in a close relationship with
the other does indeed seem to subvert the seemingly fundamental distinction of self from other.

Our model posits that this apparent subversion by close relationships
of the self–other distinction is due, specifically, to the other becoming part
of the self—to the self changing such that the self includes the other in its
very makeup. That is, we hypothesize that the knowledge structures of
close others actually share elements (or activation potentials) with the
knowledge structures of the self (Aron et al., 1991; Aron & Fraley, 1999;
Smith et al., 1999). For example, one's own and a close other's traits may
actually be confused or interfere with each other.

To test this idea, we evaluated the patterns of response latencies in
making me/not me decisions (i.e., "Does the trait describe me?") about
traits previously rated for their descriptiveness of self and of spouse (Aron
et al., 1991, Study 3 and follow-up). We found that for traits on which the
self matched the partner (the trait was true of both or false of both), me/
not-me responses were faster than when a trait was mismatched for self
and partner (was true for one but false for the other). Further, in another
study (Aron & Fraley, 1999), we found that the magnitude of this effect

correlates substantially with self-report measures of relationship quality, including predicting increases in self-reported closeness over a 3-month period. Using this same match–mismatch response-time paradigm, Smith et al. (1999) replicated both the overall difference between close and nonclose others and the correlation with the magnitude of self-reported closeness to the close other. Smith and colleagues eloquently articulated why such patterns may result: "If mental representations of two persons . . . overlap so that they are effectively a single representation, reports on attributes of one will be facilitated or inhibited by matches and mismatches with the second " (p. 873).

In another series of studies (Mashek, Aron, & Boncimino, 2003), participants rated one set of traits for self, a different set of traits for a close other, and still other traits for one or more nonclose others, such as media personalities. Participants were then given a surprise recognition task in which they were asked to indicate, for each trait, for which person they had rated it. The analysis focused on confusions—traits on which the participant remembered having rated the trait for one person when the participant had actually rated the trait for a different person. Results were consistent with predictions. For example, if participants did not correctly recognize a trait as having been originally rated for the self, they were more likely to remember it as having been rated for the partner than as having been rated for the media personality. Similarly, if participants did not correctly recognize a trait as having been originally rated for the partner, they were more likely to remember it as having been rated for the self than as having been rated for the media personality. These results were replicated in two follow-up studies and were unchanged after controlling for a variety of potential confounds, such as for any tendency to recall traits in general as having been rated for self or partner and for valence and extremity of ratings.

Finally, people seem to *perceive* close others as overlapped with self. In a series of studies, we asked participants to describe their closest relationship using the Inclusion of Other in the Self (IOS) Scale (Aron, Aron, & Smollan, 1992). This IOS Scale consists of seven pairs of circles overlapping to different degrees; the respondent selects the pair of circles (the degree of overlap) that best describes his or her relationship with a particular person. The scale appears to have levels of reliability, as well as of discriminant, convergent, and predictive validity, that match or exceed other measures of closeness—measures that are typically more complex and lengthy. For example, Agnew et al. (1998) found that the IOS scale completed for a particular relationship correlated strongly with the number of plural pronouns ("we," "us," "our") in the participant's free description of the relationship. The IOS Scale also correlates with scores on various other indirect measures of including other in the self, such as the match–mismatch response-time paradigm (e.g., Aron & Fraley, 1999).

Since its development, the scale has been used effectively in a number of studies of relationships (Agnew, Loving, Le, & Goodfriend, 2004). It seems plausible that this measure has been so successful because the metaphor of overlapping circles representing self and other corresponds to how people actually process information about self and close others.

A Note on Self-Expansion Motivation

Before concluding this first half of the chapter on our basic conceptual framework, it is important to note that much of our work regarding including other in the self has focused on the role of inclusion of other in the self as part of the larger self-expansion model (Aron & Aron, 1986; Aron et al., 2001). This model posits that people seek to expand their potential self-efficacy (i.e., ability to accomplish desired goals). It further argues that one way people seek to expand their potential efficacy is through close relationships. This is because closeness in a relationship expands the self by including in the self the resources, perspectives, and identities of the relationship partner.

This view has a number of important implications for understanding relationships. For example, Aron, Paris, and Aron (1995), in two prospective longitudinal studies, demonstrated that entering a new relationship (operationalized as falling in love) expands the self in the sense that one's spontaneous self-description increases in diversity, and in the sense of an increase in perceived self-efficacy. Taking a quite different angle, Fraley and Aron (2004) demonstrated that feelings of self-expansion mediated the effect of shared humorous activities on interpersonal attraction; and Aron, Steele, and Kashdan (2004), in two experiments, supported the hypothesis from the model that under conditions in which people are confident of reciprocation of their liking, they are most attracted to others who have dissimilar interests (and thus offer greater opportunities for expanding the self by including them in the self). We briefly consider some of our most active lines of research relating to the motivational aspects in one of the subsections in the second half of this chapter.

CURRENT NEW DIRECTIONS

Is Including Other in the Self Different from Familiarity and Similarity?

A recent focus of our work that relates to basic theory is the extent to which including other in the self can be distinguished from familiarity or similarity. That is, one possible interpretation of the various results we have reviewed showing smaller (or absent) self–other differences for close others is that close others are more familiar or more similar to the self.

Indeed, we would be surprised if familiarity and similarity do not play an important role in this process. It seems highly probable that one way in which people probably recognize anything as part of themselves is by its familiarity and similarity to other aspects of themselves. Further, familiarity and similarity are inevitably confounded with interpersonal closeness. We are likely to be most familiar with those to whom we are close because we usually spend more time with close others and do a wider variety of activities with close others (Berscheid, Synder, & Omoto, 1989), thus appreciating them in more situations. We are more likely to be similar to close others because we are likely to select similar individuals as relationship partners (e.g., Byrne, 1971) and because close relationship partners become more similar over time (e.g., Zajonc, Adelmann, Murphy, & Niedenthal, 1987).

Nevertheless, we have recently argued that inclusion of others in the self seems to be conceptually and empirically distinguishable from both familiarity and similarity (Aron, Mashek, & Aron, 2004).

Familiarity

Inclusion of others in the self and familiarity seem clearly quite different conceptually. Inclusion of another person in the self has to do with aspects of the other person treated as if they were one's own; familiarity has to do with how much exposure to and attention one has given to those aspects of the other person. Further, several findings suggest that familiarity does not account for the various results we have reviewed regarding including close others in the self. First, as part of their meta-analysis of self-reference findings, Symons and Johnson (1997) reported a near-zero mean difference in effect sizes when comparing studies where the other-referent was familiar versus studies where the other-referent was not familiar. However, they found a significant and substantial mean difference in effect sizes when comparing studies where the other-referent was intimate versus studies where the other-referent was not intimate. Second, in their source-confusion-memory studies, Mashek et al. (2003, Studies 2 and 3) compared confusions between self and one's closest friend with confusions between self and one's closest parent, when parents were more familiar (by virtue of one's long history with them) but were rated as less close. Mashek and her colleagues found significantly more confusions with the friends than with the parents. Finally, studies using the match–mismatch response-time effect have found consistently large correlations with subjectively reported closeness (Aron et al., 1991; Aron & Fraley, 1999; Smith et al., 1999), but near-zero correlations with reported familiarity and with variables that would seem to be relatively objective indicators of familiarity, such as number of different activities shared with other, amount of time spent with other, and relationship length (Aron et al., 1991; Aron & Fraley, 1999).

Similarity

Like familiarity, similarity seems distinguishable conceptually from including another person in the self. For example, including another person in the self also means including the aspects of the other that are different from the self. That is, including another person in the self refers to the elements of the other (resources, perspectives, identities) being available to and part of the structure and content of self; similarity refers to the elements of the other sharing descriptive features with those of the self. (Indeed, in the context of the motivational implications of our model, one would presumably prefer a potential partner whose resources are different from one's own, since having access to such resources would maximally expand the self beyond that to which one already has access; Aron et al., 2003.) Empirically, in the cognitive bias imaging recall study, participants rated similarity to the close other, and correlations of the effect with rated similarity were small and not significant (Aron et al., 1991, Studies 2a and 2b). Also, in the source-confusion memory experiments (Mashek et al., 2003), the greater effect for close friend than close parent held up even though ratings of friends' traits were less similar to self than were ratings of parents' traits; nor was the difference in confusions between these targets affected by partialing out ratings of similarity.

Identifying Neural Substrates of the Connection of Self and Close Others

Another new direction that relates to basic issues is examining the neural substrates of including other in the self. There is growing evidence from cognitive neuroscience (e.g., Keenan, 2003) that judgments related to self may engage specific neural systems, primarily in prefrontal areas, that differ from those engaged by judgments about others. Other work, including developmental psychology and neuropsychology in the context of theory of mind (e.g., Baron-Cohen, 1995) and comparative psychology in the context of self-awareness in primates (e.g., Gallup, 1970) lead to similar conclusions. In this context, the idea and supporting research regarding close others being "included in the self" considered in the first half of this chapter suggest that neural systems preferentially engaged for judgments regarding self when compared to those regarding others in general may also be preferentially engaged for judgments regarding close others when compared to others in general.

To date three preliminary findings lend support to this suggestion. First, Kircher et al. (2001) conducted a functional magnetic resonance imaging (fMRI) study in which participants viewed facial photographs of themselves, their romantic partner, or an unknown face. Many areas of activation differed between self and the partner, when each was compared to an unknown face; but there was at least one area that was clearly active for both self versus unknown face and partner versus unknown face. Second, Lichty et al. (2003) conducted an fMRI study in which participants performed a memory task for a series of randomly repeated names that included their own first name, the first name of a close other, and a common and uncommon first name in U.S. culture (but one that did not correspond to anyone close to the participant). Lichty and her colleagues found several areas that were clearly active for both self versus common and uncommon names and for close other versus common and uncommon names. Finally, we have been conducting an fMRI study (Aron & Keenan, 2004) in which participants rate trait adjectives for their applicability to self, spouse, and two nonclose others (media personalities). A key preliminary within-subject analyses of data from the first five usable subjects focused on regions of significant activation that are the same for self and spouse, but which are not in the same location for nonclose others. (That is, this analysis attempts to identify unique regions of self–close other commonalities.) The results were that there were more such self–close other common areas than would be expected by chance (given the number of regions of significant activation of each type overall).

These various data lend preliminary support to the suggestion that processing of self and close others shares at least some key neural circuits, providing unique triangulating evidence in relation to the behavioral and cognitive studies reviewed in the first half of this chapter. As research develops in this area, the specific brain localizations of such overlaps, as well as the conditions in which they are and are not found, should provide important new insights into what it means to include another person in the self.

Feeling "Too Close" to a Relationship Partner

Other new directions in relation to the including-other-in-the-self model focus on its potential contribution to understanding previously unstudied relationship topics. One example is recent work by Mashek and her colleagues (Mashek & Aron, 2004; Mashek & Sherman, 2004) that extends the inclusion-of-other-in-the-self model to understand instances in which a person feels "too close," that is, where the person feels too interconnected with the other. In such a situation, there is a discrepancy between what one sees as one's *actual* closeness (what one sees as the degree of inclusion of other in the self) and one's *desired* closeness with the partner. Thus, as one indicator in our research to date on feeling "too close," we compare (1) a person's rating on the IOS Scale (the overlapping circles measure of closeness discussed earlier) completed for his or her relationship with the partner, to (2), their rating on the IOS Scale completed for his or her "desired" relationship with the partner. "Feeling too close" is then operationalized as rating actual higher than desired.

Over the course of a semester, as many as 57% of dating undergraduates reported feeling too close as measured in this way (Mashek & Sherman, 2004). The participants Mashek and Sherman interviewed often used words to describe this experience such as "suffocating," "smothering," and "overwhelming." Further, across samples, the general pattern of correlations between feeling too close and relationship quality is quite clear. People who are as close as they want to be (i.e., people whose actual closeness equals their desired closeness) report exceptionally high relationship quality. However, the relationship quality of people who desire less closeness is about equally low as that of people who desire more closeness. This pattern is found across a wide variety of relationship quality measures including satisfaction, commitment, and passionate love. Preliminary data also show that the same pattern appears when looking at attachment avoidance: people who want either more or less closeness are more avoidant than people whose actual and desired closeness are equivalent.

Based on a review of biographical and clinical descriptions of feeling too close, Mashek and Sherman (2004) identified two key themes about what seems to precipitate feelings of too much closeness with a romantic partner: (1) the partner threatens personal control and (2) the partner threatens personal identity. Several theoretical models from social and clinical psychology are relevant to these two processes. Those models especially relevant to the control theme include self-determination theory (Ryan & Deci, 2000), attachment theory (Bowlby, 1969), and various ideas from the power-and-control literature (e.g., French & Raven, 1959). Each of these perspectives suggests that the self (and its development) can be influenced detrimentally when others limit our ability to control our own environment. Those models especially relevant to the identity theme include optimal distinctiveness theory (Brewer & Pickett, 1999) and object relations theory (e.g., Stierlin, 1976). Both of these perspectives hint at the notion that overinclusion in the dyad (i.e., being unable to differentiate self from other) may lead to feeling too close.

In recent research (Mashek & Aron, 2004), we have found consistent moderate-sized correlations between feeling too close and feeling undesired control by the partner. These correlations were found across all three samples studied (romantic relationships in two student samples and long-term marriages in a community sample), were not qualified by gender, held up across different measurement methods, and remained after partialing out reported relationship quality. The next steps in this research program are to examine the loss-of-identity hypothesis, test both hypothesized mechanisms experimentally and longitudinally, test the generalizability of results across methodologically diverse measures of including other in the self (such as the match–mismatch response-time paradigm for self, partner, and desired partner), and further explore the mechanisms specifically in relation to the various relevant theoretical models.

Rate of Self-Expansion

As noted earlier, some of our most important current research efforts regarding including other in the self have been in the context of the larger self-expansion model (Aron & Aron, 1986; Aron et al., 2001). One recent line of work in this regard focuses on the *rate* of self-expansion. Rapid expansion of the self, as often occurs when forming a new romantic relationship, should result in high levels of excited positive affect. This notion is consistent with Carver and Scheier's (1990) argument about the impact on affective state of rapid movement toward goals. Indeed, Lewandowski and Aron (2002) have developed a measure of experienced self-expansion in close relationships, the Self-Expansion Questionnaire (SEQ). The SEQ shows strong internal consistency, is unifactorial, and has demonstrated strong construct validity in terms of its links to key variables as predicted by the self-expansion model.

However, most of our recent attention has been focused on a prediction from this aspect of the model that the quality of long-term relationships benefits from participating together in activities that are novel and challenging. That is, novelty and challenge are thought to create a sense of self-expansion, which, as noted above, creates a highly desirable affective state. When this positive affective state is associated with a romantic partner, the desirability of the state becomes linked with that person, enhancing the quality of the relationship. In a series of surveys and laboratory experiments, Aron, Norman, Aron, McKenna, and Heyman (2000) found consistent increases in love and satisfaction when long-term relationship partners participated together in novel and challenging activities. In some of our current studies, Lewandowski and Aron (2004) demonstrated that this effect was due specifically to the novelty and challenge of the activities and not to the arousal they created; Aron, Norman, and Aron (2004) showed that the effect only occurs when the novelty and challenge is experienced in a context in which the partner is salient; and Strong and Aron (2004) found that relationship quality was specifically associated with excited positive affect but not with low levels of negative affect. These various studies do not focus directly on including other in the self. However, they are testing a principle (the effect of novelty and challenge) that in practice is thought usually to occur as a result of rapid inclusion of other in self, as, for example, when people first fall in love or when one of the partners in a relationship undergoes a major self-change.

Including Ingroups in the Self

Smith and Henry (1996) first proposed that the inclusion-of-other-in-the-self model could be extended to groups. In their study, they adapted the Aron et al. (1991) match–mismatch response-time paradigm to study links between representations of the self and the ingroup. Their finding was consistent with that found for the relation of self to close others (e.g., Aron et al., 1991): there was significantly faster response times when making me/ not-me responses for traits that were the same for self and ingroup (true of both or false of both) versus traits that were different for self and ingroup. Further research has replicated this effect (McLaughlin-Volpe, 2004; Otten, 2002; Smith, 2002; Smith et al., 1999).

Subsequently, Tropp and Wright (2001) developed a measure of the degree of ingroup identification in the context of inclusion of the ingroup in the self, adapting the overlapping-circle IOS Scale to produce the Inclusion of the Ingroup in the Self Scale (IIS Scale). In the IIS Scale, pairs of circles represent varying degrees of overlap between the self and a specified ingroup. A series of studies using responses from samples of women and ethnic minority groups supported the construct validity, the concurrent and discriminant validity, and the test–retest reliability of the IIS Scale. Most important, it appears that the IIS Scale may capture the essence of the self–ingroup connection that underlies the construct of ingroup identification (see Tropp & Wright, 2001, for an extended discussion).

Finally, just as research has demonstrated that the degree of interpersonal closeness moderates the overlap effects for self and individual others using the match–mismatch response-time paradigm (Aron & Fraley, 1999; Smith et al., 1999), Tropp and Wright predicted that ingroup identification should moderate the match–mismatch response-time effect for ingroups. The results supported this prediction (Tropp & Wright, 2001, Study 1). Participants who were strongly identified with the ingroup (as indicted by high IIS Scale scores) responded significantly slower when deciding whether a trait was applicable to self when previous ratings of the self and ingroup on the trait were inconsistent than when previous ratings of the self and ingroup on the trait were consistent. In contrast, participants with low identification with the ingroup evidenced virtually no difference between traits that were or were not similarly descriptive of the ingroup when deciding whether a trait was applicable to the self. This pattern suggests that for people low in ingroup identification, the ingroup is not adequately included in the self-concept to produce the self–ingroup confusion found among those high in ingroup identification.

Our model of ingroup identification also considers motivation: Why do people join and identify with groups? The self-expansion motive proposed as the stimulus for including others in the self also provides a potential reason for the development of ingroup identification. One way to acquire the resources, perspectives, and identities that enhance one's ability to accomplish goals is to join and identify with relevant social groups. Thus, ingroup identification (including the ingroup in the self) is, at least in part, the result of basic self-expansion motives: we include groups in the self because doing so increases our ability to meet the demands of our world and achieve our goals.

There are a number of other proposed motives for ingroup identification. These include the self-enhancement motive (see Rubin & Hewstone, 1998), the need for distinctiveness and inclusion (Brewer & Pickett, 1999), and the need to reduce subjective uncertainty (Hogg, 2001). Elsewhere (Wright, Aron, & Tropp, 2002) we have considered the similarities and distinctions between the self-expansion motive and each of these alternatives. Generally, we conclude that, despite their different pedigrees (intergroup relations and social identity for these other motives, and interpersonal relationships and intimacy for self-expansion), the idea of including other in the self fits nicely into social psychology's general understanding of ingroup identification, and the self-expansion model provides novel and potentially useful explanations for ingroup identification processes. That is, although consistent with some aspects of other motivational models of ingroup identification, the self-expansion perspective yields a number of divergent hypotheses about why people join groups and why some group memberships have such a strong influence on thoughts, attitudes, and actions.

Including Other in the Self and the Intergroup Contact Effect

Another application to groups of our model of closeness as including the other in the self focuses on the *intergroup contact effect* (Allport, 1954), the idea that contact with a member of an outgroup can lead to reduced prejudice toward that outgroup. Specifically, we have suggested, based on our model, that intergroup contact is most likely to reduce prejudice when it involves a close intimate friendship with an outgroup member (Aron & McLaughlin-Volpe, 2001; Wright et al., 2002). Specifically, we reasoned as follows: Ordinarily, in self's conception of the world, my ingroup is part of myself and outgroups are not part of myself. Thus, I spontaneously treat ingroup members, to some extent, like myself, including feeling empathy for their troubles, taking pride in their successes, and generously sharing resources with them. Outgroup members, because they are not part of myself, receive none of these advantages. However, what happens when one forms a friendship with an outgroup partner? Under these circumstances, we argue, the outgroup member—and hence to some extent the outgroup member's group identity, of which one inevitably becomes aware— becomes part of the self. That is, the representation of the outgroup comes to share elements with the representation of the self. The effect, we argue, is to undermine negative outgroup attitudes. Others have pointed to the specific role of friendship (e.g., Cook, 1984; Pettigrew & Tropp, 2000), but have not focused on the role of closeness or articulated particular mediating psychological mechanisms for why friendship should have a special effect.

Several studies, by ourselves and others, using a variety of nonexperimental and experimental methods, support the proposition that contact with a member of an outgroup is much more effective in reducing prejudice when one has a close versus a less close relationship with that outgroup member (e.g., McLaughlin-Volpe, 1998; Pettigrew, 1997; Wright & Van Der Zande, 1999). Other theoretical approaches might be applied to understand these effects, such as generalization of positive affect, dissonance, or balance theories. But such approaches do not articulate a mechanism to explain the generalization from the outgroup partner to the outgroup partner's group—an articulation that is explicitly provided by the model of closeness as inclusion of other in the self. Further, McLaughlin-Volpe (2004) has recently shown that the closeness effects are directly mediated by including other in the self. In her study, including an outgroup member in the self, as measured by the match–mismatch response-time paradigm, predicted less outgroup stereotyping. Most important, this effect was significantly mediated by including the outgroup in the self, as also measured by the match–mismatch response-time paradigm.

Finally, the closeness as including-other-in-the-self model has led to the prediction of a new phenomenon, the extended (or vicarious) contact effect (Wright, Aron, McLaughlin-Volpe, & Ropp, 1997). The idea here is that a reduction in prejudice can occur as a result of mere knowledge that an ingroup member has a close relationship with an outgroup member. The logic is that when someone who is in my ingroup, and thus part of myself, is known to have an outgroup person as part of that person's self, the effect is that, to some extent, I begin to see members of that group as part of myself. Thus, the ingroup–outgroup distinction, vital to producing negative intergroup attitudes, is directly diminished by the connection of the outgroup member to an ingroup member. Also, negative attitudes toward the outgroup are reduced by this indirect connection of the outgroup with the self. This hypothesis has so far received support in a series of surveys and experiments (Wright et al., 1997); in a study of schoolchildren in Finland (Liebkind & McAlister, 1999); and in a recent field experiment involving Protestants and Catholics in Northern Ireland (Paolini, Hewstone, Cairns, & Voci, 2004). The latter study also demonstrated including other in the self as the mediated mechanism.

Including Communities in the Self

As we have described throughout this chapter, people can certainly feel connected to individuals (e.g., Aron et al., 1992) and groups (e.g., Tropp & Wright, 2001). However, a new direction for our model is that such inclusion may also extend to communities.

Recently, Mashek, Meyer, Cannaday, and Tangney (2003) successfully adapted the IOS Scale to measure including communities in the self. Further, using this measure, Mashek et al. (2004) have been exploring jail in-mates' sense of connectedness to the criminal community and to the com-munity at large. This work with inmates has yielded several provocative results that seem unlikely to have been found using other approaches. Some of the results of this research also provide the first support for previ-ously untested central predictions from our model of including others in the self.

For example, Mashek et al. (2004) found that connectedness to the community at large was associated with low levels of criminogenic beliefs (e.g., sense of entitlement, lack of appreciation for the ripple effects of crime) and elevated levels of character strength (e.g., integrity, willingness to forgive); correspondingly, connectedness to the criminal community was associated with endorsement of criminogenic beliefs and a lack of charac-ter. These results are directly parallel to findings reviewed in previous sections regarding including in the self the perspectives and identities of individuals and groups, thus extending this approach directly to the com-munity level. More important from a theoretical point of view, the results regarding connectedness to the criminal community are the first direct evi-dence in any domain that in the process of including others in the self peo-ple may also include negative aspects of those others. This has interesting implications in a variety of other areas of application of the inclusion-of-other-in-the-self model. For example, Lewandowski (2002) suggested that the inclusion in the self of negative aspects of relationship partners may ex-plain why some individuals do better after a relationship loss. That is, when one comes to include less of another in the self (due to relationship loss), one may benefit if what had been included was detrimental to the self's interests.

As another example, Mashek et al. (2004) found that, when consid-ered in isolation, neither connectedness to the community at large nor connectedness to the criminal community were significantly associated with typical indicators of psychological health (e.g., low depression, low anxiety, high self-esteem). However, being connected to *both* the commu-nity at large and the criminal community was substantially associated with high depression, high anxiety, low self-esteem, and high drug problems. Such an effect would be predicted from our model because two conflicting elements are included in the self. However, these findings represent the first direct demonstration of such an effect in any domain of including others in the self. (The idea of distress from including conflicting elements in the self follows directly from cognitive dissonance theory. But cognitive dissonance theory only applies once one assumes that communities and their values become included in the self as cognitive elements that can be dissonant.) This result also has important implications for other domains of applica-tion of our model. For example, the motivation to reduce distress from conflicting inclusions may be one way in which including an outgroup member in the self reduces prejudice to the outgroup (as described in the previous subsection on contact effects).

CONCLUSION

In this chapter we first described our basic model of including others in the self and summarized supporting research; we then briefly described several new directions of applying this idea. A core message is that it can be misleading to consider the self as a knowledge structure separate from the knowledge structures of others. Rather, we hope this chapter has demonstrated that a fruitful way of understanding interpersonal cognition is in terms of self-related cognition being fundamentally intertwined with cognition regarding other individuals, groups, and communities.

REFERENCES

Agnew, C. R., Loving, T. J., Le, B., & Goodfriend, W. (2004). Thinking close: Measuring relational closeness as perceived self-other inclusion. In D. Mashek & A. Aron (Eds), *Handbook of closeness and intimacy* (pp. 103–115). Mahwah, NJ: Erlbaum

Agnew, C. R., Van Lange, P. A. M., Rusbult, C. E., & Langston, C. A. (1998). Cognitive interdependence: Commitment and the mental representation of close relationships. *Journal of Personality and Social Psychology, 74,* 939–954.

Ahuvia, A. (1993). *I love it!: Towards a unifying theory of love across diverse love objects.* Unpublished doctoral dissertation, Northwestern University, Evanston, IL.

Allport, G. (1954). *The nature of prejudice.* Reading, MA: Addison-Wesley.

Aron, A. (2003). Self and close relationships. In M. R. Leary & J. P. Tangney (Eds.), *Handbook of self and identity* (pp. 442–461). New York: Guilford Press.

Aron, A., & Aron, E. N. (1986). *Love as the expansion of self: Understanding attraction and satisfaction.* New York: Hemisphere.

Aron, A., Aron, E. N., & Norman, C. (2001). The self expansion model of motivation and cognition in close relationships and beyond. In M Clark & G. Fletcher (Eds.), *Blackwell handbook in social psychology: Vol. 2. Interpersonal processes* (pp. 478–501). Oxford, UK: Blackwell.

Aron, A., Aron, E. N., & Smollan, D. (1992). Inclusion of Other in the Self Scale and the structure of interpersonal closeness. *Journal of Personality and Social Psychology, 63,* 596–612.

Aron, A., Aron, E. N., Tudor, M., & Nelson, G. (1991). Close relationships as including other in the self. *Journal of Personality and Social Psychology, 60,* 241–253.

Aron, A., & Fraley, B. (1999). Relationship closeness as including other in the self: Cognitive underpinnings and measures. *Social Cognition, 17,* 140–160.

Aron, A., & Keenan, J. P. (2004). *Including close others in the self: An fMRI study.* Preliminary data.

Aron, A., Mashek, D., & Aron, E. N. (2004). Closeness as including other in the self. In D. Mashek & A. Aron (Eds.), *Handbook of closeness and intimacy* (pp. 27–41). Mahwah, NJ: Erlbaum.

Aron, A., & McLaughlin-Volpe, T. (2001). Including others in the self: Extensions to own and partner's group memberships. In C. Sedikides & M. B. Brewer (Eds.), *Individual self, relational self, and collective self: Partners, opponents, or strangers?* (pp. 89–109). Philadelphia: Psychology Press.

Aron, A., Norman, C. C., & Aron, E. N. (2004). *Couple participation in self-expanding activities and relationship quality: Is shared participation necessary?* Manuscript in preparation.

Aron, A., Norman, C. C., Aron, E. N., McKenna, C., & Heyman, R. (2000). Couples' shared participation in novel and arousing activities and experienced relationship quality. *Journal of Personality and Social Psychology, 78,* 273–283.

Aron, A., Paris, M., & Aron, E. N. (1995). Falling in love: Prospective studies of self-concept change. *Journal of Personality and Social Psychology, 69,* 1102–1112.

Aron, A., Steele, J., & Kashdan, T. (2004). *When opposites attract: A test of the self-expansion model.* Manuscript in preparation.

Bakan, D. (1966). *The duality of human existence: Isolation and commitment in Western man.* Boston: Beacon Press.

Baldwin, M. W. (1992). Relational schemas and the processing of social information. *Psychological Bulletin, 112,* 461–484.

Baron-Cohen, S. (1995). *Mindblindness: An essay on autism and theory of mind.* Cambridge, MA: MIT Press.

Beach, S. R., Tesser, A., Fincham, F. D., Jones, D. J., Johnson, D., & Whitaker, D. J. (1998). Pleasure and pain in doing well, together: An investigation of performance-related affect in close relationships. *Journal of Personality and Social Psychology, 74,* 923–938.

Belk, R. W. (1988). Possessions and the extended self. *Journal of Consumer Research, 15,* 139–168.

Berscheid, E., Snyder, M., & Omoto, A. M. (1989). The Relationship Closeness Inventory: Assessing the closeness of interpersonal relationships. *Journal of Personality and Social Psychology, 57,* 792–807.

Bowlby, J. (1969). *Attachment and loss: Vol. 1. Attachment.* New York: Basic Books.

Brewer, M. B., & Pickett, C. L. (1999). Distinctiveness motives as a source of the social self. In T. R. Tyler, R. M. Kramer, & O. P. John (Eds.), *The psychology of the social self* (pp. 47–69). Mahwah, NJ: Erlbaum.

Buber, M. (1937). *I and thou.* New York: Scribners.

Byrne, D. (1971). *The attraction paradigm.* New York: Academic Press.

Carver, C., & Scheier, M. (1990). Principles of self-regulation, action, and emotion. In E. T. Higgins & R. M. Sorrentino (Eds.), *Handbook of motivation and cognition: Foundations of social behavior* (Vol. 2, pp. 3–52). New York: Guilford Press.

Cialdini, R. B., Brown, S. L., Lewis, B. P., Luce, C., & Neuberg, S. L. (1997). Reinterpreting the empathy–altruism relationships: When one into one equals oneness. *Journal of Personality and Social Psychology, 73,* 481–494.

Clark, M. S., & Mills, J. (1979). Interpersonal attraction in exchange and communal relationships. *Journal of Personality and Social Psychology, 37,* 12–24.

Clark, M. S., & Mills, J. (1993). The difference between communal and exchange relationships: What it is and is not. *Personality and Social Psychology Bulletin,* *19,* 684–691.

Collins, N. L., & Read, S. J. (1994). Cognitive representations of attachment: The content and function of working models. In K. Bartholomew & D. Perlman (Eds.), *Advances in personal relationships* (Vol. 5, pp. 53–90). London: Jessica Kingsley.

Cook, S. W. (1984). Cooperative interaction in multiethnic contexts. In N. Miller & M. B. Brewer (Eds.), *Groups in contact: The psychology of desegregation* (pp. 155–185). New York: Academic Press.

Cooley, C. H. (1902). *Human nature and the social order.* New York: Scribners.

Fraley, B., & Aron, A. (2004). Shared humor and rapport between strangers. *Personal Relationships, 11,* 61–78.

French, J. R. P., & Raven, B. H. (1959). The bases of social power. In D. Cartwright (Ed.), *Studies in social power.* Ann Arbor: University of Michigan Press.

Gallup, G. G. (1970). Chimpanzees: Self-recognition. *Science, 167,* 86–87.

Gardner, W. L., Gabriel, S., & Hochschild, L. (2002). When you and I are "we," you are not threatening: The role of self-expansion in social comparison. *Journal of Personality and Social Psychology, 82,* 239–251.

Heider, F. (1958). *The psychology of interpersonal relations.* New York: Wiley.

Hogg, M. A. (2001). Subjective uncertainty reduction through self-categorization: A motivational theory of social identity processes. *European Review of Social Psychology, 11,* 223–255.

Ickes, W., Tooke, W., Stinson, L., Baker, V., & Bissonnette, V. (1988). Naturalistic social cognition: Intersubjectivity in same-sex dyads. *Journal of Nonverbal Behavior, 12,* 58–84.

James, W. (1948). *Psychology.* Cleveland: Fine Editions Press. (Original work published 1890)

Jones, E. E., & Nisbett, R. (1971). The actor and the observer: Divergent perceptions of the causes of behavior. In E. E. Jones, D. E. Kannouse, H. H. Kelley, R. E. Nisbett, S. Valins, & B. Weiner (Eds.), *Attribution: Perceiving the causes of behavior* (pp. 79–94). Morristown, NJ: General Learning Press.

Jung, C. G. (1959). Marriage as a psychological relationship. In V. S. DeLaszlo (Ed.) & F. C. Hull (Trans.), *The basic writings of C. G. Jung* (pp. 531–544). New York: Modern Library. (Original work published 1925)

Keenan, J. P. (2003). *The face in the mirror: The search for the origins of consciousness.* New York: HarperCollins.

Kelley, H. H., & Thibaut, J. W. (1978). *Interpersonal relationships: A theory of interdependence.* New York: Wiley.

Kircher, T. T. J., Senior, C., Phillips, M. L., Rabe-Hesketh, S., Benson, P. J., Bullmore, E. T., Brammer, M., Simmons, A., Bartels, M., & David, A. S. (2001). Recognizing one's own face. *Cognition, 78,* B1–B15.

Konrath, S. H., & Ross, M. (2003). *Our glories, our shames: Expanding the self in temporal self appraisal theory.* Paper presented at the American Psychological Society conference, Atlanta, GA.

Lewandowski, G. W. Jr. (2002). *Relationship dissolution and the self-concept: The effects of interpersonal closeness and self-expansion.* Unpublished doctoral dissertation, State University of New York at Stony Brook.

Lewandowski, G. W., Jr. & Aron, A. (2002). *The Self-Expansion Scale.* Paper presented at the third annual meeting of the Society of Personality and Social Psychology, Savannah, GA.

Lewandowski, G. W. Jr., & Aron, A. (2004). *Self-expansion versus arousal in promoting relationship quality in long-term relationships.* Manuscript under review.

Lichty, W., Chyou, J., Anderson, A. K., Ghahremanni, D. G., Yamahuchi, Y., & Gabrieli, J. D. E. (2003, November). *What's in a name: Neural correlates related to self and self-relevance.* Paper presented at the Society for Neuroscience Conference, New Orleans.

Liebkind, K., & McAlister, A. L. (1999). Extended contact through peer modeling to promote tolerance in Finland. *European Journal of Social Psychology, 29, 765–780.*

Lord, C. G. (1980). Schemas and images as memory aids: Two modes of processing social information. *Journal of Personality and Social Psychology, 38, 257–269.*

Lord, C. G. (1987). Imagining self and others: Reply to Brown, Keenan, and Potts. *Journal of Personality and Social Psychology, 53, 445–450.*

MacKay, L., McFarland, C., & Buehler, R. (1998, August). *Affective reactions to performances in close relationships.* Paper presented at the annual meeting of the American Psychological Association, San Francisco.

Mashek, D. J., & Aron, A. (2004). *Feeling controlled and feeling "too close" in relationships.* Manuscript in preparation.

Mashek, D. J., Aron, A., & Boncimino, M. (2003). Confusions of self and close others. *Personality and Social Psychology Bulletin, 29, 382–392.*

Mashek, D., Meyer, P., Cannaday, L., & Tangney, J. (2003, February). *Seeing oneself as part of the criminal community: Self-community overlap and the moral emotions of incarcerated offenders.* Poster presented at the meeting of the Society for Personality and Social Psychology, Los Angeles.

Mashek, D., & Sherman, M. (2004). Feeling too close to intimate others. In D. Mashek & A. Aron (Eds.), *Handbook of closeness and intimacy* (pp. 343–356). Mahwah, NJ: Erlbaum.

Mashek, D., Stuewig, J., Furukawa, E., & Tangney, J. (2004). *Connectedness to the criminal community and to the community at large: Psychological and behavioral correlates.* Manuscript under review.

Maslow, A. H. (1967). A theory of metamotivation: The biological rooting of the value-life. *Journal of Humanistic Psychology, 7, 93–127.*

McCall, G. J. (1974). A symbolic interactionist approach to attraction. In T. L. Huston (Ed.), *Foundations of interpersonal attraction* (pp. 217–231). New York: Academic Press.

McFarland, C., Buehler, R., & MacKay, L. (2001). Affective responses to social comparisons with extremely close others. *Social Cognition, 19, 547–586.*

McLaughlin-Volpe, T. (1998). *Social interactions with members of ethnic outgroups and ethnic prejudice: A diary study.* Unpublished master's thesis, State University of New York at Stony Brook.

McLaughlin-Volpe, T. (2004). *The intergroup contact effect as including an outgroup other in the self.* Unpublished doctoral dissertation, State University of New York at Stony Brook.

Mead, G. H. (1934). *Mind, self, and society.* Chicago: University of Chicago Press.

Medvene, L. J., Teal, C. R., & Slavich, S. (2000). Including the other in self: Implications for judgments of equity and satisfaction in close relationships. *Journal of Social and Clinical Psychology, 19,* 396–419.

Merleau-Ponty, M. (1945). *Phenomenologie de la perception.* Paris: Gallimard.

O'Mahen, H. A., Beach, S. R. H., & Tesser, A. (2000). Relationship ecology and negative communication in romantic relationships: A self-evaluation maintenance perspective. *Personality and Social Psychology Bulletin, 26,* 1343–1352.

Otten, S. (2002). I am positive and so are we: The self as a determinant of favoritism towards novel ingroups. In J. P. Forgas & K. Williams (Eds.), *The social self: Cognitive, interpersonal and intergroup perspectives* (pp. 273–292). Philadelphia: Psychology Press.

Paolini, S., Hewstone, M., Cairns, E., & Voci, A. (2004). Effects of direct and indirect cross-group friendships on judgments of Catholics and Protestants in Northern Ireland: The mediating role of an anxiety-reduction mechanism. *Personality and Social Psychology Bulletin, 30,* 770–786.

Pettigrew, T. F. (1997). Generalized intergroup effects on prejudice. *Personality and Social Psychology Bulletin, 23,* 173–185.

Pettigrew, T. F., & Tropp, L. (2000). Does intergroup contact reduce prejudice?: Recent meta-analytic findings. In S. Oskamp (Ed.), *Reducing prejudice and discrimination: Social psychological perspectives* (pp. 93–114). Mahwah, NJ: Erlbaum.

Reik, T. (1944). *A psychologist looks at love.* New York: Farrar & Reinhart.

Reis, H. T., & Shaver, P. (1988). Intimacy as interpersonal process. In S. Duck (Ed.), *Handbook of personal relationships: Theory, research and interventions* (pp. 367–389). Chichester, UK: Wiley.

Rubin, M., & Hewstone, M. (1998). Social identity theory's self-esteem hypothesis: A review and some suggestions for clarification. *Personality and Social Psychology Review, 2,* 40–62.

Runciman, W. G. (1966). *Relative deprivation and social justice.* Berkeley, CA: University of California Press.

Rusbult, C. E., & Arriaga, X. B. (2000). Interdependence in personal relationships. In W. Ickes & S. Duck (Eds.), *The social psychology of personal relationships* (pp. 79–108). Chichester, UK: Wiley.

Ryan, R. M., & Deci, E. L. (2000). Self-determination theory and the facilitation of intrinsic motivation, social development, and well-being. *American Psychologist, 55,* 68–78.

Sande, G. N., Goethals, G. R., & Radloff, C. E. (1988). Perceiving one's own traits and others': The multifaceted self. *Journal of Personality and Social Psychology, 54,* 13–20.

Schlenker, B. R., & Britt, T. W. (2001). Strategically controlling information to help friends: Effects of empathy and friendship strength on beneficial impression management. *Journal of Experimental Social Psychology, 37,* 357–372.

Schultz, P. W. (2002). Inclusion with nature: Understanding the psychology of human–nature interactions. In P. Schmuck & P. W. Schultz, *The psychology of sustainable development* (pp. 61–78). New York: Kluwer.

Schutz, A. (1970). *On phenomenology and social relations.* Chicago: University of Chicago Press.

Sedikides, C., Olsen, N., & Reis, H. T. (1993). Relationships as natural categories. *Journal of Personality and Social Psychology, 64,* 71–82.

Sivadas, E., & Machleit, K. A. (1994). A scale to determine the extent of object incorporation in the extended self. *American Marketing Association, 5*, 143–149.

Smith, E. (2002). Overlapping mental representations of self and group: Evidence and implications. In J. P. Forgas & K. Williams (Eds.), *The social self: Cognitive, interpersonal and intergroup perspectives* (pp. 21–35). Philadelphia: Psychology Press.

Smith, E., Coates, S., & Walling, D. (1999). Overlapping mental representations of self, in-group, and partner: Further response time evidence and a connectionist model. *Personality and Social Psychology Bulletin, 25*, 873–882.

Smith, E., & Henry, S. (1996). An in-group becomes part of the self: Response time evaluation. *Personality and Social Psychology Bulletin, 22*, 635–642.

Stapel, D. A., & Koomen, W. (2001). I, we, and the effects of others on me: How self-construal level moderates social comparison effects. *Journal of Personality and Social Psychology, 80*, 766–781.

Stierlin, H. (1976). The dynamics of owning and disowning: Psychoanalytic and family perspectives. *Family Process, 15*, 277–289.

Strong, G., & Aron, A. (2004, July). *Positive and negative affect variation and association with experienced relationship quality.* Paper presented at International Association for Relationship Research Conference, Madison, WI.

Symons, C. S., & Johnson, B. T. (1997). The self-reference effect in memory: A meta-analysis. *Psychological Bulletin, 121*(3), 371–394.

Tajfel, H., & Turner, J. C. (1979). An integrative theory of intergroup conflict. In W. G. Austin & S. Worchel (Eds.), *The social psychology of intergroup relations* (pp. 33–47). Monterey, CA: Brooks/Cole.

Tesser, A. (1988). Toward a self-evaluation maintenance model of social behavior. In L. Berkowitz (Ed.), *Advances in experimental social psychology* (Vol. 11, pp. 288–338). San Diego, CA: Academic Press.

Tropp, L. R., & Wright, S. C. (2001). Ingroup identification as inclusion of ingroup in the self. *Personality and Social Psychology Bulletin, 27*, 585–600.

Wright, S. C., Aron, A., McLaughlin-Volpe, T., & Ropp, S. A. (1997). The extended contact effect: Knowledge of cross-group friendships and prejudice. *Journal of Personality and Social Psychology, 73*, 73–90.

Wright, S. C., Aron, A., & Tropp, L. R. (2002). Including others (and groups) in the self: Self-expansion and intergroup relations. In J. P. Forgas & K. Williams (Eds.), *The social self: Cognitive, interpersonal and intergroup perspectives* (pp. 343–363). Philadelphia: Psychology Press.

Wright, S. C., & Van Der Zande, C. C. (1999). *Bicultural friends: When cross-group friendships cause improved intergroup attitudes.* Paper presented at the annual meeting of the Society for Experimental Social Psychology, St. Louis, MO.

Zajonc, R. B., Adelmann, P. K., Murphy, S. T., & Niedenthal, P. M. (1987). Convergence in the physical appearance of spouses: An implication of the vascular theory of emotional efference. *Motivation and Emotion, 11*, 335–346.

10

Mental Representations of Attachment Security

Theoretical Foundation
for a Positive Social Psychology

MARIO MIKULINCER *and* PHILLIP R. SHAVER

Social psychology, like its sister discipline clinical psychology, has devoted much more attention to the problematic than to the admirable qualities of the "social animal." Whether this is because science is supported by national governments in order to solve social problems or because human perception naturally tilts investigators, like everyone else, toward threats that arouse negative rather than positive affect, we cannot say. A brief look at the cumulative record of social psychology confirms, however, that our predecessors were more concerned with racism, aggression, violence, destructive obedience, mindless conformity, failure to assist others, egotistical self-enhancement, and biased social cognition than with sympathy, tolerance, kindness, support, healthy autonomy, and accurate self- and social perception. From time to time, an alternative, more optimistic, more hopeful, actualization-oriented approach to psychology emerges—for example, the "humanistic psychology" movement of the 1950s and 1960s or today's "positive psychology" movement (Aspinwall & Staudinger, 2003; Seligman, 2002). But this reaching toward positivity seems frivolous or elitist to many people in the field, and after a while positivity tends to give way again to a focus on human misery and misbehavior.

Along with the emphasis on threats, deficits, defenses, and distortions goes social psychology's persistent preference for nondevelopmental theories. Somewhat oddly for a *social* discipline, social psychology tends to study individuals who resemble Rousseau's vision of the presocialized "savage": arriving seemingly from nowhere, as solitary adults, they enter into brief laboratory scenarios where they interact with various stimuli or simulated minimal social situations. Little attention is given to adults' personalities and previous social experiences. One would never guess from reading social-psychological texts that people are born into and generally remain connected to nuclear and extended families, live in distinctive neighborhoods and cultures, get married and have families of their own, and continue to develop across the lifespan. Social psychologists sometimes behave as if focusing on these aspects of the social animal would violate an important taboo and suddenly transport them out of social psychology, into an uncomfortably alien intellectual realm such as developmental or personality psychology, family sociology, or anthropology.

In the present chapter we consider the possibility that social psychology has unwittingly focused most of its attention on the defensive processes that characterize relatively insecure, rather than securely attached, people—that is, people with a history of inadequate support from attachment figures rather than those who have been well treated. If so, it is likely that a more balanced consideration of the behavior, motivational tendencies, and cognitive propensities of secure and insecure people will help to create a social psychology that is compatible with the vision inherent in the humanistic psychology of the past (e.g., Rogers, 1961) and the present-day positive psychology movement, while placing these movements on a deeper theoretical foundation. In particular, we think recent research on human attachments and their cognitive representations provides a strong and generative foundation for a positive, health- and growth-oriented social psychology. In explaining this foundation, we use Rogers's (1961) now somewhat neglected theory as a touchstone, as seems to be happening in other areas of social psychology where a deeper conception of self-esteem and well-being is being sought (e.g., Kernis, 2003).

ATTACHMENT THEORY: BASIC CONCEPTS

In his exposition of attachment theory, Bowlby (1982/1969, 1973, 1980) placed great emphasis on mental representations of attachment security (i.e., expectations that key people will be available and supportive in times of need) as supports for constructively coping with life's problems, maintaining emotional equanimity and stability, and forming mature, intimate, and mutually beneficial relationships. In the following pages we focus on these mental representations and examine what is known about their effects on social motives, cognitions, and behaviors. We propose that chronic

tions with the environment, results in activation of the attachment system when a potential or actual threat is encountered. This activation is manifested through efforts to seek and/or maintain actual or symbolic proximity to external or internalized attachment figures. Once the attachment system is activated, a person, in effect, asks whether or not an attachment figure is sufficiently available and responsive. An affirmative answer results in the appropriate functioning of the attachment system, characterized by reinforced mental representations of attachment security and consolidation of security-based strategies of affect regulation (Shaver & Mikulincer, 2002). These strategies are aimed at alleviating distress, fostering supportive intimate relationships, and increasing both perceived and actual personal and social adjustment.

Perceptions of attachment figures as unavailable or insensitive result in attachment insecurity, which compounds the distress already aroused by the appraised threat. This state of insecurity forces a decision about the viability of proximity seeking as a protective strategy. When proximity seeking is appraised as viable or essential—because of attachment history, self-concept, temperament, or contextual cues—people adopt *hyperactivating attachment strategies*, which include intense appeals to attachment figures and continued reliance on them as a source of comfort. Hyperactivation of the attachment system involves increased vigilance to threat-related cues and a reduction in the threshold for detecting cues of attachment figures' unavailability—the two kinds of cues that activate the attachment system (Bowlby, 1973). As a result, even minimal threat-related cues are easily detected, the attachment system is chronically activated, psychological pain related to the unavailability of attachment figures is exacerbated, and doubts about one's ability to achieve relief and attain a sense of security are heightened. These concomitants of attachment system hyperactivation account for many of the psychological correlates of attachment anxiety (see Mikulincer & Shaver, 2003, for an extensive review).

Appraising proximity seeking as unlikely to alleviate distress results in the adoption of *attachment-deactivating strategies*, manifested in distancing oneself from stimuli and events that activate the attachment system and making attempts to handle distress alone. These strategies involve dismissal of threat- and attachment-related cues, suppression of threat- and attachment-related thoughts and emotions, and repression of threat- and attachment-related memories. These tendencies are further reinforced by adoption of a self-reliant attitude that decreases dependence on others and discourages acknowledgment of personal faults or weaknesses. These aspects of deactivation account for the psychological manifestations of avoidant attachment (again, see Mikulincer & Shaver, 2003, for a review).

Our model provides a guide for delineating the cognitive, affective, and relational behaviors associated with attachment system functioning in adulthood. The module that monitors attachment figure availability and promotes a sense of attachment security is related to optimal functioning of the attachment system and helps explain the key benefits of interacting with security-enhancing attachment figures: healthy personality development, favorable psychological functioning, and good social and personal adjustment. The module that monitors the viability of proximity seeking and determines the adoption of hyperactivating or deactivating strategies is related to the specific defensive measures used by insecurely attached people to regulate distress and manage doubts about their self-worth and others' good intentions, as well as the specific emotional and relational problems that result from anxious and avoidant forms of attachment. In the next section, we focus on the attachment-figure-availability component of our model, the resulting representations of attachment security, and the positive effects they have on a person's social motives, cognitions, and behaviors.

MENTAL REPRESENTATIONS OF ATTACHMENT SECURITY

In our model, appraisal of attachment-figure availability automatically activates mental representations of attachment security. These representations include both declarative and procedural knowledge organized around a relational prototype or script (Waters, Rodrigues, & Ridgeway, 1998). This script includes something like the following if–then propositions: If I encounter an obstacle and/or become distressed, I can approach a significant other for help; he or she is likely to be available and supportive; I will experience relief and comfort as a result of proximity to this person; I can then return to other activities. Once activated, this script serves as a guide for adaptively regulating one's own cognitive and affective processes.

Representations of attachment security include three core sets of declarative beliefs, which play a central role in maintaining emotional stability and personal adjustment. The first set of beliefs concerns the appraisal of life problems as manageable, which helps a person maintain an optimistic and hopeful stance regarding distress management. These beliefs are a result of positive interactions with sensitive and available attachment figures, during which individuals learn that distress is manageable, external obstacles can be overcome, and the course and outcome of most threatening events are at least partially controllable. Adult attachment studies provide extensive support for a connection between mental representations of attachment security and hopeful, optimistic beliefs. Specifically, secure individuals, as identified by self-report measures, are consistently found to appraise a wide variety of stressful events in less threatening terms than insecure people, either anxious or avoidant, and to hold more optimistic expectations about their ability to cope with sources of distress (e.g., Berant, Mikulincer, & Florian, 2001; Mikulincer & Florian, 1995; Radecki-Bush, Farrell, & Bush, 1993).

The second kind of declarative knowledge included in representations of attachment security is positive beliefs about others' intentions and traits. Again, these positive representations are a result of interactions with available attachment figures, during which individuals learn about the sensitivity, responsiveness, and goodwill of their primary relationship partners. Numerous studies have shown that individuals who score low on attachment anxiety and avoidance (i.e., securely attached persons) possess a relatively positive view of human nature (e.g., Collins & Read, 1990; Hazan & Shaver, 1987), describe relationship partners using positive trait terms (e.g., Feeney & Noller, 1991; Levy, Blatt, & Shaver, 1998), perceive partners as supportive (e.g., Davis, Morris, & Kraus, 1998; Ognibene & Collins, 1998), and feel trusting toward partners (e.g., Collins & Read, 1990; Hazan & Shaver, 1987; Simpson, 1990). In addition, securely attached people have positive expectations concerning their partners' behavior (e.g., Baldwin, Fehr, Keedian, & Seidal, 1993; Baldwin et al., 1996; Mikulincer & Arad, 1999) and tend to explain a partner's negative behavior in relatively positive terms (e.g., Collins, 1996; Mikulincer, 1998a).

The third kind of declarative knowledge included in security-maintaining representations is beliefs about one's own worth, competence, and mastery. During interactions with sensitive, available attachment figures, individuals learn to view themselves as active, strong, and competent, because they can effectively mobilize a partner's support and overcome threats that activate attachment behavior. Moreover, they can easily perceive themselves as valuable, lovable, and special—thanks to being valued, loved, and regarded as special by a caring attachment figure. Research has consistently shown that such positive self-representations are characteristic of securely attached persons. Compared to anxiously attached persons, securely attached people report higher self-esteem (e.g., Bartholomew & Horowitz, 1991; Mickelson, Kessler, & Shaver, 1997), view themselves as competent and efficacious (e.g., Brennan & Morris, 1997; Cooper, Shaver, & Collins, 1998), describe themselves in positive terms, and exhibit small discrepancies between actual self-representations and self-standards (Mikulincer, 1995).

Representations of attachment security also involve procedural knowledge concerned with affect regulation and coping effectively with stress. This knowledge facilitates the use of what Epstein and Meier (1989) called "constructive ways of coping," that is, active attempts to manage problematic situations and restore emotional equanimity by seeking support and solving problems in ways that do not generate negative side effects. This knowledge stems from interactions with security-providing attachment figures, interactions in which secure individuals learn that their own actions can often reduce distress and solve important problems, and that turning to others when threatened is an effective way to bolster coping capacity.

Adult attachment studies provide extensive support for an association between attachment security and support seeking. Several investigators have reported a positive association between self-reports of secure attachment and the self-reported tendency to seek support in times of need (e.g., Larose, Bernier, Soucy, & Duchesne, 1999; Ognibene & Collins, 1998). Similar findings have emerged from studies examining self-reported reactions to a specific stressor (e.g., Berant et al., 2001; Radecki-Bush et al., 1993). The same positive association has been observed in studies examining actual support-seeking behavior in stressful naturalistic and laboratory situations (e.g., Fraley & Shaver, 1998; Simpson, Rholes, & Nelligan, 1992). For example, Simpson et al. (1992) told participants they would be exposed to a frightening procedure; the investigators then unobtrusively observed and coded participants' actual behavior while they were interacting with their romantic partner. Secure participants, as compared with insecure ones, exhibited little hesitation in seeking proximity to, and comfort and reassurance from, their partner.

The association between secure attachment and constructive, problem-focused coping has also been documented. For example, self-reports of attachment security have been associated with reliance on problem-focused coping strategies in studies involving a wide variety of stressors (e.g., Lussier, Sabourin, & Turgeon, 1997; Mikulincer & Florian, 1998). Moreover, people who classify themselves as securely attached tend to deal with interpersonal conflicts in close relationships by compromising and creatively integrating their own and their partner's positions (e.g., Carnelley, Pietromonaco, & Jaffe, 1994), as well as by openly discussing the problem and resolving the conflict (e.g., Simpson, Rholes, & Phillips, 1996).

Like other cognitive-affective schemas (Baldwin, 1992), representations of attachment security are closely related to affective nodes in a person's semantic memory network. Specifically, these representations have strong links with positive affect, because anticipated positive affect is an integral part of the prototypical relational script (i.e., proximity maintenance results in relief). In support of this view, research has shown that secure attachment is positively associated with self-report measures of joy and happiness (e.g., Magai, Hunziker, Mesias, & Culver, 2000; Simpson, 1990). Our own recent studies have also shown that various priming techniques (e.g., subliminal presentation of security-related words, visualization of the faces of available attachment figures) designed to heighten the accessibility of representations of attachment security result in the elicitation of positive emotions during an experimental session (Mikulincer, Gillath, et al., 2001; Mikulincer & Shaver, 2001). In addition, these priming techniques infuse even formerly neutral stimuli with positive affect without participants being aware of the underlying process. Mikulincer, Hirschberger, Nachmias, and Gillath (2001) reported that the subliminal presentation of security-related pictures or the names of people who were nominated by participants as security-enhancing attachment figures (as compared with subliminal presentation of neutral stimuli) led to higher liking ratings of unknown Chinese ideographs.

On the whole, research consistently indicates that both chronic and contextual (including manipulated) activation of mental representations of attachment security consolidates positive mental representations of others, a stable sense of self-efficacy and self-esteem, and reliance on constructive ways of coping, which in turn facilitates emotional strength and stability even in times of stress (see Mikulincer & Florian, 1998, and Mikulincer & Shaver, 2003, for reviews). In our view, people with security-supporting mental representations of attachment experiences tend to feel generally safe and protected without having to activate defensive strategies. They can interact with others in a confident and open manner without being driven by defensive social motives and strategies aimed at protecting a fragile or false self-concept. Moreover, they can devote mental resources that otherwise would be employed in preventive, defensive maneuvers to more growth-oriented, promotion-focused activities that contribute to the broadening of their perspectives and capacities and facilitate the development of autonomy, self-actualization, and a fully functioning personality. In the following sections, we review evidence concerning the positive changes that chronic or contextual activation of representations of attachment security produce in social motives and cognitions.

EVIDENCE THAT ATTACHMENT SECURITY REDUCES THE NEED FOR DEFENSIVE MOTIVES AND COGNITIONS

In this section, we review evidence that the chronic or contextual activation of representations of attachment security reduces a *prevention orientation*—a motivational stance involving a search for emotional safety and security and the avoidance of negative, painful outcomes (Higgins, 1998)—and attenuates *defensive motivations* aimed at protecting a person's self, identity, or knowledge structures. We organize this section according to the specific defensive tendencies examined thus far by adult attachment researchers: need for self-enhancement, needs for consensus and uniqueness, intergroup biases, defense of knowledge structures, and defense of cultural worldviews in the face of death reminders. We begin our discussion of each of these defensive tendencies with a brief theory-derived account supporting the attenuating effects of attachment security, after which we review key findings.

The Need for Self-Enhancement

Self-enhancement, the tendency to distort self-appraisals so as to maintain the most favorable self-view, is considered by social psychologists to be one of the basic motivations that guide the regulation of cognitive and affective processes (e.g., Fiske & Taylor, 1991). Research has consistently shown that this motivation leads people to exaggerate positive appraisals of their abilities and traits, dismiss and easily forget negative information about the self, seek positive feedback about the self, attribute positive outcomes to the self and negative outcomes to external forces (self-serving attributions), and positively bias appraisals and expectations of control and success (see Fiske & Taylor, 1991, and Taylor & Brown, 1988, for reviews). These positive distortions of the self-image are viewed as adaptive means of maintaining emotional stability and mental health (e.g., Taylor & Brown, 1988). It has also been suggested, however, that they have negative side effects, including self-deception, egocentrism, and even violence (e.g., Bushman & Baumeister, 1998).

In contrast to the view that such self-enhancement strategies are necessary for healthy functioning, we maintain that chronic or contextual activation of representations of attachment security allows a person to function adaptively without these distorting practices. As reviewed earlier, representations of security involve feelings of being loved and accepted by others and possessing special and valuable qualities within oneself. These feelings constitute part of an authentic sense of self-worth (Kernis, 2003) or what Rogers (1961) called the "real self": positive self-perceptions derived from the positive regard others have actually exhibited over the course of a person's development. In other words, securely attached people can find comfort, reassurance, and strength in authentic, solidly grounded feelings of self-worth while confronting threats. Because they are able to feel good about themselves even under threatening circumstances, there is less need for defensive inflation of self-esteem or rejection of negative feedback about the self.

In our view, interactions with available, caring, and loving attachment figures in times of need constitute the most important form of personal protection and the primary source of an authentic, stable sense of self-worth. Accordingly, we view the activation of representations of attachment security as default inner resource that supersedes self-enhancement needs and renders self-enhancement maneuvers less necessary. We also view reliance on defensive self-enhancement as an indication that a person has been forced by social experiences to transact with the environment without adequate representations of attachment security and has had to struggle for a sense of self-worth, despite experiencing serious doubts about being lovable and possessing good inner qualities.

If this view is correct, social psychologists have focused on, and theoretically enshrined as universal, motivational tendencies that are more characteristic of insecurely than of securely attached people, and perhaps especially of the more avoidant ones who deactivate their attachment system and compulsively seek self-reliance. This is not to say that social psychologists have studied only insecurely attached people, or that there is a sharp demarcation between categorically secure and insecure people. We do mean to suggest, however, that if attachment measures were included in studies like most of the classic ones that define the field of experimental social psychology, interactions (i.e., moderation effects) would be obtained, indicating that the field's negative depiction of human beings as selfish, defensive, and biased would apply more robustly to relatively insecure than to relatively secure study participants. We believe, moreover, that the induction of heightened security in such experiments would eliminate or greatly reduce the classic effects of defensive self-enhancement, just as the induction of greater insecurity would augment them. The social-psychological laboratory in itself is likely to induce greater than usual insecurity, involving, as it does, an environment pervaded by cool neutrality if not distance, and increased uncertainty, evaluation, and dependency or loss of personal control.

Adult attachment research already provides strong support for these still unconventional ideas. For example, Mikulincer (1995) measured the accessibility of positive and negative self-relevant traits in a Stroop task and examined the level of integration among people's different self-aspects. He found that people who classified themselves as securely attached had ready access to both positive and negative self-attributes and possessed a highly integrated self-organization. Only the participants who classified themselves as avoidant had a defensive self-organization, which included poor access to negative self-attributes and low integration among these attributes and other self-aspects.

In another series of four studies, Mikulincer (1998b) found that defensive self-inflation was most characteristic of avoidant individuals, especially under threatening conditions, and that secure individuals made relatively stable and unbiased self-appraisals even when confronted with self-relevant threats. Participants in these studies were exposed to various kinds of threatening or neutral situations, and appraisals of self were measured with self-report scales and other subtler cognitive techniques, such as reaction times for trait recognition. Participants who classified themselves as securely attached showed no notable difference in their self-appraisal between neutral and threatening conditions. In contrast, avoidant participants made more explicit and implicit positive self-appraisals following threatening, as compared with neutral, situations.

Mikulincer (1998b) also noted that introducing contextual factors that inhibit defensive self-enhancement tendencies (a "bogus pipeline" device that measures "true feelings about things" or the presence of a friend who knew the participants) had no effect on secure persons' self-appraisals. However, these factors inhibited avoidant participants' endorsement of a more positive self-view following threatening conditions. This pattern of findings implies that secure people's positive self-appraisals are rooted in a solid sense of self-worth, whereas avoidant people's positive self-appraisals are attempts to compensate for feelings of rejection, abandonment, or unlovability.

Similar findings have been obtained in recent studies examining attachment style differences in self-serving attributions (e.g., Kogot, 2002; Man & Hamid, 1998). As compared with their securely attached counterparts, avoidant individuals attributed positive outcomes to more internal, stable, global, and controllable causes, and negative outcomes to more external, unstable, specific, and uncontrollable causes. Kogot (2002) also found that avoidant students who failed an actual academic examination attributed the failure to less internal causes and were more likely to dismiss the diagnosticity of the failure and to blame others for it, compared with secure students who failed the same exam.

Attachment style differences have also been found in reactions to self-relevant feedback from a romantic partner (Brennan & Bossom, 1998). Securely attached people sought their partner's feedback and showed favorable and accepting reactions to it. That is, they were relatively open to their partner's feedback and tended to use it to adjust their self-appraisals and create a more accurate self-conception. Again, only avoidant people reacted defensively, being averse to partner feedback, preferring partners who did not know them and reacting to feedback dismissingly or indifferently.

Two recent studies provide interesting evidence regarding the effects on self-enhancement tendencies of contextually activated representations of attachment security (Arndt, Schimel, Greenberg, & Pyszczynski, 2002; Schimel, Arndt, Pyszczynski, & Greenberg, 2001). In these studies, participants were primed with representations of security-enhancing attachment figures (thinking about an accepting and loving other) or with other mental representations, and their use of specific self-enhancement strategies was assessed. Schimel et al. (2001) focused on a defensive bias in social comparison: searching for more social comparison information when it suggested that others scored worse than oneself than when it suggested that others outperformed oneself (Pyszczynski, Greenberg, & LaPrelle, 1985). Arndt et al. (2002) focused on defensive self-handicapping: emphasizing factors that can impair one's performance so as to avert the damage to self-esteem that can result from attributing negative outcomes to lack of ability (Berglas & Jones, 1978). In both studies, momentary strengthening of representations of attachment security weakened the tendencies to search for self-enhancing social comparison information and make self-handicapping attributions. Arndt and Schimel (2003) concluded that activation of representations of security-enhancing attachment figures "promotes a more secure feeling of self-esteem that is less vulnerable and thus less in need of psychological maneuvers to sustain it" (p. 29).

Adult attachment studies also suggest ways in which securely attached people can maintain a stable sense of self-worth without pursuing defensive self-enhancement strategies. For example, Mikulincer (1998b) found that securely attached people recalled more self-attributes, both positive and negative, in threatening than in neutral situations. This finding suggests a self-affirmation process in which the secure person's self-representations serve as an inner anchor for dealing with threats. Instead of distorting and inflating their self-conception, secure individuals seem to affirm a stable self-view by keeping active in memory more self-attributes, both positive and negative.

We (Mikulincer & Shaver, 2004) recently proposed that some components or subroutines of the self that originate in interactions with available attachment figures (*security-based self-representations*) underlie the maintenance of self-worth and emotional equanimity in times of stress. Specifically, we focused on (1) representations of the self derived from how a person sees and evaluates him- or herself during interactions with an available attachment figure (*self-in-relation-with-a-security-enhancing-attachment figure*), and (2) representations of the self derived from identification with features and traits of a caring, supportive attachment figure (*self-caregiving representations*). We hypothesized that these representations would become accessible during encounters with threats; have a soothing, comforting effect on the person; and render the pursuit of defensive self-enhancement strategies unnecessary.

To test these expectations, we conducted two separate two-session studies. In the first session, we asked participants to generate traits that described a security-enhancing attachment figure and their self-in-relation-with-this-figure. In the second session, we exposed participants to either a threatening or a neutral condition, noted the accessibility of various categories of traits within their self-descriptions, and then assessed their current emotional and cognitive state. As predicted, securely attached participants reacted to the threat condition with heightened accessibility of security-based self-representations: they rated traits that they originally used to describe a security-enhancing attachment figure or the self-in-relation-with-this-figure as more descriptive of their current self following threatening than following neutral conditions. This heightened accessibility of security-based self-representations was not observed among insecurely attached persons. More important, security-based self-representations had a soothing effect: the higher the accessibility of these self-representations, the more positive was a participant's emotional state following a threat and the less frequent were task-related worries and other interfering thoughts. Thus, it appears that securely attached individuals can mobilize caring qualities within themselves—qualities modeled on those of their attachment figures—as well as representations of being loved and valued, and these representations can provide real comfort, allowing a person to feel worthy and unperturbed without engaging in defensive forms of self-enhancement.

The Needs for Consensus and Uniqueness

Beyond self-enhancement, social psychologists have long recognized two additional motives that affect the way people perceive social reality. On the one hand, due to the subjective, interpretational nature of the knowledge they gather about themselves and the world (Kruglanski, 1989), people may feel insecure about the appropriateness of their social behavior and the correctness of their feelings and beliefs. As a result, they tend to seek *consensual validation*, evidence that their beliefs and behaviors are shared with others and that their knowledge is supported by relevant groups and institutions (e.g., Festinger, 1954). On the other hand, people also wish to distinguish themselves from others, stand out, emphasize the uniqueness of their beliefs and behaviors, and assert their individuality (e.g., Snyder & Fromkin, 1980).

These two motives distort social perception in two ways, creating both false consensus and false uniqueness. Whereas the need for consensual validation leads people to overestimate the extent to which their beliefs and behaviors are typical of those held by others (Marks & Miller, 1987), the need to stand out leads people to underestimate self–other similarity in traits, opinions, and behaviors (Snyder & Fromkin, 1980). The false-consensus bias provides a sense of security regarding the correctness of one's behaviors and beliefs and creates an illusory sense of belonging to a larger collective (Fiske & Taylor, 1991). The false-uniqueness bias increases distinctiveness, and when it involves a more positive perception of the self than of others, it can also serve the goal of self-enhancement (Tesser, 1988).

Given our understanding of the role of representations of attachment security, we would expect the activation of these representations to attenuate false-consensus and false-uniqueness biases and allow people to maintain more accurate interpretations of social reality. With regard to false consensus, given that security representations establish a sense of connectedness, belonging, protection, and support from others (Lifton, 1979), securely attached people should not urgently need to amplify their symbolic connections with others by imagining false self–other similarity. In addition, attachment figure availability makes people less anxious about holding erroneous beliefs or engaging in inappropriate behaviors. Experiencing, or having experienced, attachment figures as loving and approving allows secure people to be less afraid of criticism or rejection when they make cognitive or behavioral mistakes or reveal personal weaknesses. With regard to false uniqueness, representations of attachment security involve confidence in having something unique and special within oneself, which renders unnecessary any defensive effort to portray oneself as unique. In fact, secure people feel unique and distinct and can assert their individuality even when they are closely involved with a relationship partner (Feeney, 1999).

When people lack the emotional security provided by attachment figure availability, they are likely to attempt to compensate by defensively biasing social perception to bolster a false sense of consensus or uniqueness. In the case of avoidant individuals, who wish to deactivate the attachment system, maintain distance from others, and view themselves more positively than they view others, efforts are likely to be directed toward increasing distinctiveness, uniqueness, and devaluation of others. In contrast, in the case of anxiously attached people, who hyperactivate the attachment system and want desperately to be loved and accepted by others, compensatory efforts are likely to be directed toward increasing the sense of connectedness and belongingness, which can be accomplished in part by creating a false sense of consensus.

Studies from our laboratories provide initial support for these ideas. In a series of six studies, Mikulincer, Orbach, and Iavnieli (1998) found that securely attached people were more accurate in assessing self–other similarity than were insecurely attached people. Specifically, anxious individuals were more likely than their secure counterparts to perceive others as similar to themselves and to show a false-consensus bias in both trait and opinion descriptions. In contrast, avoidant individuals were more likely than secure individuals to perceive others as dissimilar to them and to exhibit a false-distinctiveness bias. Mikulincer et al. (1998) also found that anxious individuals reacted to threats by generating a self-description that was more similar to a partner's description and by recalling more partner traits that matched their own. In contrast, avoidant individuals reacted to the same threats by generating a self-description that was less similar to a partner's description and by forgetting more traits that they and their partner shared. Notably, secure individuals' self-descriptions and recall of partners' traits were not affected by threats, revealing once again that they can handle threats without distorting reality.

Following up these experiments, Mikulincer and Horesh (1999) found that secure people's representations of others were relatively unbiased by the projective mechanisms that underlie false consensus and false uniqueness effects. That is, people with a secure attachment style were less prone than their insecure counterparts to project onto others features that defined themselves or that they denied having. Avoidant participants defensively projected their own unwanted traits onto others, which increased self–other differentiation and, by comparison, enhanced their sense of self-worth. Anxiously attached participants projected their own traits onto others, which increased their sense of self–other similarity, compatibility, and closeness. Whereas avoidant individuals perceived in others the traits of their own unwanted selves, anxious individuals perceived duplicates of their own actual traits.

Intergroup Biases

Social psychologists have extensively documented another defensive bias in social perception: the tendency to perceive one's own social group (ingroup) as better than others (e.g., Allport, 1954; Devine, 1995). This tendency has been documented in studies of ingroup favoritism, derogation of members of other groups (outgroup members), and prejudice toward people who are different from oneself. According to social identity theory (Tajfel & Turner, 1986), intergroup bias serves a self-protective function, maintenance of self-esteem (We, including I, are better than them). Unfortunately, this method of maintaining self-esteem depends on emphasizing real or imagined ways in which the ingroup and outgroups differ, and especially on emphasizing ways in which the ingroup can be perceived as better (Tajfel & Turner, 1986).

This tendency seems likely to be especially characteristic of insecure people. A person who can maintain a sense of value by virtue of possessing salient representations of attachment security should have less need to fear and disparage outgroup members. In his account of human behavioral systems, Bowlby (1982/1969) stated that activation of the attachment system is closely related to innate fear of strangers and that attachment figure availability mitigates this innate reaction and fosters a more tolerant attitude toward unfamiliarity and novelty. In addition, as reviewed earlier, securely attached people tend to maintain high, stable self-esteem (what Kernis, 2003, calls "optimal" or "authentic" self-esteem) without relying on defensive derogation of other people.

In a recent series of five studies, we (Mikulincer & Shaver, 2001) provided preliminary evidence for the attenuating effects of attachment security on intergroup bias. Correlational findings indicated that the higher a person's sense of chronic attachment security, the weaker his or her hostile responses to a variety of outgroups (as defined by secular Israeli Jewish students): Israeli Arabs, ultra-Orthodox Jews, Russian immigrants, and homosexuals. Experimental findings indicated that various priming techniques—subliminal presentation of security-related words such as "love" and "proximity," evocation via guided imagery of the components of the attachment security script, and visualization of the faces of security-enhancing attachment figures—heightened the sense of attachment security and eliminated negative responses to outgroups. These effects were mediated by threat appraisal and were found even when participants were led to believe that they had failed a cognitive task or that their national group had been insulted by an outgroup member. That is, experimentally augmented attachment security reduced the sense of threat created by encounters with outgroup members and thus rendered unnecessary any efforts to derogate or distance oneself from them.

These findings should not be interpreted, however, as implying that attachment security inhibits ingroup identification or encourages an individualistic ideology. This interpretation would contradict Bowlby's (1988) portrayal of attachment security as promoting a sense of togetherness, as well as Smith, Murphy, and Coats's (1999) documentation of a positive association between secure attachment and identification with social groups. Brewer (1999) recently broke the assumed connection between ingroup love and outgroup hatred, showing that attachment to one's ingroup does not require hostility toward outgroups. In our studies, attachment security reduced outgroup hostility without diminishing ingroup favorability.

The Defense of One's Knowledge Structures

Social psychologists have extensively studied what they believe to be a human tendency to protect and defend existing knowledge structures even if they are incorrect or misleading and contribute to faulty decisions and actions (e.g., Fiske & Taylor, 1991; Kruglanski, 1989). This defensive tendency is related to self-esteem maintenance and motivated by a need to deny that one holds erroneous beliefs or has done something stupid or wrong. This self-defensive motivation causes what Kruglanski (1989) called "epistemic freezing" and is manifested in cognitive closure and rigidity; preference for secure, stable knowledge; and rejection of information that heightens ambiguity and challenges the validity of one's existing beliefs.

To us, this seems likely to be another overgeneralization that applies more accurately to insecure than to secure people. Theoretically, attachment security should foster openness to new information and accommodation of one's knowledge structures when evidence indicates that accommodation is called for. Being confident in their ability to deal with distress, securely attached people should be able to incorporate new evidence at the price of experiencing a temporary state of confusion or ambiguity. Such cognitive unclarity should not threaten the solid foundation of their general sense of competence, lovability, and control. They should generally realize that this state, like other challenging experiences, is reversible and that they have the necessary skills to reorganize parts of their knowledge structures without succumbing to total disorganization or disintegration. Moreover, they should be comforted by the thought that others will love and accept them even if they revise some of their opinions, decisions, or actions.

In contrast, lack of attachment security results in fragile views of self and world that make incorporation of new evidence threatening and potentially disorganizing. Because insecurely attached people lack a sense of mastery in dealing with distress, they may interpret confusion and ambiguity as highly threatening, causing them to block the inflow of new and challenging information. They may mistake knowledge stability for increased security, even if faulty knowledge leads to poor decisions and regrettable actions.

Research provides good evidence that attachment security attenuates the need for rigid cognitive structures. For example, Mikulincer (1997,

Study 3) found that secure people scored lower than insecure people on self-report measures of cognitive closure, intolerance of ambiguity, and dogmatic thinking. In another study, Mikulincer (1997, Study 4) focused on the *primacy effect*—the tendency to make judgments on the basis of early information and to ignore later data—and found that both anxious and avoidant individuals were more likely than secure individuals to rate a target person based on the first information received. In a third study, Mikulincer (1997, Study 5) examined stereotype-based judgments, that is, the tendency to judge a member of a group based on a generalized notion about the group rather than on exploration of new information about the member. Anxious and avoidant individuals tended to evaluate the quality of an essay based on the supposed ethnicity of the writer: the more positive the stereotype of the writer's ethnic group, the higher the grade assigned to the essay. In contrast, secure individuals were relatively unaffected by ethnic stereotypes.

Based on these findings, Mikulincer and Arad (1999) examined attachment style differences in the revision of knowledge about a relationship partner following behavior on the part of the partner that seemed inconsistent with this knowledge. Compared to insecure persons, secure individuals were more likely to revise their baseline perception of the partner after being exposed to expectation-incongruent information about the partner's behavior. Moreover, the contextual activation of attachment security representations (visualizing a supportive other) increased cognitive openness and led even chronically anxious and avoidant people to revise their conception of a partner based on new information (Mikulincer & Arad, 1999).

Defending Cultural Beliefs in the Face of Death

Another broad theory of social cognition and behavior—terror management theory (Greenberg, Pyszczynski, & Solomon, 1997)—claims that the needs for self-esteem, consensus, uniqueness, and knowledge stability as well as intergroup biases are consequences of death anxiety. Human beings' knowledge that they are destined to die, coexisting with strong wishes to perceive themselves as special, important, and immortal, makes it necessary for them to engage in self-promotion, to defend their cultural worldview, and to deny their animality. Extensive research has shown that experimentally induced death reminders heighten death-thought accessibility and lead to more positive reactions to ideas and people that validate cultural worldviews, more negative reactions to moral transgressors, more hostile and derogatory responses to outgroup members, a heightened sense of social consensus regarding one's own beliefs, more stereotypic thinking, and more intense self-esteem strivings (see Greenberg et al., 1997, for a review).

Although worldview validation has been assumed to be a normative defensive response to universal existential threats (Greenberg et al., 1997), studies from our laboratory suggest that this response is more characteristic of insecurely than of securely attached individuals. For example, Mikulincer and Florian (2000) found that experimentally induced death reminders lead to more severe judgments and punishments of moral transgressors only among insecurely attached people, either anxious or avoidant. Securely attached people did not recommend harsher punishments for transgressors following a mortality salience induction. In a subsequent study, Caspi-Berkowitz (2003) examined the effects of mortality salience on willingness to endanger one's life in order to defend important cultural values, and observed that only insecurely attached people reported higher willingness to die for a cause. Securely attached people were not affected by death reminders and were generally averse to endanger life to protect cultural values.

Interestingly, our studies have also revealed how securely attached people react to death reminders. Mikulincer and Florian (2000) reported that secure people reacted to mortality salience with an increased sense of symbolic immortality—a transformational, constructive strategy that, while not solving the unsolvable problem of death, leads a person to invest in his or her children's care and to engage in creative, growth-oriented activities whose products will live on after death. Secure people have also been found to react to mortality salience with heightened attachment needs: a more intense desire for intimacy in close relationships (Mikulincer & Florian, 2000) and greater willingness to engage in social interactions (Taubman Ben-Ari, Findler, & Mikulincer, 2002). Caspi-Berkowitz (2003) also found that secure people reacted to death reminders by strengthening their desire to care for others. In her study, participants were presented with hypothetical scenarios in which a relationship partner (e.g., spouse) was in danger of death, and the participants were asked about their willingness to endanger their own life to save the life of the partner. Securely attached persons reacted to death reminders with heightened willingness to sacrifice themselves. Insecurely attached persons were generally averse to this kind of sacrifice and reacted to death reminders with even lesser willingness to save others' lives.

These findings imply that, even when faced with their biological finitude, securely attached people maintain a secure psychological foundation. They seem to adhere to the attachment security script even when coping with the threat of death (seeking proximity to others), heighten their sense of connectedness and togetherness, and symbolically transform the threat into an opportunity to contribute to others and grow personally. It therefore seems to us that being part of a loving, accepting, valued world—having strong emotional and caring bonds with others—is a primary source of self-transcendence (being part of a larger entity that transcends one's own biological self), which promotes a sense of symbolic immortality and overrides needs for worldview validation and self-promotion. Defensive, distorting reactions to mortality seem to result from recurrent failures of attachment figures to accomplish their protective, supportive, anxiety-buffering task. As a result of such failures, many people lack a sense of continuity and connection to the world, and are unable to rely on a solid psychological foundation that sustains vitality even in the face of mortality concerns. As a result, insecure people cling to particular cultural worldviews and derogate alternative views in a desperate attempt to enhance their impoverished selves and achieve some sense of value and meaning that can overpower their fear of death and insignificance.

A Two-Level Model of Psychological Defenses

The findings reviewed in the preceding section are at odds with social psychological models that equate defensiveness with mental health and lack of defensiveness with psychopathology. In fact, attachment security has been related to both mental health and lack of defensiveness, supporting studies by Shedler, Mayman, and Manis (1993), John and Robins (1994), and others who have challenged the view that authentic self-esteem requires self-enhancing biases and "positive illusions" (Taylor & Brown, 1988). Our findings fit a two-level model of psychological defenses, a model rooted in attachment theory. At the primary level, attachment figure availability and the resulting sense of attachment security are natural building blocks of a secure, solid, and stable psychological foundation. At this level, representations of attachment security act as resilience resources that maintain emotional equanimity and effective psychological functioning without requiring other defensive maneuvers. A second level of defenses is required when a person fails to form secure attachments and is unable to construct a secure, solid, stable foundation that allows undistorted coping with threats. For an insecurely attached person, many everyday experiences threaten the sense of safety and one's tenuous hold on life, self, identity, and knowledge of the world. At this level, a prevention motivational orientation and the use of biased, distorting defenses can sometimes compensate for the absence of attachment security, create a façade of self-esteem and efficacy, and contribute some degree of adjustment. At this level, defensiveness may actually contribute to mental health, whereas lack of defensiveness, or a breakdown of defenses, may increase the likelihood of serious psychopathology.

As we have shown, however, this seemingly positive contribution of defensiveness is achieved at the cost of cognitive rigidity, distorted perception of social reality, and an increase in interpersonal and intergroup conflict. These negative side effects are not entailed by the use of defenses at the first, more basic level. At this primary level, attachment security promotes mental health while allowing for accurate social perception; a compassionate, loving attitude toward others, even those who are different from oneself; and cognitive openness and flexibility. As a result, the protective action of attachment security does not collide with natural processes of growth and self-actualization. Rather, attachment security enables and accelerates these processes and contributes to development of a fully functioning personality. In the next section, we review evidence concerning these growth-enhancing benefits of attachment security.

EVIDENCE THAT ATTACHMENT SECURITY PROMOTES GROWTH AND DEVELOPMENT OF A FULLY FUNCTIONING PERSONALITY

In this section, we explore the possibility that attachment security facilitates a person's advancement toward positive personal and social states, self-expansion (Aron & Aron, 1997), and the actualization of his or her natural talents. In our model (Mikulincer & Shaver, 2003), attachment figure availability initiates what we, following Fredrickson (2003), called a "broaden and build" cycle of attachment security, which, beyond building a person's resilience, also broadens his or her perspectives and capacities. According to Bowlby (1982/1969), the unavailability of attachment figures inhibits the activation of other behavioral systems, because a person without an attachment figure's protection and support tends to be so focused on attachment needs and feelings of distress that he or she lacks the attention and resources necessary to engage in non-attachment-related activities. Only when an attachment figure is available and a sense of attachment security is restored can a person devote full attention and energy to other behavioral systems. Moreover, being confident that support is available when needed, securely attached people can take risks and engage in autonomy-promoting activities. This is what causes us to believe that attachment security is essential for the development of what Rogers (1961) called a "fully functioning personality." To make this theoretical connection clear, we will use Rogers's (1961) definitional features of the fully functioning person to organize our review of the evidence concerning the importance of attachment security for achieving full functionality.

One definitional quality of the fully functioning person is *openness to experience*, the capacity to listen to one's feelings, to experience what is going on within oneself, and to reflect on one's own thoughts and feelings. Openness to experience also involves richness of information about the self and the ability to accept both positive and negative emotions and cognitions. In Rogers's (1961) words, a fully functioning person "is more open to his feelings of fear and discouragement and pain. He is also more open to his feelings of courage and tenderness, and awe. He is free to live his feelings subjectively, as they exist in him, and also free to be aware of these feelings" (p. 188).

Attachment security provides a foundation for openness to experience. According to Cassidy (1994), interactions with available, sensitive, and responsive attachment figures provide a context in which a child can openly and flexibly experience, organize, and express emotions and understand their functions and benefits. In these interactions, one learns that emotional signals evoke appropriate responses from attachment figures and that open and direct communication of distress results in effective caregiver interventions. As a result, secure people learn to feel comfortable exploring and learning about emotions; they view emotions and emotional expressions as useful contributors to growth and adjustment. Also contributing to secure people's openness to experience is their *self-reflective capacity*, their ability to think about and understand mental states (Fonagy, Steele, Steele, Moran, & Higgit, 1991). According to Fonagy et al. (1991), positive interactions with attachment figures result in an increased capacity to understand emotions. Fonagy et al. (1991) conceptualized the security-enhancing attachment figure as able "to reflect on the infant's mental experience and re-present it to the infant translated into the language of actions the infant can understand. The baby is, thus, provided with the illusion that the process of reflection of psychological processes was performed within its own mental boundaries" (p. 207).

Evidence is accumulating for a positive association between attachment security and the acknowledgment and display of emotions. With regard to the acknowledgment of emotions, Mikulincer and Orbach (1995) reported that, as compared with avoidant participants, those who classified themselves as securely attached were more willing and able to access painful memories and to reexperience the accompanying negative affect. With regard to the display of emotions, studies using either self-report or behavioral measures of self-disclosure have shown that securely attached people are more likely to appropriately disclose personal feelings to significant others and express their emotions more openly than insecure participants (e.g., Collins & Read, 1990; Feeney, 1999; Mikulincer & Naschon, 1991).

Attachment studies have also shown that both chronic and contextual activation of representations of attachment security facilitate exploration and acceptance of one's feelings. In an in-session analysis of brief psychotherapy, Mallinckrodt, Porter, and Kivlighan (2003) found that clients who developed secure attachments to their therapists engaged in greater depth of exploration during the early phases of therapy. In several studies, self-reports of secure attachment have been associated with higher scores on self-acceptance scales (e.g., Bartholomew & Horowitz, 1991; Shaver et al., 1996). Recently, Mikulincer and Rom (2003) primed participants with representations of either a security-enhancing attachment figure (thinking about a supportive other) or a relationship partner who did not accomplish attachment functions, and found that attachment-security priming led to heightened self-acceptance even among chronically insecure persons.

Another core quality of the fully functioning person, according to Rogers (1961), is *existential living*, enjoying the flow of current experiences and living fully at every moment. This quality involves spontaneity, cognitive flexibility, and an ability to adaptively change one's beliefs about self and world according to incoming information. It "means that one becomes a participant in and an observer of the ongoing process of organismic experience, rather than being in control of it" (Rogers, 1961, p. 188).

As reviewed in the previous section, attachment security facilitates cognitive openness and adaptive revision of knowledge structures in response to new evidence. That is, for secure people, there is no need for rigid cognitive structures or for imposing such structures on one's current experiences. This heightened flexibility has been documented in the ways secure people cope with stress (Berant et al., 2001; Miller, 1996). For example, Berant et al. (2001) found that securely attached women who gave birth to a child with a mild or severe congenital heart defect (CHD) showed higher levels of well-being and a more positive appraisal of motherhood than insecurely attached mothers. However, whereas secure mothers of infants with *mild* CHD dealt with the problematic situation by relying on problem-solving strategies, secure mothers of infants with a - *severe* CHD relied on cognitive distancing strategies. That is, secure mothers seemed to maintain their well-being and adjust to their motherhood tasks by flexibly employing different coping strategies according to the severity of the external demands. As a result, they could rely on distancing coping whenever the suppression of painful thoughts about the infant's severe CHD was the most adaptive way to mobilize internal and external resources for caring for a vulnerable baby. Insecure mothers did not exhibit the same degree of coping flexibility.

Research also provides initial evidence for the contribution of attachment security to two other aspects of existential living: *savoring one's good moments and capitalizing on the experience of positive affect*. With regard to the capacity to fully enjoy one's transactions with the environment, two week-long diary studies, focused on feelings experienced during daily social interactions, revealed that secure participants experienced more positive emotions than insecure participants (Pietromonaco & Feldman Barrett, 1997; Tidwell, Reis, & Shaver, 1996). Secure individuals' relatively more positive emotional tone has also been noted in studies of sexual activities (e.g., Tracy, Shaver, Albino, & Cooper, 2003), friendship (Mikulincer & Selinger, 2001), marital interactions (see Feeney, 1999, for a review), and group interactions (Rom & Mikulincer, 2003). Several studies have also found that secure attachment is associated with higher scores on scales assessing expression of positive emotions and lower scores on scales assessing control over positive emotions—the tendency to bottle up positive emotions and conceal them from a relationship partner (see Feeney, 1999, for a review).

With regard to capitalizing on current positive experiences, Mikul-incer and Sheffi (2001) found that attachment security allows people to take advantage of the enhanced cognitive functioning made possible by positive affect. In three separate studies, participants were exposed to posi-tive or neutral affect inductions, following which their breadth of mental categorization and ability to solve problems creatively were assessed. The beneficial effects of the positive affect induction on cognitive functioning were observed only among people who scored relatively low on attach-ment anxiety and avoidance. These secure individuals reacted to positive affect by adopting more liberal and inclusive criteria when categorizing se-mantic stimuli and by performing better on a creative problem-solving task. In contrast, avoidant participants were not affected by positive affect inductions, and anxiously attached participants actually reacted to positive affect with *impaired* creativity and a narrowing of mental categories. We interpret these results as indicating that secure people's openness to emo-tional experience allows them to treat positive affect as a relevant input for cognitive processing (a signal that "all is going well"), which allows them to "loosen" their cognitive strategies and explore unusual associations. Avoidant people seem to ignore affective signals of safety, and anxious people somehow turn them into signs of trouble rather than safety. Secure people's enhanced creativity may help them find new and unusual ways to deal with events, enjoy tasks, and maintain a positive mood.

Two other characteristics of the fully functioning person are *organis-mic trusting*—the ability to trust one's feelings, thoughts, and sensations, and to make decisions based on what one feels is right rather than being driven by uncontrollable external forces—and *experiential freedom*, the feeling that one is free to choose among alternative courses of actions and take responsibility for one's choices. According to Rogers (1961), these qualities indicate that a fully functioning person has a strong sense of au-thenticity, personal responsibility, and self-determination. Accordingly, he or she can find personal meaning, coherence, and value in his or her ac-tions and believe that what happens depends on oneself.

Although adult attachment studies have not systematically examined the contribution of attachment security to organismic trusting and experi-ential freedom, there is some evidence linking the activation of attachment security to a person's sense of personal meaning, coherence, and self-deter-mination. Mikulincer and Rom (2003) conducted two studies in which they primed participants who had previously completed an attachment-style scale with representations of either a security-enhancing attachment figure (thinking about a supportive other) or a relationship partner who did not accomplish attachment functions, and then assessed self-reports of personal meaning and sense of coherence, defined as the tendency to per-ceive the world as understandable and life as "making sense" (Antonovsky, 1987). Lower scores on attachment anxiety and avoidance (secure attachment) were associated with higher levels of personal meaning and coherence. Moreover, as compared to the neutral-priming control condition, attachment security priming led to a heightened sense of meaning and coherence even among chronically insecure participants.

Studies examining the extent to which a person's goals and plans are internally, autonomously regulated also point to the importance of social interactions with supportive others (see Ryan & Deci, 2000, for a review). For example, Ryan, Stiller, and Lynch (1994) found that children who felt securely attached to parents and teachers displayed heightened internal, autonomous regulation of school-related behaviors. Furthermore, some studies have established a link between attachment security and *intrinsic motivation*, the inherent tendency to extend and exercise one's capacities, and to enjoy exploration and learning (Elliot & Reis, 2003; Ryan & Deci, 2000). For example, Hazan and Shaver (1990) reported that securely attached people were more likely than insecure ones to perceive work as an opportunity for learning, and Elliot and Reis (2003) found that self-reports of attachment security were associated with stronger endorsement of mastery goals in academic settings (goals focused on learning and expansion of one's capacities). Interestingly, Mikulincer and Rom (2003) assessed the endorsement of these goals following the priming of representations of either a security-enhancing attachment figure (thinking about a supportive other) or a relationship partner who did not serve attachment functions. Findings revealed that the security-priming condition led to heightened endorsement of mastery goals at the beginning of an academic course.

The final characteristic of a fully functioning person, according to Rogers (1961), is *creativity*, the ability to produce new and effective thoughts, actions, and objects, and the willingness to contribute to the growth and actualization of others. This characteristic involves real participation in the world, a sense of generativity, and the endorsement of prosocial values and goals that orient a person toward maintenance and enhancement of others' welfare and protection and improvement of physical and social surroundings.

With regard to generativity, self-reports of attachment security are associated with better functioning in conflictual interpersonal interactions (e.g., Simpson et al., 1996), more creative problem solving (Mikulincer & Sheffi, 2000), better maintenance of task performance following an uncontrollable failure (Mikulincer & Florian, 1998), and better instrumental and socioemotional functioning during group interactions (Rom & Mikulincer, 2003). The sense of attachment security is also positively associated with adaptive interpersonal functioning and the ability to maintain satisfactory, stable close relationships (see Feeney, 1999, for a review).

Adult attachment studies have also demonstrated that attachment security promotes genuine altruistic concern for others' welfare. Secure mothers, for example, are more caring and supportive in interactions with their children (e.g., Crowell & Feldman, 1991; Rholes, Simpson, & Blakely, 1995). Secure people are more sensitive than their insecure counterparts to romantic partners' needs and behave more supportively toward their partner during distressing interactions (e.g., Collins & Feeney, 2000; Kunce & Shaver, 1994). In a series of five experiments, Mikulincer, Gillath, et al. (2001) found that scoring low on attachment anxiety and avoidance (i.e., being securely attached) was associated with more empathic, compassionate responses to others' needs. Moreover, the contextual activation of attachment security representations increased reports of altruistic empathy. In three other studies, Mikulincer et al. (2003) reported that self-reports of attachment security and contextual activation of attachment security representations were associated with stronger endorsement of values of universalism (concern for the welfare of all people) and benevolence (concern for the welfare of close persons). Recent studies in our laboratories also reveal that self-reports of attachment security are related to volunteerism, altruistic helping, and other-regarding virtues such as gratitude and forgiveness (Shaver & Mikulincer, 2003).

CONCLUDING COMMENTS

In recent years, under the banner of "positive psychology," there has been a resurgence of interest in such issues as personal authenticity, self-actualization, virtuous and compassionate behavior, and optimal self-esteem and self-development (e.g., Aspinwall & Staudinger, 2003; Kernis, 2003; Seligman, 2002). To date, while interesting, this turn toward positive psychology has seemed to us to lack a coherent theoretical foundation. A variety of investigators are exploring important phenomena, such as authentic self-esteem, optimism, compassion, gratitude, and forgiveness, but without much grounding in a general understanding of the human mind and its roots in close interpersonal relationships. We may be biased by tunnel vision and overcommitment to a theory we have found useful for generating novel research findings, Bowlby's (1982/1969) attachment theory, but so far the theory has certainly proved to be a rich source of hypotheses and insights. We have attempted to show here, by reviewing findings related to differences between more and less secure people, that the human portrait painted by the rest of social psychology—of frightened, selfish, biased, defensive information processors—is more appropriate for insecure than for secure people. This is perhaps a natural outcome of focusing on human problems and foibles instead of human potentials and strengths. It may also be an unintended consequence of cool, "objective," interpersonally distancing, and somewhat threatening laboratory contexts.

With respect to many of the social and psychological phenomena we have examined, similar findings have been obtained by studying either (1) correlates of dispositional attachment security, which has been demonstrated by a large body of research (see Cassidy & Shaver, 1999, for reviews) to be at least largely a product of attachment history (i.e., accumulated experiences with previous attachment figures), or (2) contextually primed representations of attachment security. In most of the studies establishing parallels between dispositional and contextual activation of security, experimental enhancement of security works as well for insecure as for secure people, suggesting that the attachment system itself is similar in all people. It therefore seems possible that chronic application of security-enhancing influences could move an insecure person toward security, with important consequences for mental health and prosocial behavior. This is presumably what therapists like Rogers (1961) and Bowlby (1988) were attempting to do, and what they described in compatible but somewhat different theoretical languages. (What Rogers called "unconditional positive regard," supplied by parents or a therapist, Bowlby called available, sensitive, responsive caregiving and provision of a safe haven and secure base.)

The integration we seek between what is valid in bias- and distortion-oriented social psychology (as it applies to insecure individuals) and what is valid in contemporary research on growth- and virtue-oriented social processes would be facilitated by further consideration of chronic and contextual activation of *insecurity*-related self- and social representations. For ethical and therapeutic reasons, our work has focused primarily on the induction and consequences of enhanced security, but it would be useful either to conduct similar studies involving the temporary strengthening of insecure representations or, at least, to reconceptualize many of the landmark studies of mainstream social psychology in those terms—that is, as explorations of the biasing effects of chronic or temporary insecurity.

If we think about the ways in which people are recruited to violent terrorist movements (as described, for example, by Stern, 2003)—a necessarily important topic given today's social climate—it seems likely that such recruitment targets people who are chronically insecure because of previous abuse, trauma, or humiliation, and that their behavior is progressively brought into line with the aims of terrorist groups or religious cults by alternately heightening their sense of insecurity and then reducing it through group solidarity exercises, praise from cult leaders, and applause for feats of violence against threatening enemies. Thus, it is important not to forget or ignore the important insights of "negative" social psychology while making room for a greater emphasis on positive possibilities. After all, if we try to look at social reality objectively, it is marked by conflicts, atrocities, and examples of defensive narcissism as well as by moving examples of human compassion, altruism, and personal strength. We need a coherent theoretical framework for conceptualizing the full range of human potential, from negative to positive.

ACKNOWLEDGMENT

Preparation of this chapter was facilitated by a grant from the Fetzer Institute.

REFERENCES

Ainsworth, M. D. S., Blehar, M. C., Waters, E., & Wall, S. (1978). *Patterns of attachment: Assessed in the Strange Situation and at home.* Hillsdale, NJ: Erlbaum.

Allport, G. W. (1954). *The nature of prejudice.* Reading, MA: Addison-Wesley.

Arndt, J., & Schimel, J. (2003). Will the real self-esteem please stand up?: Toward an optimal understanding of the nature, functions, and sources of self-esteem. *Psychological Inquiry, 14,* 27–31.

Arndt, J., Schimel, J., Greenberg, J., & Pyszczynski, T. (2002). The intrinsic self and defensiveness: Evidence that activating the intrinsic self reduces self-handicapping and conformity. *Personality and Social Psychology Bulletin, 28,* 671–683.

Aron, A., & Aron, E. N. (1997). Self-expansion motivation and including other in the self. In S. Duck (Ed.), *Handbook of personal relationships: Theory, research, and interventions* (2nd ed., pp. 251–270). New York: Wiley.

Antonovsky, A. (1987). The salutogenic perspective: Toward a new view of health and illness. *Advances, 4,* 47–55.

Aspinwall, L. G., & Staudinger, U. M. (Eds.). (2003). *A psychology of human strengths: Fundamental questions and future directions for a positive psychology.* Washington, DC: American Psychological Association.

Baldwin, M. W. (1992). Relational schemas and the processing of social information. *Psychological Bulletin, 112,* 461–484.

Baldwin, M. W., Fehr, B., Keedian, E., & Seidel, M. (1993). An exploration of the relational schemata underlying attachment styles: Self-report and lexical decision approaches. *Personality and Social Psychology Bulletin, 19,* 746–754.

Baldwin, M. W., Keelan, J. P. R., Fehr, B., Enns, V., & Koh Rangarajoo, E. (1996). Social-cognitive conceptualization of attachment working models: Availability and accessibility effects. *Journal of Personality and Social Psychology, 71,* 94–109.

Bartholomew, K., & Horowitz, L. M. (1991). Attachment styles among young adults: A test of a four-category model. *Journal of Personality and Social Psychology, 61,* 226–244.

Berant, E., Mikulincer, M., & Florian, V. (2001). The association of mothers' attachment style and their psychological reactions to the diagnosis of infant's congenital heart disease. *Journal of Social and Clinical Psychology, 20,* 208–232.

Berglas, S., & Jones, E. (1978). Drug choice as a self-handicapping strategy in response to noncontingent success. *Journal of Personality and Social Psychology, 36,* 405–417.

Bowlby, J. (1973). *Attachment and loss: Vol. 2. Separation: Anxiety and anger.* New York: Basic Books.

Bowlby, J. (1980). *Attachment and loss: Vol. 3. Sadness and depression.* New York: Basic Books.

Bowlby, J. (1982). *Attachment and loss: Vol. 1. Attachment* (2nd ed.). New York: Basic Books. (First edition published 1969)

Bowlby, J. (1988). *A secure base: Clinical applications of attachment theory.* London: Routledge.

Brennan, K. A., & Bosson, J. K. (1998). Attachment-style differences in attitudes toward and reactions to feedback from romantic partners: An exploration of the relational bases of self-esteem. *Personality and Social Psychology Bulletin, 24,* 699–714.

Brennan, K. A., Clark, C. L., & Shaver, P. R. (1998). Self-report measurement of adult attachment: An integrative overview. In J. A. Simpson & W. S. Rholes (Eds.), *Attachment theory and close relationships* (pp. 46–76). New York: Guilford Press.

Brennan, K. A., & Morris, K. A. (1997). Attachment styles, self-esteem, and patterns of seeking feedback from romantic partners. *Personality and Social Psychology Bulletin, 23,* 23–31.

Brewer, M. B. (1999). The psychology of prejudice: Ingroup love or outgroup hate? *Journal of Social Issues, 55,* 429–444.

Bushman, B. J., & Baumeister, R. F. (1998). Threatened egotism, narcissism, self-esteem, and direct and displaced aggression: Does self-love or self-hate lead to violence? *Journal of Personality and Social Psychology, 75,* 219–229.

Carnelley, K. B., Pietromonaco, P. R., & Jaffe, K. (1994). Depression, working models of others, and relationship functioning. *Journal of Personality and Social Psychology, 66,* 127–140.

Caspi-Berkowitz, N. (2003). *Mortality salience effects on the willingness to sacrifice one's life—The moderating role of attachment orientations.* Unpublished doctoral dissertation, Bar-Ilan University, Ramat Gan, Israel.

Cassidy, J. (1994). Emotion regulation: Influence of attachment relationships. In N. A. Fox & J. J. Campos (Eds.), The development of emotion regulation: Biological and behavioral considerations. *Monographs of the Society for Research in Child Development, 59,* 228–249.

Cassidy, J., & Shaver, P. R. (Eds.). (1999). *Handbook of attachment: Theory, research, and clinical applications.* New York: Guilford Press.

Collins, N. L. (1996). Working models of attachment: Implications for explanation, emotion, and behavior. *Journal of Personality and Social Psychology, 71,* 810–832.

Collins, N. L., & Feeney, B. C. (2000). A safe haven: An attachment theory perspective on support seeking and caregiving in intimate relationships. *Journal of Personality and Social Psychology, 78,* 1053–1073.

Collins, N. L., & Read, S. J. (1990). Adult attachment, working models, and relationship quality in dating couples. *Journal of Personality and Social Psychology, 58,* 644–663.

Cooper, M. L., Shaver, P. R., & Collins, N. L. (1998). Attachment styles, emotion regulation, and adjustment in adolescence. *Journal of Personality and Social Psychology, 74,* 1380–1397.

Crowell, J. A., & Feldman, S. S. (1991). Mothers' working models of attachment relationships and mother and child behavior during separation and reunion. *Developmental Psychology, 27,* 597–605.

Davis, M. H., Morris, M. M., & Kraus, L. A. (1998). Relationship-specific and global perceptions of social support: Associations with well-being and attachment. *Journal of Personality and Social Psychology, 74,* 468–481.

Devine, P. G. (1995). Prejudice and out-group perception. In A. Tesser (Ed.), *Advanced social psychology* (pp. 466–524). New York: McGraw-Hill.

Elliot, A. J., & Reis, H. T. (2003). Attachment and exploration in adulthood. *Journal of Personality and Social Psychology, 85*, 317–331.

Epstein, S., & Meier, P. (1989). Constructive thinking: A broad coping variable with specific components. *Journal of Personality and Social Psychology, 57*, 332–350.

Feeney, J. A. (1999). Adult romantic attachment and couple relationships. In J. Cassidy & P. R. Shaver (Eds.), *Handbook of attachment: Theory, research, and clinical applications* (pp. 355–377). New York: Guilford Press.

Feeney, J. A., & Noller, P. (1991). Attachment style and verbal descriptions of romantic partners. *Journal of Social and Personal Relationships, 8*, 187–215.

Festinger, L. (1954). A theory of social comparison processes. *Human Relationships, 1*, 117–140.

Fiske, S. T., & Taylor, S. E. (1991). *Social cognition.* New York: McGraw-Hill.

Fonagy, P., Steele, M., Steele, H., Moran, G. S., & Higgit, P. (1991). The capacity for understanding mental states: The reflective self in parent and child and its significance for security of attachment. *Infant Mental Health Journal, 12*, 201–218.

Fraley, R. C., & Shaver, P. R. (1998). Airport separations: A naturalistic study of adult attachment dynamics in separating couples. *Journal of Personality and Social Psychology, 75*, 1198–1212.

Fraley, R. C., & Shaver, P. R. (2000). Adult romantic attachment: Theoretical developments, emerging controversies, and unanswered questions. *Review of General Psychology, 4*, 132–154.

Fredrickson, B. L. (2001). The role of positive emotions in positive psychology: The broaden-and-build theory of positive emotions. *American Psychologist, 56*, 218–226.

Greenberg, J., Pyszczynski, T., & Solomon, S. (1997). Terror management theory of self-esteem and cultural worldviews: Empirical assessments and conceptual refinements. In M. P. Zanna (Ed.), *Advances in experimental social psychology* (Vol. 29, pp. 61–141). San Diego, CA: Academic Press.

Hazan, C., & Shaver, P. R. (1987). Romantic love conceptualized as an attachment process. *Journal of Personality and Social Psychology, 52*, 511–524.

Hazan, C., & Shaver, P. R. (1990). Love and work: An attachment-theoretical perspective. *Journal of Personality and Social Psychology, 59*, 270–280.

Higgins, E. T. (1998). Promotion and prevention: Regulatory focus as a motivational principle. In P. M. Zanna (Ed.), *Advances in experimental social psychology* (Vol. 30, pp. 1–46). New York: Academic Press.

John, O. P., & Robins, R. W. (1994). Accuracy and bias in self-perception: Individual differences in self-enhancement and the role of narcissism. *Journal of Personality and Social Psychology, 66*, 206–219.

Kernis, M. H. (2003). Toward a conceptualization of optimal self-esteem. *Psychological Inquiry, 14*, 1–26.

Kogot, E. (2002). *Adult attachment style and cognitions, affect, and behavior in achievement settings.* Unpublished doctoral dissertation, Bar-Ilan University, Ramat Gan, Israel.

Kruglanski, A. W. (1989). *Lay epistemology and human knowledge: Cognitive and motivational bases.* New York: Plenum Press.

Kunce, L. J., & Shaver, P. R. (1994). An attachment-theoretical approach to caregiving in romantic relationships. In K. Bartholomew & D. Perlman (Eds.), *Advances in personal relationships* (Vol. 5, pp. 205–237). London, UK: Jessica Kingsley.

Larose, S., Bernier, A., Soucy, N., & Duchesne, S. (1999). Attachment style dimensions, network orientation, and the process of seeking help from college teachers. *Journal of Social and Personal Relationships, 16*, 225–247.

Lazarus, R. S., & Folkman, S. (1984). *Stress, appraisal, and coping.* New York: Springer.

Levy, K. N., Blatt, S. J., & Shaver, P. R. (1998). Attachment styles and parental representations. *Journal of Personality and Social Psychology, 74*, 407–419.

Lifton, R. J. (1979). *The broken connection.* New York: Simon & Schuster.

Lussier, Y., Sabourin, S., & Turgeon, C. (1997). Coping strategies as moderators of the relationship between attachment and marital adjustment. *Journal of Social and Personal Relationships, 14*, 777–791.

Magai, C., Hunziker, J., Mesias, W., & Culver, L. C. (2000). Adult attachment styles and emotional biases. *International Journal of Behavioral Development, 24*, 301–309.

Mallinckrodt, B., Porter, M. J., & Kivlighan, D. M. Jr. (2003). *Client attachment to therapist, depth of in-session exploration, and object relations in brief psychotherapy.* Manuscript submitted for publication.

Man, K., & Hamid, P. N. (1998). The relationship between attachment prototypes, self-esteem, loneliness, and causal attributions in Chinese trainee teachers. *Personality and Individual Differences, 24*, 357–371.

Marks, G., & Miller, N. (1987). Ten years of research on the false-consensus effect: An empirical and theoretical review. *Psychological Bulletin, 102*, 72–90.

Mickelson, K. D., Kessler, R. C., & Shaver, P. R. (1997). Adult attachment in a nationally representative sample. *Journal of Personality and Social Psychology, 73*, 1092–1106.

Mikulincer, M. (1995). Attachment style and the mental representation of the self. *Journal of Personality and Social Psychology, 69*, 1203–1215.

Mikulincer, M. (1997). Adult attachment style and information processing: Individual differences in curiosity and cognitive closure. *Journal of Personality and Social Psychology, 72*, 1217–1230.

Mikulincer, M. (1998a). Attachment working models and the sense of trust: An exploration of interaction goals and affect regulation. *Journal of Personality and Social Psychology, 74*, 1209–1224.

Mikulincer, M. (1998b). Adult attachment style and affect regulation: Strategic variations in self-appraisals. *Journal of Personality and Social Psychology, 75*, 420–435.

Mikulincer, M., & Arad, D. (1999). Attachment working models and cognitive openness in close relationships: A test of chronic and temporary accessibility effects. *Journal of Personality and Social Psychology, 77*, 710–725.

Mikulincer, M., & Florian, V. (1995). Appraisal of and coping with a real-life stressful situation: The contribution of attachment styles. *Personality and Social Psychology Bulletin, 21*, 406–414.

Mikulincer, M., & Florian, V. (1998). The relationship between adult attachment styles and emotional and cognitive reactions to stressful events. In J. A. Simpson & W. S. Rholes (Eds.), *Attachment theory and close relationships* (pp. 143–165). New York: Guilford Press.

Mikulincer, M., & Florian, V. (2000). Exploring individual differences in reactions to mortality salience: Does attachment style regulate terror management mechanisms? *Journal of Personality and Social Psychology, 79*, 260–273.

Mikulincer, M., Gillath, O., Halevy, V., Avihou, N., Avidan, S., & Eshkoli, N. (2001). Attachment theory and reactions to others' needs: Evidence that activation of the sense of attachment security promotes empathic responses. *Journal of Personality and Social Psychology, 81,* 1205–1224.

Mikulincer, M., Gillath, O., Sapir-Lavid, Y., Yaakobi, E., Arias, K., Tal-Aloni, L., & Bor, G. (2003). Attachment theory and concern for others' welfare: Evidence that activation of the sense of secure base promotes endorsement of self-transcendence values. *Basic and Applied Social Psychology, 25,* 299–312.

Mikulincer, M., Hirschberger, G., Nachmias, O., & Gillath, O. (2001). The affective component of the secure base schema: Affective priming with representations of attachment security. *Journal of Personality and Social Psychology, 81,* 305–321.

Mikulincer, M., & Horesh, N. (1999). Adult attachment style and the perception of others: The role of projective mechanisms. *Journal of Personality and Social Psychology, 76,* 1022–1034.

Mikulincer, M., & Nachshon, O. (1991). Attachment styles and patterns of self-disclosure. *Journal of Personality and Social Psychology, 61,* 321–331.

Mikulincer, M., & Orbach, I. (1995). Attachment styles and repressive defensiveness: The accessibility and architecture of affective memories. *Journal of Personality and Social Psychology, 68,* 917–925.

Mikulincer, M., Orbach, I., & Iavnieli, D. (1998). Adult attachment style and affect regulation: Strategic variations in subjective self-other similarity. *Journal of Personality and Social Psychology, 75,* 436–448.

Mikulincer, M., & Rom, E. (2003). *An attachment perspective on positive psychology—Evidence that attachment security promotes meaning, coherence, and self-determination.* Manuscript in preparation.

Mikulincer, M., & Selinger, M. (2001). The interplay between attachment and affiliation systems in adolescents' same-sex friendships: The role of attachment style. *Journal of Social and Personal Relationships, 18,* 81–106.

Mikulincer, M., & Shaver, P. R. (2001). Attachment theory and intergroup bias: Evidence that priming the secure base schema attenuates negative reactions to outgroups. *Journal of Personality and Social Psychology, 81,* 97–115.

Mikulincer, M., & Shaver, P. R. (2003). The attachment behavioral system in adulthood: Activation, psychodynamics, and interpersonal processes. In M. P. Zanna (Ed.), *Advances in experimental social psychology* (Vol. 35, pp. 53–152). San Diego, CA: Academic Press.

Mikulincer, M., & Shaver, P. R. (2004). Security-based self-representations in adulthood: Contents and processes. In W. S. Rholes & J. A. Simpson (Eds.), *Adult attachment: Theory, research, and clinical implications* (pp. 159–195). New York: Guilford Press.

Mikulincer, M., & Sheffi, E. (2000). Adult attachment style and cognitive reactions to positive affect: A test of mental categorization and creative problem solving. *Motivation and Emotion, 24,* 149–174.

Miller, J. B. (1996). Social flexibility and anxious attachment. *Personal Relationships, 3,* 241–256.

Ognibene, T. C., & Collins, N. L. (1998). Adult attachment styles, perceived social support, and coping strategies. *Journal of Social and Personal Relationships, 15,* 323–345.

Pierce, T., & Lydon, J. (1998). Priming relational schemas: Effects of contextually activated and chronically accessible interpersonal expectations on responses to a stressful event. *Journal of Personality and Social Psychology, 75,* 1441–1448.

Pietromonaco, P. R., & Feldman Barrett, L. (1997). Working models of attachment and daily social interactions. *Journal of Personality and Social Psychology, 73,* 1409–1423.

Pyszczynski, T., Greenberg, J., & LaPrelle, J. (1985). Social comparison after success and failure: Biased search for information consistent with a self-serving conclusion. *Journal of Experimental Social Psychology, 21,* 195–211.

Radecki-Bush, C., Farrell, A. D., & Bush, J. P. (1993). Predicting jealous responses: The influence of adult attachment and depression on threat appraisal. *Journal of Social and Personal Relationships, 10,* 569–588.

Rholes, W., Simpson, J. A., & Blakely, B. S. (1995). Adult attachment styles and mothers' relationships with their young children. *Personal Relationships, 2,* 35–54.

Rogers, C. R. (1961). *On becoming a person.* Boston: Houghton Mifflin.

Rom, E., & Mikulincer, M. (2003). Attachment theory and group processes: The association between attachment style and group-related representations, goals, memory, and functioning. *Journal of Personality and Social Psychology, 84,* 1220–1235.

Ryan, R. M., & Deci, E. L. (2000). Self-determination theory and the facilitation of intrinsic motivation, social development, and well-being. *American Psychologist, 55,* 68–78.

Ryan, R. M., Stiller, J., & Lynch, J. H. (1994). Representations of relationships with teachers, parents, and friends as predictors of academic motivation and self-esteem. *Journal of Early Adolescence, 14,* 226–249.

Schimel, J., Arndt, J., Pyszczynski, T., & Greenberg, J. (2001). Being accepted for who we are: Evidence that social validation of the intrinsic self reduces general defensiveness. *Journal of Personality and Social Psychology, 80,* 35–52.

Seligman, M. E. P. (2002). *Authentic happiness: Using the new positive psychology to realize your potential for lasting fulfillment.* New York: Free Press.

Shaver, P. R., & Clark, C. L. (1994). The psychodynamics of adult romantic attachment. In J. M. Masling & R. F. Bornstein (Eds.), *Empirical perspectives on object relations theory (Empirical studies of psychoanalytic theories,* Vol. 5, pp. 105–156). Washington, DC: American Psychological Association.

Shaver, P. R., & Hazan, C. (1993). Adult romantic attachment: Theory and evidence. In D. Perlman & W. Jones (Eds.), *Advances in personal relationships* (Vol. 4, pp. 29–70). London: Jessica Kingsley.

Shaver, P. R., & Mikulincer, M. (2002). Attachment-related psychodynamics. *Attachment and Human Development, 4,* 133–161.

Shaver, P. R., & Mikulincer, M. (2003, May). *Attachment, compassion, and altruism.* Paper presented at the Conference on Compassionate Love, Normal, IL.

Shaver, P. R., Papalia, D., Clark, C. L., Koski, L. R., Tidwell, M., & Nalbone, D. (1996). Androgyny and attachment security: Two related models of optimal personality. *Personality and Social Psychology Bulletin, 22,* 582–597.

Shedler, J., Mayman, M., & Manis, M. (1993). The illusion of mental health. *American Psychologist, 48,* 1117–1131.

Simpson, J. A. (1990). Influence of attachment styles on romantic relationships. *Journal of Personality and Social Psychology, 59,* 871–980.

Simpson, J. A., Rholes, W. S., & Nelligan, J. S. (1992). Support seeking and support giving within couples in an anxiety-provoking situation: The role of attachment styles. *Journal of Personality and Social Psychology, 62,* 434–446.

Simpson, J. A., Rholes, W. S., & Phillips, D. (1996). Conflict in close relationships: An attachment perspective. *Journal of Personality and Social Psychology, 71,* 899–914.

Smith, F. R., Murphy, J., & Coats, S. (1999). Attachment to groups: Theory and measurement. *Journal of Personality and Social Psychology, 77,* 94–110.

Snyder, C. R., & Fromkin, H. L. (1980). *Uniqueness: The human pursuit of difference.* New York: Plenum Press.

Stern, J. (2003). *Terror in the name of God: Why religious militants kill.* New York: HarperCollins.

Tajfel, H., & Turner, J. C. (1986). The social identity theory of intergroup behavior. In S. Worchel & W. Austin (Eds.), *Psychology of intergroup relations* (pp. 7–24). Chicago: Nelson.

Taubman-Ben-Ari, O., Findler, L., & Mikulincer, M. (2002). The effects of mortality salience on relationship strivings and beliefs: The moderating role of attachment style. *British Journal of Social Psychology, 41,* 419–441.

Taylor, S. E., & Brown, J. D. (1988). Illusion and well-being: A social psychological perspective on mental health. *Psychology Bulletin, 103,* 193–210.

Tesser, A. (1988). Toward a self-evaluation maintenance model of social behavior. In L. Berkowitz (Ed.), *Advances in experimental social psychology* (Vol. 21, pp. 181–227). New York: Academic Press.

Tidwell, M. C. O., Reis, H. T., & Shaver, P. R. (1996). Attachment, attractiveness, and social interaction: A diary study. *Journal of Personality and Social Psychology, 71,* 729–745.

Tracy, J. L., Shaver, P. R., Albino, A. W., & Cooper, M. L. (2003). Attachment styles and adolescent sexuality. In P. Florsheim (Ed.), *Adolescent romance and sexual behavior: Theory, research, and practical implications* (pp. 137–159). Mahwah, NJ: Erlbaum.

Waters, H. S., Rodrigues, L. M., & Ridgeway, D. (1998). Cognitive underpinnings of narrative attachment assessment. *Journal of Experimental Child Psychology, 71,* 211–234.

11

The Four Basic Social Bonds

Structures for Coordinating Interaction

ALAN PAGE FISKE *and* NICK HASLAM

HOW MANY WAYS TO COORDINATE?

People observe objects and persons, categorize and remember them, make inferences and plans about them. A large body of research has explored how people cognize others (S. Fiske 2004). But people do more than cognize each other, they coordinate. They create relationships that are intrinsically motivating, that evoke emotions, and that they constantly evaluate with respect to shared models of how people *should* coordinate with each other. The structures and mechanisms of social relationships are distinct from the psychological structures and mechanisms of individual persons—and the characteristics of relationships are not simply combinations of the characteristics of the individuals that engage in them. Social relationships are distinct entities that must be analyzed at their own level, as forms of motivated coordination.

How many ways are there for people to coordinate activity? Any anthropologist can list innumerable systems. But how do humans generate these bewilderingly diverse and complex systems of sociality? Relational models theory (RMT) posits that human relationships and social systems are culture-specific implementations of just four elementary relational models in various combinations (Fiske 1991, 1992, 2004a). The relational models (RMs) are communal sharing (CS), authority ranking (AR), equality matching EM), and market pricing (MP). These four models are the structures out of which people construct, understand, evaluate, sanction, and motivate most joint activities.

These models are manifest, for example, when a group or dyad makes a joint decision: there are four basic ways to proceed. They can seek a consensus of the group as a whole, the chief can decide (and delegate minor aspects of the decision), people can vote, or they can use a market mechanism based on utilities or prices. Likewise, when a group or dyad organizes to accomplish some task, they have four alternatives: they can all simply pitch in without assigning individual responsibilities, an authority can give orders down a chain of command, everyone can do an equal share (or take turns), or participants can be compensated in proportion to the amount they each complete. The same models are the fundamental frameworks for moral judgment: treat each person's needs and suffering as your own, do what the gods or your elders command, treat each person equally, or give every person their due in proportion to what they deserve. Humans use these same four modes of coordination to organize nearly every aspect of every social domain. Consider the social meanings of land. Land can be a shared commons, the domain or fief of a lord, a marker of equal status (such as eligibility to vote), or a commercial investment. When people transfer goods or services, they can give a gift without expecting any specific return; they can pay tribute in fealty to a superior (or, inversely, bestow a benefit to a subordinate as a gesture of largesse); they can make a balanced, quid-pro-quo exchange; or they can sell and purchase at market rates.

The RMs comprise an implicit repertoire or menu of components for the construction of relationships. Most enduring, multifaceted dyads, groups, and institutions are composites—as are all communities and societies. So when I invite you to dinner, we share the food and drink; it's ours to consume together, without keeping track of who gets how much (CS). If I am making a soufflé, as expert and host I may direct you in assisting me (AR). At the same time, this meal creates an obligation for you to invite me over (EM). Of course, I bought the food I prepare (MP). Or suppose we are soldiers in a platoon. We care about each other's welfare and may be ready to sacrifice our lives for each other, we work to achieve the mission assigned to our unit, we uphold the platoon's reputation (CS). Yet one of us is the sergeant, commanding the platoon in accord with the orders he receives; if he dies, then our relative ranks determine succession to command (AR). We serve equal tours of duty, take turns standing guard, draw straws to see who goes out alone to reconnoiter, expect equal treatment from our sergeant, and trade favors (EM). If one of us gets cigarettes, he can barter or sell them to others; we bribe the supply officer for beer; we expect commendation and respect in proportion to our performance; we take a very utilitarian attitude toward achieving our combat objective, calculating how we can have the best chance of achieving it with the least risk; and we try to use our scarce ammunition most efficiently (MP).

Of course, people do not always coordinate: There are *null* interactions in which people do not orient their action to a joint (or putatively joint) model of the meaning of their actions. People may make individual decisions or act independently; they may think and act without reference to any moral standard; they may use land without evaluating the social implications of their use. People ordinarily act without taking into account any relationship with most other humans on earth, and sometimes they act without coordinating even with those in close proximity. A person running down the sidewalk avoids lampposts, trees, dogs, trashcans, and other humans, but this collision avoidance is not social—unless they keep to the right, or think they should, or think others should. A soldier under fire who ducks behind a corpse is not acting socially, even if the body turns out to be alive.

Sometimes people take into account others' social expectations purely for the purpose of conning or exploiting them, without any intrinsically social motivation, and without any concern about evaluating the action in moral terms. Psychopaths do this all the time. They may make use of others' moral sentiments without feeling in any way bound by them. People steal, rape, and coerce others, using fear, force, or control over material resources. These are *asocial* interactions, in which other people are merely a means to some other end. There is no relationship in the sense we mean here when people manipulate other humans as if they were tools or draft animals in asocial interactions. Nor is there a relationship in the *null* case when people simply ignore others' sociality entirely.

Each culture implements the four RMs in many distinct ways and in different combinations. In a particular culture, a given aspect of a given domain of sociality may be organized by any of the RMs, and the way each aspect is organized may change historically. In many cultures, elders used to decide who married whom (AR) and many other aspects of marriage used to be based on AR as well. But now in many cultures marriages are formed through love (CS), and are often sustained in an EM framework.

Even when two cultures use the same RM, they are likely to implement it differently. When Americans encounter a severe misfortune such as death or a debilitating injury, they typically interpret their suffering in RM terms. They may make sense of it by concluding, "That's the price I paid for having so much fun riding my motorcycle at high speed all these years." Americans also often say, "God has his reasons—it is not for us to try to make sense of them" (AR). Or they may say, "I've had a wonderful life; compared to other folks, I've had more than my share of good things, but things even out in the long run" (EM). Misfortune may also lead to the eventual discovery of unity, perhaps in a survivor's support group with others who have shared the same misfortune (CS).

The Moose (pronounced *MOH*-say) of Burkina Faso also use these four RMs to make sense of their suffering, but they have very different cultural implementations of the RMs. Like Americans, in a vague way they

attribute many deaths and misfortunes to a high god, a distant and inscru-
table one. More specifically, however, in some misfortunes they perceive
the wrath of their ancestors, using various methods of divination to determine why their ancestors are angry and what sacrifices or offerings to
make to propitiate them (AR). Divination shows Moose that other suffering and deaths are due to the malevolence of sorcerers who are envious of
people who have more good fortune and consequently attempt to even the
score (EM). Moose occasionally discover that people have died because
they, or someone else in their kin group, violated a communal norm, causing them to suffer the immanent collective consequences (CS). To my
knowledge, Moose rarely, if ever, make sense of misfortune in terms of any
kind of cost or payment (MP).

As these examples illustrate, the four RMs govern relationships with
humans, gods, and spirits—even animals. And culture provides the necessary guidance in implementing them. Even when the same RM operates in
two cultures, their implementations of it may be quite distinct. Compared
to Americans, Moose much more freely share food and work with their
kin, but almost never share personal history, plans, or feelings. Moose vil-
lagers are perfectly comfortable paying for or selling sex under appropriate
circumstances, but would not consider selling land or laboring for pay in
the village—although most Moose men work as wage laborers in the Ivory
Coast for years at a time. A Moose man shares work and harvests with all
of his wives, but never eats or drinks with any of them. As this illustrates,
cultural precepts, prototypes, or precedents are essential for completing the
RMs, each of which only partially determines a coordination structure that
is open-ended and indeterminate. The coordination of any specific aspect
of any activity depends on socially transmitted cultural complements that
specify which RMs to use, and how, when, where, and with whom they
operate.

A BRIEF REVIEW OF RELATIONAL MODELS THEORY

The four RMs are easy to define. Communal sharing (CS) is an equivalence
relation, in which people attend to something important they have in common. People in each group are the same in respect to the matter at hand;
outsiders are different. Authority ranking (AR) is a linear hierarchy in
which people are asymmetrically differentiated in the current context.
Equality matching (EM) is a relationship in which people keep track of additive differences, with even balance as the reference point. Market pricing
(MP) is based on a socially meaningful proportionality, where the ratio
may concern monetary value, utility, efficiency, effort, merit, or anything
else. CS is the core framework for parks or roads, love and close friendship, ethnicity and ethnic cleansing. AR is manifest in military hierarchies,

corporate chains of command, government offices, seniority systems, and wars of conquest to extend the dominion of a head of state. EM organizes turn taking, lotteries, the framework of games and sports, co-ops, and eye-for-an-eye vengeance. MP operates whenever people are concerned with cost–benefit analysis, utility calculations, efficient utilization of manpower, prices, wages, rents, interest, tithes, and taxes.

These are the four fundamental forms. There are other idiosyncratic patterns of coordination that appear here and there in human life, but there are only four fundamental RMs that generate coordination systems in every domain of sociality in every culture. The four RMs are "fundamental" in the sense that people use them to plan and construct action; to anticipate and interpret others' actions; to encode, process, and remember social experience; to evaluate and sanction their own and others' action. They also are "fundamental" because they are intrinsically motivated— they are inherently meaningful. And they are "fundamental" because they are the building blocks that, operationalized in innumerable combinations, organize most of social life. Moreover, they operate at all levels of social coordination; hence we use the term "relationships" to encompass coordination in dyads, groups, networks, communities, and societies. Just as four basic forces generate the complex and varied structures of the physical universe, four basic social bonds generate the complex and varied structures of the social universe.

Each of the four RMs is a distinct structure, but analytically, from a theoretical perspective, they are related in a sort of Guttman scale (Fiske, 1991, pp. 207–223). The simplest social distinction is to consider whether a person is the same or different with respect to the relevant aspect of whatever people are coordinating; this is the only meaningful distinction in CS. In AR, people recognize equivalent ranks, but if there is a difference, people consider also the direction of the difference: Who is higher? In EM, people are aware of whether they are equivalent (balanced), as well as the direction of any imbalance (e.g., whose turn it is); they are also aware of the additive obligation outstanding: how many turns you owe me, or how many points you are ahead and I have to score to beat you. In MP, people are concerned about equality, who owes or is ahead of whom, and the amount of the difference, but also the ratio: this latté costs $3.05, while the pay for this hour of labor is $6.50. Indeed, money is precisely the abstract representation of the ratio value of every commodity in proportion to all others. It is noteworthy that these are the same four relational structures that we see in the four classic scales of measurement: nominal, ordinal, interval, and ratio.

RMT arose as a synthesis of several theories of the basic forms of sociality. The original inspirations were Weber's (1922/1978) analysis of three forms of legitimation of political authority, Piaget's (1932/1973) characterization of three stages of moral development, and Ricoeur's

(1967) history of three forms of Christian theodicy. The theory was also influenced by several binary theoretical contrasts, including Tönnies (1887/
1988) *Gemeinschaft* and *Gesellschaft*, Durkheim's comparison of mechan-
ical and organic solidarity, and Douglas's (1978) grid-group matrix. RMT
grew to incorporate classic economic typologies, especially Polanyi's (1968)
characterization of householding, redistribution, and markets; Sahlins's
(1965) cross-cultural comparison of forms of exchange; Udy's (1970) studies of systems of labor recruitment; and (after the original publication of
the theory) Williamson's (1975) comparison of markets and hierarchies,
with Ouchi's (1980) addition of clans. While RMT thus encompasses the
distinctions proposed by many major theories, what sets RMT apart is that
earlier theories did not recognize that people use the same structures to
coordinate action in virtually all aspects of sociality. Moreover, many earlier theories identified only two or occasionally three of the elementary
forms. And none of them explained how elementary coordination structures generate complex and culturally distinctive social systems. Furthermore, no earlier theories attempted to integrate relational and societal
structures; semiotics and ontogeny; natural selection and culture; cognition, motivation, and emotion; and psychobiology.

RESEARCH SUPPORT FOR RELATIONAL MODELS THEORY

RMT began life as an attempt to synthesize social theories characterizing
the elementary forms of relationships, and specifically to make sense of
patterns of social life among the Moose. However, it was never intended to
serve only as a theoretical integration or as an interpretive tool for
ethnographers. Rather, Fiske (1991) developed RMT as an account of how
people cognize (and motivate, enact, and coordinate) their relationships.
To test the basic propositions of this account, we brought RMT into the
social psychological laboratory, conducting an extensive series of studies
during the 1990s. These studies employed a wide and innovative variety of
methods, which we believe is a notable strength of our work. This work
addressed two broad questions. First, we asked whether the proposed
structure of people's understandings of social relationships matched the
four RMs (i.e., do people implicitly or explicitly think about relationships
in these four ways, and are they really distinct?). Second, we asked whether
the RMs *influence* social cognition and help to explain psychological processes and practices. Studies on these two questions are reviewed below.

RMT makes three basic structural claims: (1) that there are four basic
models governing social relationships, (2) that these RMs are best understood as discrete categories, and (3) that their core features match Fiske's
formulation. None of these claims is self-evident. Theorists have proposed
classifications containing from two categories and upward, and many have

eschewed categories altogether, describing differences among relationships in terms of continuous dimensions. The three structural claims of RMT therefore require thorough empirical validation. Such validation would involve demonstrating that the features of the RMs covary into four distinct and irreducible latent variables in multivariate analyses of relationships, and that these latent variables are better modeled as discontinuous categories than as continuous dimensions.

In the first attempt to assess whether the RMs represent four distinct structures, Haslam (1995) conducted an exploratory factor analysis of undergraduates' ratings of their personal relationships on features of the RMs and of four resource classes (Foa & Foa, 1974). Two bipolar factors emerged (CS vs. MP and EM vs. AR), with EM items falling closer to CS items than to MP items, suggesting that the factors were not independent. Items for each RM loaded in a consistent pattern on the factors, whereas resource-class items did not. The failure of this analysis to yield four distinct factors may have been due to its inclusion of resource-class items and its use of exploratory methods. Consequently, Haslam and Fiske (1999) conducted a confirmatory factor-analytic study. Nonstudent adults rated their personal relationships on items assessing the RMs across multiple social domains. Findings strongly supported RMT's proposed structure. A model representing the RMs as two bipolar factors (CS vs. MP and AR vs. EM) yielded a markedly inferior fit to a model that represented them as four distinct factors. A model in which these factors were free to intercorrelate, consistent with the expected covariation of some RMs as a function of cultural norms, fitted better still, and all items loaded highly on their correct factor.

Although this confirmatory factor-analytic work is encouraging, it fails to do justice to the claim that the RMs are discrete categories that reflect incommensurable relational grammars. Factor analysis assumes that variation is continuous, consistent with dimensional models of relationships (e.g., Wish, Deutsch & Kaplan, 1976). To test between dimensional and categorical models of relationships, we conducted two studies using taxometric methods (Meehl, 1992). In the first study (Haslam, 1994a), participants rated a sample of their personal relationships on items assessing the RMs. Taxometric analyses of these items yielded strong support for the discreteness of all four RMs. Very few relationships did not clearly belong to one of these categories—supporting the RMs' exhaustiveness—and many relationships belonged to more than one category, consistent with Fiske's (1991) claims. In a second study (Haslam, 1999), another sample of relationships was gathered, rated on a different set of items assessing the RMs, and subjected to more comprehensive taxometric analyses. These analyses replicated the earlier findings that the RMs are discontinuous.

The studies reviewed above show that cognitive structures resembling the RMs exist, but not that the RMs map people's intuitive relational understandings. RMT would be boosted if the RMs also capture the intuitive organization of relationships. We therefore conducted a study assessing this intuitive organization by having participants do free sorting or similarity ratings of their own relationships (Haslam & Fiske, 1992). Participants also classified these relationships using five relationship taxonomies: the RMs, resource classes (Foa & Foa, 1974), the communal versus exchange dichotomy (Mills & Clark, 1984), role expectations (Parsons & Shils, 1951), and social orientations (MacCrimmon & Messick, 1976). The extent to which participants' relationship groupings mapped onto these taxonomies was then examined. The RMs were associated with the groupings as strongly as the role expectations and resource classes and more strongly than the other two classifications. The RMs covered a multidimensional relational attribute space derived from the five classifications particularly well, uniquely capturing the crucial authority- and equality-related aspects of relationships. Intuitive relationship groupings were best modeled by about four categories, consistent with RMT. Thus, RMT offers a particularly strong account of people's intuitive understandings of their relationships.

A second study (Haslam, 1994b) assessed intuitive relational understandings in a different manner. Participants rated the prototypicality of a sample of hypothetical relationships, or chose which of several forms of behavior of one interactant—described in terms of interpersonal circle octants (Kiesler, 1983)—would be most appropriately paired with a specific form of behavior of a second interactant. The fit to these data of three alternative structures—based on dimensions (warmth and dominance), laws (complementarity and symmetry; Wiggins, 1980), or the AR and CS categories—was then compared. The categories modeled the prototypicality rating and choice data more powerfully and economically than the alternatives. Again, RMT appears to make good sense of people's intuitive understandings of relationships.

Our research makes a strong case for the structural claims of RMT. The confirmatory factor-analytic and taxometric studies support the existence of four RMs irreducible to more basic structures, and Haslam and Fiske (1992) indicate that four RMs may be sufficient to account for intuitive understandings of relationship types. Additional models might exist, but the finding that the RMs govern all but a small minority of relationships—most of which are probably asocial or null relationships—suggests that no indispensable fifth model is waiting to be discovered. The taxometric studies and Haslam (1994b) rebut any reduction of the RMs to simpler dimensions. The factor-analytic and taxometric studies confirm the coherence of the RMs, demonstrating systematic covariance among items intended to tap diverse aspects of each RM. Finally, when we have compared the RM taxonomy to its alternatives, RMT has tended to fare well (Haslam, 1994a, 1994b, 1995; Haslam & Fiske, 1992).

Validating RMT's structural claims was a necessary but preliminary step in our research program, as the theory's true test is whether it can account for interpersonal cognition and behavior. The first paper to demonstrate this capacity (Fiske, Haslam, & Fiske, 1991) reported seven studies of inadvertent social errors in which one person is mistakenly substituted for another (i.e., misnamed, misrecalled, or incorrectly targeted for an interpersonal act). In each study, participants recorded personal examples of these errors using diary methods, describing each error, who figured in it, and what RM they employed with each person involved. In all studies participants tended to substitute people with whom they related in the same manner (i.e., using the same RM). These relational effects were more robust than those of such variables as the age, social role, race, and name similarity of the substituted individuals, and were statistically independent of them. The RM effects were also stronger than those of alternative relational taxonomies (i.e., resource classes [Foa & Foa, 1974] and the communal vs. exchange distinction [Mills & Clark, 1984]). Only gender rivaled RM as a determinant of slips. Further analyses showed that participants substituted acquaintances designated by the same culturally available role term largely because they shared with these acquaintances the same kind of relationship. Thus the "deeper" relational structures were more important and basic for social cognition than the colloquial role categories. In a second paper, Fiske (1993) replicated the earlier studies with participants from four diverse cultures (Bengali, Chinese, Korean, and Vai from West Africa). RM effects were substantial in every sample, demonstrating an impressive level of cross-cultural validity for the RMs and their influence on social cognition.

In a follow-up to the error studies, Fiske and Haslam (1997) examined intentional substitutions, in which an initially intended interactant was replaced with another when the former was unavailable or the participant changed plans. Using the same diary methods for collecting naturally occurring substitutions, Fiske and Haslam again found that participants substituted interactants with whom they had the same kind of relationship. Although substitutability was also predicted by interactants' personal attributes—gender, ethnicity, and age, but generally not personality—their effects again appeared to reflect the participants' demographically differentiated patterns of affiliation rather than cognitive equivalence. The findings of the study therefore offer further support for the role of the RMs in determining social equivalence.

Further evidence for the wide-ranging role of the RMs in interpersonal cognition comes from a study of social memory. Fiske (1995) had two samples of participants freely list their acquaintances by name and subsequently classify them according to relational properties (RMs, resources, communal vs. exchange, role term, situations in which they interacted), and according to personal attributes (gender, age, race). The extent to which the order of recall of the acquaintances was clustered into "runs" by each of these characteristics was then compared. Recall order was most powerfully determined by the relational characteristics, all of which yielded stronger clustering values than all of the personal attributes, with social situation preeminent. The RMs yielded the strongest effect of the relational taxonomies, once again demonstrating their influence on social cognition in a new methodology and cognitive task.

These studies of social errors, social substitutions, and recall of acquaintances all demonstrate that the RMs organize many aspects of interpersonal cognition and behavior across a variety of domains and methodologies. More abstractly, the studies indicate that interpersonal cognition—whether it involves the naming or representation of persons, recall of social episodes or individuals, or formulation of interpersonal intentions—is powerfully influenced and guided by the nature of people's relationships with their interactants, rather than simply by the personal attributes that inhere in them, such as gender, age, race, or personality. Much social cognition truly is "thinking about relationships" (Fiske & Haslam, 1996).

ADDITIONAL RESEARCH ON RELATIONAL MODELS THEORY

Our program of research demonstrates that RMT has solid credentials as an account of interpersonal cognition. However, RMT has been employed in many other lines of research, conducted by scholars from a wide variety of disciplines. A comprehensive review of this work is beyond the scope of this chapter (see Haslam, 2004), but a small sample can convey an impression of the range of phenomena that RMT illuminates. This selection ranges from neuroscience to organizational behavior, and from the psychology of groups to family studies.

A study by Iacoboni et al. (2004) illustrates the discoveries that can be made using neuroscientific methods to illuminate RMT. Using functional magnetic resonance imaging (fMRI), they investigated the brain regions activated by observation of CS and AR relationships depicted in 36 professionally produced movie clips. They compared the brain regions activated by observing these interactions with the regions active in a baseline condition when subjects saw only a blank screen, and also with regions active when subjects observed segments of the movies showing only one person alone. In both comparisons, surprisingly, CS and AR clips activated brain regions that were essentially the same at the level of spatial resolution of whole-brain fMRI. The regions activated included the temporal poles, inferior frontal cortices, superior temporal cortices, and extrastriate areas. Moreover, watching the CS and AR interactions activated the dorsomedial prefrontal cortex and the medial parietal cortex (precuneus). These latter two regions are among the brain regions that have been identified as constituting the "default state" network that is tonically active when subjects have no particular task to perform, and that becomes *less* active when performing most nonsocial cognitive tasks. Indeed, the dorsomedial prefrontal and medial parietal cortex have never been activated together in comparison to a resting baseline in any of the thousands of cognitive neuroscience experiments conducted in scanners. Even social cognition experiments that involve processing attributes of individuals or making inferences about persons have not reported activating these regions beyond their resting levels. This suggests that the dorsomedial prefrontal and medial parietal cortex are components of a system that may be dedicated to processing social *relationships*, a system that ruminates (consciously or unconsciously) about social relations whenever there are no nonsocial tasks to perform. This supports the core axiom of RMT, that humans are fundamentally and pervasively social animals, oriented toward relationships, not just persons.

Iacoboni et al.'s (2004) work is about as "micro" in focus as research on interpersonal cognition can be. Work by Connelley (Connelley & Folger, 2004) goes to the opposite end of the spectrum, examining processes at the level of organizational culture and collective action. Connelley conducted focus groups within a Fortune 100 manufacturing firm that had recently attempted to expand the hiring of women and minority group members. This initiative produced an angry backlash from the existing workforce, along with misunderstanding and distrust from the targeted employees, who complained about hiring, performance evaluation, and promotion decisions, and whose retention rates were poor. Connelley showed that three groups of employees—the white male "establishment," and the white female and African American targeted minorities—thought about workplace relationships and human resource systems in ways that corresponded to different RMs. The white males conducted their work lives according to a CS model in which ingroup solidarity and consensus-driven decision making tended to define other employees as outsiders and deprive them of consultation and informal networking. The white females preferred an MP definition of the work environment, with competence and efficiency governing the allocation of rewards along meritocratic lines. African Americans favored the strict parity of an EM model, supporting definite hiring and promotion targets. Connelley's study shows how the RMs clarify the fault lines of a deep organizational conflict, and how the "choice" of a relational stance may be at least partially strategic and positional, motivated in response to a prevailing ethos that does not serve one's relational goals.

Connelley's research investigates collective phenomena in a particular situated context, but other researchers have used RMT to examine laypeople's generalized understandings of groups. Lickel, Hamilton and Sherman (2001) used the RMs to investigate people's intuitive "theories" of groups, starting from an empirically derived classification of four group types: "intimacy groups" (e.g., families), "task groups" (e.g., work teams), "social categories" (e.g., women), and "loose associations" (e.g., classical music lovers). They showed that people expect different RMs to predominate among members of different types of group, so people draw strong inferences from group types to likely relational norms and vice versa. Intimacy groups are associated with CS and to a lesser extent with EM relations, task groups with AR and to a lesser extent MP and EM relations, and loose associations with MP relations. Social categories (such as men) were not perceived to have a consistent relational model. Lickel et al. (2001) also found that intragroup relationships plainly figure prominently in lay theories of groups. For example, participants judged that groups organized in a CS fashion were the most unified, coherent, and entity-like, and they made the strongest judgments of collective responsibility for CS groups when one member committed a wrongdoing.

Lickel and colleagues' (2001) work shows how people hold organized expectations about the relational processes operating within groups, categories, and networks. Research by Goodnow (2004) showed in a more contextualized way how implementations of RMs influence justice perceptions within actual households. Goodnow found that RMT helped to clarify the distribution of work responsibilities among family members, and the strains that divisions of labor produce. Decisions regarding work distributions depended crucially on the RMs that members believed should apply to their family relationships, and these RMs were implemented in varied ways as a function of age and family role. The RMs also clarified the tensions that family members experienced when their work contributions were not treated in a manner that they judged to be appropriate. Goodnow (2004) found that parents and children often made distinctions between different kinds of relationships, and reacted negatively when they felt "relationship errors" had been made: Mothers sometimes felt that children treated them like maids, and children sometimes used expressions such as "I'm not your slave" and "You're not paying me," all of which imply the inappropriateness of a perceived definition of the parent–child relationship. Goodnow's analysis shows in vivid detail how relational definitions are negotiated and implemented within families, and how interpersonal cognition within this context is both complex and emotionally saturated.

RMT also provides a deeper understanding of two major violations of economic rationality known as the "endowment effect" and "mental accounting." People typically demand a much higher price to sell an item in their possession than they are willing to pay to acquire it, and people compartmentalize their assets into discrete, nonfungible categories. Kahneman and Tversky (1984) explained the endowment effect in terms of loss aversion: the negative utility of parting with an object is greater than the positive utility of gaining it. They theorized that mental accounting results from cognitive heuristics people employ because of their limited mental capacities. However, McGraw, Tetlock, and Kristel (2003) hypothesized that RMT offers an alternative or complementary explanation: people are offended by the idea of selling an object acquired in a non-MP relationship, valuing objects in the framework of the social relationships they symbolize and mediate. A woman would not want to sell her engagement ring and could not easily put a meaningful price on it; finding his favorite teacher's watch at an auction, a person would value it beyond its market value; money received from a business is more readily spent while money received as a gift from a parent, friend, or academic supervisor is likely to be set aside for special uses. McGraw et al. (2003) conducted four studies of selling and spending decisions and reactions to the possibility of selling relationally meaningful objects. All four studies generally supported their hypotheses. People were uncomfortable with MP transactions of EM and AR objects, and even more offended by the prospect of commoditizing objects representing CS relationships. People were distressed and confused when asked to set MP values on objects embedded in CS, AR, or EM relationships; the dollar values they set varied erratically, with a long tail.

The five lines of research sketched here barely scratch the surface of RMT-inspired work, but they show how the theory has an unusually broad sweep as an account of interpersonal cognition and behavior, with applications in neuroscience, management studies, and social and consumer psychology. This short list is not exhaustive—later sections of the chapter present research in the domains of personality and clinical psychology, for example—but shows that this relational approach to interpersonal processes can yield insights across the social and behavioral sciences.

DISTINCTIVE ASPECTS OF THE RELATIONAL MODELS THEORY APPROACH TO INTERPERSONAL COGNITION

RMT is obviously not alone as an account of interpersonal cognition and behavior. Indeed, the chapters of this volume attest to the rich variety of theoretical and methodological approaches that are available. It is therefore worth stepping back and asking how RMT is distinctive. How does the approach that we are presenting here differ in its focus, scope, and basic assumptions from alternative approaches, and how does it complement them? We argue that RMT is distinctive in four main ways, which we briefly discuss in turn below. First, we propose that it encompasses cordial and conflictual interactions within a single conceptual framework. Second, we propose that RMT takes culture seriously, and is therefore particularly apt as a framework for ethnographic and cross-cultural research. Third, we propose that RMT takes a somewhat broader view of human relationships than many psychological approaches, which commonly restrict their focus either to close relationships or to interactions with strangers. Finally, we argue that RMT differs from many psychological approaches to the study of interpersonal cognition in taking a thoroughly relational approach, whereas many of its alternatives are implicitly or explicitly individualistic.

As we suggest, RMT applies a common theoretical framework to interpersonal conflict and coordination. If moral obligations, social motives, and emotions are concomitants of implementing RMs, then many kinds of violence can be understood as null or asocial interactions. The existence of a relationship that both parties regard as meaningful, valid, and morally binding is the only intrinsic bar to harming each other. In the absence of a relationship, there is nothing to prevent simply using other people as a means to ulterior ends without intrinsic regard for their well-being. For example, if I don't feel that I have anything essential in common (CS) with something or any obligation to respect or protect it (AR), there is no reason not to chop up a tree or a piece of meat or a living person. Thus it is crucial to discover precisely how social relationships are constituted: What creates a relationship among persons? (See below, and Fiske, 2004b.)

However, RMT highlights the fact that aggression and conflict are often organized forms of sociality—for example, ethnic cleansing to create pure homogeneity (CS), fighting for dominance or asserting dominion (AR), tit-for-tat revenge and arms races (EM), and rationally calculated strategies to maximize kill ratios (MP). RMT also provides a potential explanation for discord and conflict across and within cultures: when people implement different RMs, or implement the same RM according to different rules or parameters, coordination fails, leading to anger and recrimination. If you expect to divide the work evenly, but I treat the task as CS, then you'll be offended when I don't take my turn, and I'll be offended when you don't step in and take care of things for a few days while I'm busy or the work can benefit from your special expertise.

Several lines of research have demonstrated the capacity of RMT to clarify interpersonal conflict. Connelley and Folger's (2004) work on conflict associated with diversity initiatives within a large organization has been described above. Vodosek (2003) collected data on culturally diverse chemistry research groups. He looked at groups composed of participants who had the same RM expectations for their work process and for the benefits that resulted from their work, and compared them with groups whose participants implemented different relational mods for the work process and its products. Groups whose participants were implementing discrepant RMs had less positive attitudes toward the group and were less affectively committed to it, less satisfied, and more inclined to quit. In a similar vein, Fiske and Tetlock (1997) theorize about why people resist making trade-offs across different RMs, reacting angrily to interpersonal transactions that transgress "spheres of exchange" governed by different RMs. In short,

RMT is equally adept at making sense of conflict as it is at understanding smooth coordination.

A second distinctive feature of our RMT approach is its attentiveness to culture. Unlike other approaches to interpersonal cognition, RMT was formulated in an anthropological context, developed in the course of ethnographic fieldwork, and refined through broad ethnological comparison; subsequent research on the RMs has taken pains to study people from diverse cultural backgrounds (e.g., Fiske, 1993; Whitehead, 2000). Indeed, one of the hallmarks of RMT is that it offers a conceptual framework that accounts for the cultural universals and cultural variation (Fiske, 2000). The RMs are universal but indeterminate, depending on cultural complements that specify how to implement them to organize specific aspects of particular domains of sociality. Thus unique, culturally distinctive social practices can be understood in relation to diverse social arrangements in other cultures around the world. Cultural diversity in social practices is the product of universal RMs realized through culturally distinctive "preos": precedents, prototypes, or precepts.[1] These preos of each culture specify who, when, where, how, and with respect to what each RM operates. For example, is decision making in marriage to be structured as CS, AR, EM, or MP? All decisions? Which way should a couple organize household work and the utilization of family resources (Goodnow, 2004)? But selecting an RM is not sufficient to guide action or evaluation: people also need to know how to implement the model. CS is a relational structure that consists of equivalence classes, but each culture defines the groups and determines the membership in each. AR is a linear ordering, but to use this relational structure to organize any specific aspect of any activity, each culture must rank the persons involved. EM consists of additive units, but it is not intrinsic to EM that the units be votes, or lottery chances, or turns. If the culture implements EM in collective decisions as voting, it still remains to be determined who is entitled to vote and precisely what counts as a vote. If children apply EM to the utilization of a playground swing, they have to work out what counts as a turn. When adults implement EM to organize the exchange of dinners, they have to decide what counts as a dinner that balances the dinner they received, and they must know the conventions regarding the proper interval before reciprocating: The same day? Several years later? MP consists of organizing an aspect of interaction with reference to ratios, but there is nothing in the innate human proclivity for MP that determines whether food, land, labor, or sex is for sale, or at what price. Hence the structured but indeterminate RMs require socially transmitted preos to complete them. Because the RMs are innate and universal, by learning the local preos, children, immigrants, and social scientists can comprehend the unique social practices of any culture they enter.[2]

A third distinctive feature of RMT is its attention to a broad variety of social relationships. Whereas the RMs span the full range of human sociality, some prominent approaches to the study of interpersonal processes focus almost exclusively on close or romantic relationships. Attachment theory, for example, has been extremely productive as an approach to the study of interpersonal schemas and traits, but its main focus is on how working models and attachment styles affect people's romantic relationships, supporting or sabotaging their desires for intimacy and interdependence. These relationships are undoubtedly very important, but close attachments compose only a small fraction of our everyday social bonds. Relationships based on EM or MP are unlikely to resonate very well with the attachment perspective. Likewise, authority differentials have no obvious place within the attachment framework—an omission that is shared by many approaches to interpersonal cognition and behavior.

Just as attachment and related approaches tend to focus on the intense, intimate end of the relational spectrum, some approaches within the mainstream social cognition tradition focus implicitly on interactions among strangers. Commonly this work examines the ways in which people form impressions and make judgments of others with whom they have no prior acquaintance, rather than addressing real, enduring relationships. As with the study of close relationships, this work has paid great empirical and theoretical dividends, but we would argue that both carve off relatively narrow segments of the interpersonal domain. There is a great deal of relational ground between the null relationships that hold between strangers and the intimate relationships of lovers, and one of RMT's strengths is that it covers this ground in a comprehensive fashion.

A final distinctive feature of our RMT approach to interpersonal cognition and behavior is that its level of analysis and emphasis is relational rather than individual. Many approaches to interpersonal cognition direct attention toward the attributes of individual persons, such as demographic features (e.g., gender, race, age), personality characteristics (e.g., traits, values), and mental states (e.g., attitudes, beliefs, desires). All of these attributes characterize, distinguish, and inhere in individuals. When researchers investigate how we perceive others based on their social category membership, how we infer their dispositions and thoughts (i.e., "theory of mind"), and how we represent self and others in memory, they are focusing on individual-level attributes.

RMT argues that many important processes of interpersonal cognition cannot be understood at this individual level because people are thinking about the structures and processes of interaction. People are intensely concerned and deeply knowledgeable about relationships in their own right, not simply about the features of the individuals who participate in them. We care about and cognize equality, balance, hierarchy, shared communal identity, and so on—all of which describe aspects of relationships between people that are irreducible to personal attributes. According to RMT, thinking about relationships (Fiske & Haslam, 1996) represents a distinct level of cognition from thinking about individuals, and the RMs operate at this level. To be socially competent, it is not enough to be adept at perceiving individuals' emotional states, traits, and demographic characteristics, and not sufficient to have well-organized knowledge about the properties of certain kinds of people. People must also be able to make sense of the irreducibly relational aspects of their interactions, based on organized understandings of the kinds of relationships that people enact (Haslam & Fiske, 2004). Interpersonal theorists and researchers need to pay more attention to people's relational schemas and their perceptions of relationships. Researchers need to recognize that analyses pitched at the individual level are partial analyses. Human sociality is based on shared, culturally informed models that permit people to generate actions that are socially meaningful, to coordinate their actions and evaluations, and to understand and anticipate each other. The properties and dynamics of the relationships that people jointly construct from these models are distinct from the properties and dynamics of the individuals who are relating to each other.

Our insistence that the relational level of interpersonal cognition deserves greater attention may strike some readers as ideological. Indeed, we do believe that individualistic assumptions pervade much psychological research (Fiske & Haslam, 1996) and obscure the irreducible importance of relationships. However, our position is also empirically warranted by our past and ongoing research. In many of our early studies, we found that the RMs predicted a variety of social-cognitive phenomena independently of individual-level variables. In our studies of inadvertent social errors (Fiske et al., 1991), intentional substitutions (Fiske & Haslam, 1997), and person memory (Fiske, 1995), we consistently found that these phenomena were organized by the RMs independently of, and usually at least as powerfully as, individual attributes such as gender, race, and personality. That is, the people who we tend to mistake for one another, select as social substitutes, and recall together in memory are not just those who share similar personal attributes and dispositions: they are people with whom we have the same type of relationship. The work of Iacoboni et al. (2004) underscores this point. When their participants watched videos of realistic social interactions, parts of the brain that support a "default state" of tonic activation were further activated in a way that appears to be unique to the processing of social relations and that does not occur when people think about attributes or categories of objects or persons. In short, beyond the processes involved in reading the attributes, mental states, and traits of individuals, there are special processes in cognizing relationships *among* people.

Our arguments about the importance of the relational level of analysis in interpersonal cognition also extend to interpersonal motivation. Just as some approaches to social cognition are implicitly individualistic in their exclusive focus on individual-level attributes, many social theories make the individualistic assumption that people are selfish materialists, or proximal fitness maximizers. In contrast, RMT posits that humans have evolved intrinsic motives for seeking, sustaining, sanctioning, and redressing the RMs. People are sociable in large part because relationships are inherently rewarding in themselves; the lack, threat to, loss, or transgression of relationships is inherently distressing (Fiske, 1992, Part IV). Given the heuristics and biases in human cognition, dispassionate cognition alone is insufficient to sustain valuable relationships or to motivate costly punishment of violations (Fiske, 2002). Because human fitness depends on sustaining effective participation in a myriad of long-term relationships, humans have evolved emotions that motivate them to do so.[3] Social emotions and motives—for example, love, need to belong, shame, and anger—are typically focused on processes and states of *relationships* such as exclusion, fairness, respect, loss, betrayal, punishment, or atonement.

Our aim in laying out these four distinctive features of RMT is not to suggest dogmatically that our approach is better than the alternatives but to highlight the ways in which it can complement them. The study of interpersonal cognition is probably best served by a variety of approaches, and we recognize the importance of approaches that are tailored to perception of strangers, that chiefly address close relationships, or that focus on individual-level variables. We acknowledge that theories that ignore evolution, culture, ontogeny, or neurobiology can be useful heuristics nonetheless. However, we do believe that to understand human sociality, we need to adopt a relational approach that explains how people coordinate their interaction. Such an explanation must ultimately encompass natural selection, the development of the child, the functioning of the brain, and the mechanisms of culture. This is what RMT attempts to do.

RECENT THEORETICAL AND RESEARCH DEVELOPMENTS

Up to this point we have described RMT, summarized the research evidence that supports it, and argued that it has several distinctive characteristics as an account of interpersonal cognition and behavior. RMT is also a theory in motion, however, and so we spend the rest of this chapter presenting some of our recent work and our forecasts of some of the directions in which future work will proceed. Among the recent developments of our work, two lines of progress stand out. In the first, Fiske has taken some major theoretical steps toward an understanding of how social relationships are constituted, and how people represent each RM in a distinct semiotic medium. In the second, Haslam and Fiske have attempted to show how RMT can illuminate issues that normally concern clinical and personality psychologists. This line of research and theory indicates that individual differences, both normal and abnormal, can be understood in terms of signature patterns of implementation of RMs.

The Constitution of Relationships

One of the most important—and the least studied—question in the social sciences is, How do people constitute relationships? That is, how do people create, reinforce, modulate, and terminate relationships? Another set of important but neglected questions concerns the connections among the constitution of social relationships, the ways people cognize and communicate them, the cultural reproduction of local forms of relationships, and the manner in which children discover the preos that complete the elementary RMs. Theoretical analysis and a synthesis of the extant, relevant empirical literature suggest that the constitution, cognition, communication, cultural transmission, and cultural completion of relationships compose an integrated "conformation system" (Fiske, 2004b).

The *conformation system* of a relationship is the medium in which people conduct the relationship (Fiske, 2004b). In order to coordinate—in order for people to understand each other and construct a jointly meaningful interaction—participants have to recognize the RM they both intend to use and the manner in which they intend to implement it. For example, to construct a CS relationship, participants need to identify who belongs to what groups. To construct an AR relationship, people need to know everyone's rank. They also have to be able to communicate what is going on in the relationship—to signal that they are incorporating a new person in their group, or deferring to an authority. Furthermore, people have to think about the relationship in a manner that is congruent with how they communicate about the relationship and how they are constituting it. That is, their mental representations of relationships must readily "map onto" the structures and processes of those relationships. As they enter a culture, in order to discover how to coordinate with people in a community, newcomers such as children have to grasp where each RM operates and how they are operating. That means that children must be innately, intuitively attuned to how people constitute and communicate group membership, rank, even balance, and ratios. Children and immigrants can only develop the capacity to participate in local coordination systems if they recognize them and can in turn signal to others their intent to participate in specific relationships, tapping appropriate motives and emotions. Conversely, culture consists of continuity over time and consistency through communities in the ways that people coordinate. The media for transmitting and reproducing the local implementations of the RMs are the media through which children learn to participate in them, and in which people constitute and communicate relationships. This integrated set of mediators of each RM is its conformation system. Simply stated, the conformation system is the way people understand each other, the way they connect. Moreover, it is how they commit, how they motivate each other, and how they evoke the emotions necessary to sustain enduring relationships.

Fieldwork among the Moose and systematic comparison of ethnographies from many cultures suggests that the four RMs each have distinctive and universal conformations. The conformation of CS is consubstantial assimilation, based on the perception that participants' bodies are the same or connected in some essential respect: by birth or nursing; by transfer of blood; by commensal eating or drinking; by skin-to-skin contact; by rhythmic synchronous movement; by features of face, skin, or hair. Recognition that bodies are equivalent evokes sentiments of solidarity and elicits commitments to care—it motivates people to share in other ways. People in CS relationships think of each other as sharing the identity-defining aspects of their bodies, and they communicate about their CS relationships to each other and observers using this conformation system. Children (and other newcomers) recognize core CS relationships in their lives by attending to consubstantial assimilation. Conversely, consubstantial assimilation is the medium through which the primary groups and dyads of a culture are reproduced and sustained (cf. Durkheim, 1912/ 1965). For example, intense and enduring solidarity results from initiation rituals in which adolescents sleep and bathe together, are dressed and adorned alike, dance and eat and drink special foods with each other, and are scarified or circumcised together.

In contrast, the conformation of AR consists of relations of space, magnitude, time, and force. People think and communicate about hierarchy in terms of people being above and below, greater and lesser, stronger and weaker, or preceding and following. This is reflected, for example, in plural forms of address and reference to higher ranking persons; the abasement of the body to show respect; or the elevation of superiors on a dais, hill, or higher floor. It operates when seniority is a function of temporal order of birth, arrival, or joining the group. Young children expect that people higher in rank will be bigger, stronger, go first, and be above them. Indeed, adult speakers of diverse languages talk about "superiors" as high up, big, powerful, and senior. Likewise, people indicate hierarchical positions by the relative elevation of the postures and positions they assume and the elevation and size of the abodes or offices they occupy. This is why supreme gods are far above mortals, pharaohs constructed massive pyramids, and taller candidates tend to win elections. People also assert and confer authority by taking or according positions in time and space—for example, by waiting for superiors to arrive and depart; the order of being served, beginning to eat, or speaking turns; or precedence in making choices.

The conformation of EM consists of concrete procedures such as taking turns, conducting a lottery (such as a coin flip), handing things out one by one in rounds, aligning starting points side by side so they match (as in a race), or acting in one-to-one correspondence to each other (e.g., by working in unison). These concrete operations are ostensive demonstrations of an evenly balanced relationship, so they make a relationship feel fair and commit participants to the results. This is what underlies the constitutive rules of sports and games, as well as procedures that define equal treatment under the law.

Abstract symbolism is the primary medium of MP—notably, numbers such as prices or cost–benefit ratios; the propositional language of sales, haggling, and contracts; the signals for bidding in auctions and the gestures that seal a deal; and the concept of utility. MP relations are organized with reference to ratios, an utterly abstract concept. The quintessential symbol is money, the units of which represent rates of exchange with all commodities in the market (Simmel, 1900/1990). These symbols are commitments to the terms of relationships: making a claim in a sales pitch, posting a price in an advertisement, gesturing to bid in an auction, and typing in a bid on E-Bay are binding acts. Violations of these symbolic acts evoke strong emotions, arouse moral sentiments, and motivate sanctions. What binds people to a relational commitment depends on the RM. Signing a contract commits contractor and client to the terms symbolically represented in it, while giving birth commits a mother to care for her child.

The concept of conformation systems takes RMT beyond taxonomy, making it a dynamic causal theory of the processes by which people create, transform, modulate, sustain, and terminate social relationships. If this theory of conformation systems is corroborated, it would have wide applications in everyday life, management and politics, and the clinic.

Relational Models Theory and Individual Differences

RMT was originally developed as an account of the shared schemas that allow social relationships to be coordinated and the motives that sustain relationships. The RMs were understood to be universal. Our early studies focused on demonstrating their role in normal social-cognitive processes. Relational discord, discrepancy, exploitation, and pathology were mentioned but not well addressed in the original work, as reviewers pointed out (see especially Whitehead, 1993). More recently we have begun to examine individual differences in the implementation of the RMs, with a special interest in the part that such differences might play in psychopathology. Many forms of mental disorder have prominent interpersonal elements, but attempts to capture these elements as aberrant ways of implementing relationships have barely begun. Nevertheless, our work strongly suggests that a relational approach has a great deal to contribute.

Personality disorders (PDs) are an obvious place to search for deviant relationship patterns. The interpersonal manifestations of these enduring and refractory conditions are very prominent, and their diagnostic features are laced with interpersonal features. As we have argued previously (e.g., Fiske, 1991; Haslam, 1997b), some PDs may represent inflexible aberrations in the implementation of particular RMs. In the strongest form of this argument, a PD might be caused by the absence of a particular RM, and in the weakest a PD might simply be associated with an aberrant level or manner of implementation of an RM. Predictions about the kind of aberration specific to a particular PD are not difficult to derive. For example, the schizoid personality's aloofness and detachment might be understood as the expression of unusually weak motivation for CS relationships, and the narcissist's grandiosity, need for admiration, and sense of entitlement might be viewed as expressions of underimplementation of EM and overimplementation of AR.

Haslam, Reichert, and Fiske (2002) conducted a study of aberrant use of the RMs in a nonclinical sample of people with significant levels of self-identified interpersonal problems. Participants completed self-report measures of their PD symptoms, their interpersonal problems, and their implementation of, motivation for, and difficulties with relationships governed by each of the four RMs. Numerous predicted associations between specific PDs and relational aberrations received support. Interestingly, the RMs captured distinctive interpersonal components of PDs that have no distinctive interpersonal profile on the interpersonal circle (e.g., Wiggins, 1980), the most prominent interpersonal account of PDs. They also distinguished between pairs of PDs that have identical circle profiles. For example, the circle identifies both schizoid and avoidant PDs with a pattern of cold submissiveness, but the study found them to be marked by unusually high and unusually low motivation for CS relationships, respectively.

Implementing particular RMs in deviant ways is linked to a number of PDs and may also be associated with other mental disorders (e.g., depression; see Allen & Badcock, 2003). Clinical psychologists also hope to understand the factors that predispose people to mental disorders; these vulnerability factors might be equally amenable to a relational approach. Individuals at risk for mental disorders may perceive and implement their interpersonal relationships in distinctively abnormal ways. Detecting any such abnormalities is particularly important, because the abnormalities may play a causal role in precipitating the disorder and may be suitable targets for preventive interventions.

At present, several personality constructs that confer risk for disorders such as schizophrenia and depression have been identified, although the psychological pathways along which these traits promote risk are not well understood. One study of relational correlates of these vulnerabilities recently investigated some possible pathways (Allen, Haslam, & Semedar, 2004). Allen et al. assessed a large undergraduate sample with self-report measures of vulnerability to depression, bipolar disorder, and psychosis, and also with a measure of tendencies to construe personal relationship in terms of the four RMs. Tendencies to construe several relationship types according to particular RMs were then correlated with the vulnerability measures. As expected, depression-proneness was associated with unusually high levels of CS and AR construal of family and close friend relationships, consistent with the view that depression-prone people have overheated close relationships characterized by dependency and excessive reassurance seeking (Joiner & Schmidt, 1998). People prone to bipolar disorder displayed unusually high levels of EM and CS construal within authority relationships (e.g., with employers or teachers), tending to violate the normative AR expectations that govern these relationships. Psychosis-prone students, finally, tended to approach family and close friend relations in a relatively cold and distant (low CS) manner, and to apprehend relations with peers in an unusually asymmetric manner (high AR).

Although preliminary, the findings of Allen et al.'s (2004) study are illuminating. First, young people at risk of several disabling mental disorders, and at an age when these disorders begin to emerge, show distinctive relational tendencies that distinguish them from their less vulnerable peers. Second, these patterns help to bridge trait (e.g., depression-proneness) and process (e.g., excessive reassurance seeking leading to interpersonal rejection) models of vulnerability. Third, the vulnerabilities appear to have some relational specificity, being manifested in particular relationship types. Finally, in some cases the relational patterns associated with vulnerability seem to place individuals at risk of precisely the sorts of interpersonal turmoil that might precipitate their vulnerability. Behaving in an overly familiar and egalitarian manner with a boss may create problems in the workplace for the hypomanic individual, whose behavior might be perceived as disrespectful or rude. Subordinating themselves to their friends and soliciting care and direction from them is likely to trigger the interpersonal rejection and loss that is particularly toxic for the depression-prone. An RMT-based account of vulnerability might therefore help to illuminate the mechanisms, cognitive and interactional, that result in psychopathology.

Personality factors that predispose people to mental disorders fall in between psychopathology proper and normal personality. Just as our relational approach to individual differences can help to account for the signature interpersonal abnormalities of mental disorders and their vulnerabilities, it should also be able to make sense of normal variations in personality. Any theory of interpersonal cognition and behavior should be capable of explaining how personality dispositions are expressed interpersonally. The challenge for our relational approach is to demonstrate how people who differ along normal trait dimensions differentially construe or enact their relationships.

It is important to note here that trait psychology generally gives a quite limited role to interpersonal factors. For example, accounts of the five-factor model (Costa & McCrae, 1992) commonly characterize only two of the factors, Extraversion and Agreeableness, as being substantially interpersonal. Neuroticism, Conscientiousness, and Openness are normally presented as fundamentally intrapersonal properties, representing the individual's emotional lability, self-restraint, and imaginativeness. Surprisingly, some writers in the interpersonal tradition have gone along with this restricted view of the interpersonal realm, defining as interpersonal only those traits that project robustly onto the interpersonal circle (Gurtman, 1991), whose dimensions of warmth and control map onto Agreeableness and Extraversion, respectively (Soldz, Budman, Demby, & Merry, 1993). From our relational perspective, we would expect that a considerably broader range of personality factors have important interpersonal components, and we would argue that the interpersonal circle might not be an adequate arbiter of a trait's "interpersonalness."

Only one study has examined associations between relational patterns and normal personality dimensions. Caralis and Haslam (2004) assessed a sample of psychiatric outpatients on implementation of and motives for the RMs and on the five personality factors. Consistent with expectation, a rich set of associations emerged that extended well beyond the Extraversion and Agreeableness factors. People who strongly implemented or desired CS relationships tended to be low in Neuroticism and high in Agreeableness and Conscientiousness. Tendencies to implement EM were associated with low Neuroticism and high Extraversion and Openness. Preferential use of AR was linked with high Neuroticism and low Agreeableness and Openness. In short, every personality factor was associated with a distinctive relational pattern.

This preliminary support for a relational approach to personality has several potentially important implications. First, it enlarges trait psychology's view of the interpersonal domain by refusing to fence off certain traits as "noninterpersonal." All personality dimensions are apt to have interpersonal aspects or expressions, so purely intrapersonal accounts of them fail to capture essential aspects of personality. Second, our findings reinforce the importance of the AR model, showing it to be linked to negative emotionality and disagreeable rigidity, just as our earlier work linked it to several PDs and vulnerability factors. In U.S. middle-class culture, at least, perceiving the social world in terms of rank and status differentials is associated with psychological disturbance, an observation that would not have surprised early psychoanalytic dissidents such as Alfred Adler and Erich Fromm. However, most interpersonal approaches—for example, the interpersonal circle, attachment theory, or the Structural Analysis of Social Behavior model (Benjamin, 1996)—neglect this authority dimension, and cannot readily capture tendencies to apprehend relationships in asymmetrical terms.

A third potential benefit of a relational view of personality is a more psychologically rich account of some traits. Personality psychologists are often criticized for treating traits as reified entities, and for failing to account for the cognitive structures and processes that generate behavioral regularities. Something important is gained if, instead of explaining some-one's devious and self-serving behavior by their high Machiavellianism, we account for it as an unusually strong tendency to construe their relation-ships in MP terms. The Machiavellianism explanation barely escapes circu-larity, and says nothing of psychological structures and processes. In con-trast, the MP explanation makes reference to the mediating role of an established relational schema, and makes claims about how the person in question perceives the social world. In principle, RMT might enable inno-vative relational accounts of such traits as dependency (inflexible and cul-turally excessive implementation of AR) and envy-proneness (inflexible and culturally excessive use of EM).

FROM TAXONOMY TO DYNAMICS

We have reviewed two lines of recent work that currently represent grow-ing edges of RMT. Before concluding this chapter we would also like to discuss some directions that we believe would be especially fruitful to pur-sue. We highlight the importance of new methods of measurement of the RMs. We recommend research on their ontogenetic emergence and cultural variation. And we propose exploration of discrepant implementations of RMs in relation to discord in personal relationships, organizations, and intercultural relations. We also speculate about possible RMT-based inter-ventions to alleviate these discords.

Research on any theory depends on measures of its constructs. The first measure used to study RMs consisted of paragraphs describing each model; subjects selected the paragraph that best described each of their own relationships. A more subtle instrument, the Models of Relationship Questionnaire (MORQ; Haslam & Fiske, 1999) breaks relationships down into major component domains, asking subjects to characterize, in a given relationship, decision making, exchange, the organization of work, and so forth. These measures have worked well but they are limited insofar as they require subjects to reflectively analyze their relationships. Research on RMs will be facilitated by the invention of new, less reflective measures, including some that have recently been developed. For an fMRI study (Iacoboni et al., 2004), we produced 18 very short digital movies of every-day CS interactions and 18 of AR. In this study, subjects simply watched the movies while we did fMRI scans of their brains, but the movies could be used in many other ways. We are currently using these movies in a de-velopmental study in which children match each movie to one of two car-toon line drawings; each pair of cartoons is selected from a set of figures representing either AR or CS. Another measure under development (by Mark Sergi, Fiske, and Michael Green) taps Relationships Across Domains (RAD). Participants are given a stem describing the interaction of a pair of people in one domain, then asked to decide whether the pair would coordinate in specified ways in three other domains. Each stem and each probe represent coordination in the framework of one RM. So the RAD tests implicit recognition of the RMs, along with implicit understanding that people tend to be consistent in their use of a given RM across domains (as demonstrated in Haslam & Fiske, 1999). Lotte Thomsen, Fiske, and Jim Sidanius are also developing a measure of perception of social relationships, the Circles in Relationship Configuration Arrays (CIRCA), which consists of figures in arrays representing CS, AR, and EM relationships. Participants can be asked to pick the figure that best represents how people in a nation or organization relate, or to express preferences for each configuration. CIRCA is designed especially to assess cultural differences in perceptions of and preferences for relationships, but could be used in many other ways. These instruments can and have been used to capture values, but future measures should go deeper to tap emotional and motivational components of the RMs and their conformations.

Indeed, while several cognitive aspects of the RMs have been investigated, there has been little research on their emotional and motivational components (Fiske, 2002). People can sustain social relationships only if they make sufficient effort to act in accord with the RMs and overcome selfish temptations to shirk or defect. Deficient relational motives may underlie some pathologies of sociality, including psychopathy and frontotemporal dementia; defects in relational emotions may also contribute to some personality disorders and some forms and aspects of schizophrenia. To fully understand relational motives, we need to decipher their neurochemistry—including the social experiences that trigger neurochemical emotional cascades, along with their experiential and behavioral expressions. Maternal and/or pair bonding in some mammals is mediated by oxytocin, arginine vasopressin, and cortisol, among other peptides, but the mechanisms of human social chemistry have hardly been studied. One promising point of entree is MDMA (Ecstasy—a drug often taken at raves), which temporarily produces an intense and indiscriminate CS bond (Fiske, 2004b; Olaveson, 2004).

Other understudied but promising topics include the ontogeny, evolution, and neurobiology of the RMs. RMT suggests that CS emerges in infancy, AR in the second and third years, EM at age 4, and MP by around 10 or 11. However, this developmental aspect of the theory has not yet been tested. The first systematic study of the development of understanding of the RMs (Greenfield, Pfeifer, Fiske, Lim, & Blajesko, 2004) has found that around age 7 children begin to be able to match the Iacoboni et al. (2004) videos of AR and CS to still cartoons of AR and CS, and to free sort the cartoons according to type of relationship. As expected, recognition of CS emerges earlier than recognition of AR, and complete competence in matching CS videos to cartoons is a developmental prerequisite for complete competence matching the representations of AR. (Clearly children can *participate* effectively in relationships of all types long before they can immediately apprehend what is going on in short videos or simple cartoons.)

The theory further suggests that CS is an evolved generalization of mother–offspring bonding and pair bonds or group ties, while AR is an evolutionary generalization of dominance hierarchies (see Haslam, 1997a). These hypotheses could be tested in part by comparing the neural substrates and neurochemistry of CS to those involved in primate maternal bonding and ingroup affiliation, while comparing the neuroanatomy of primate dominance behavior with that of AR. But no one has yet studied the functional anatomy of relationships in primates, and so far only one study has looked specifically at the functional anatomy of human CS and AR (Iacoboni et al., 2004). Complex social coordination has many adaptive advantages, as the social insects show, and the flexibility in implementation and combination of RMs has helped humans to adapt to more diverse environments and more ecological–technological niches than any other organism (Fiske, 2000). Yet we still have no rigorous model for the processes of natural selection that resulted in our flexible capacities and motives for the four RMs. Furthermore, virtually nothing is yet known about the neurochemistry of the RMs.

Few questions are more interesting than those concerning the nature of culture and the processes by which children develop competence to participate in their culture. And no other phenomena can provide as much insight into the processes connecting human nature and culture. Complementarity theory (Fiske, 2000) and the concept of conformations (Fiske, 2004b) offer a detailed RMT account of how children develop the capacity to coordinate with people in the communities in which they are born, and offer an analysis of the nature of cultural universals and variation. There is ethnologic support for these theories, but they need to be investigated in the lab and with systematic behavioral observation.

RMT posits that meaningful social relationships and their emotional rewards depend on the joint use of RMs to coordinate interaction. The corollary is that discrepant implementations of RMs may be a major cause of social discord and distress. This discrepancy hypothesis is supported by studies of satisfaction and hostility in organizations and groups (Connelley & Folger, 2004; Vodosek, 2002) and research on vulnerability and tendencies to psychopathology (Allen et al., 2004; Caralis & Haslam, 2004; Haslam et al., 2002). Extending this research on RM discrepancy is a high priority, given its explanatory potential. Moreover, where RM discrepancy is a source of discord, interventions might be developed, based on the established premise that everyone intuitively understands every RM and appreciates their fundamental validity. Strategies for intervention could involve explicating the RMs and helping all the participants in the interactions to articulate how they are implementing them. Participants could express how they react to what they perceive as transgressions of their own implementations, and be encouraged to acknowledge the potential validity of each other's implementations. That is, each participant could be helped to recognize that others' actions are appropriate in the framework of another intrinsically valid RM implementation, and not merely aggressive violations of the RM that they themselves are implementing. Applying jointly accepted moral and procedural standards derived from the basic RMs, it might be possible to foster tolerance and eventually find common ground for resolving discord. This basic approach to seeking comity might be adapted for mediating disharmony in close relationships, facilitating group process, improving organizational management, and ameliorating intercultural friction.

CONCLUSIONS

A valid taxonomy provides the necessary ontological foundation for science, and RMT offers a promising taxonomy for fundamental forms of social coordination. Wide-ranging empirical research in the RMT framework has consistently supported the theory, more brightly illuminating the structures of human social relations. Having provisionally identified these fundamental entities structuring human sociality, we now have the opportunity to understand their generative dynamics. We need to develop theory and collect evidence on the processes through which people create and transform relationships. Relational dynamics involves interacting processes in evolution, genetics, neurochemistry, neuroanatomy, development, psychology, cultural transmission, social practices, and institutions. This is a vast, wide-open frontier. Exploring this frontier will be intellectually exciting. And as our comprehension of relational dynamics progresses, we may discover new opportunities to address the myriad problems that beset human social relations.

ACKNOWLEDGMENT

We appreciate the cogent and helpful comments of readers of earlier drafts of this chapter: Mark Baldwin, Barbara Fiske, Marco Verweij, and Rick Wicks.

NOTES

1. It happens that the English words for most types of preos are "*p(-)r*" words: *practices*, *paragons*, *propositions*, *proverbs*, *paradigms*, *parameters*. We can't discern any etymological basis for this, but we have coined the word "preo" to reflect it.

2. RMs are probably not the only innately structured but incomplete social proclivities that must be linked to socially transmitted cultural complements. Complementarity theory (Fiske, 2000) posits that this interdependence of evolutionary and cultural transmission is the basis for language, ritual, marriage, many food and sex taboos, and probably many other cultural coordination devices.

3. The strength of these motives seems to differ, such that typically CS > AR > EM > MP. However, there is considerable cultural, individual, and dyad-specific variation in the relative and absolute strength of the motives to seek and sustain the four types of relationships.

REFERENCES

Allen, N. B., & Badcock, P. (2003). Social risk and depressed mood: Evolutionary, psychosocial, and neurobiological perspectives. *Psychological Bulletin, 129*, 887–913.

Allen, N. B., Haslam, N., & Semedar, A. (2004). *Relationship patterns associated with vulnerability to psychopathology.* Manuscript submitted for publication.

Benjamin, L. S. (1996). *Interpersonal diagnosis and treatment of personality disorders* (2nd ed.). New York: Guilford Press.

Caralis, D., & Haslam, N. (2004). Relational tendencies associated with broad personality dimensions. *Psychology and Psychotherapy: Theory, Research and Practice, 77*, 397–402.

Connelley, D., & Folger, R. (2004). Hidden bias: The influence of relational models on perceptions of fairness in human resource systems. In N. Haslam (Ed.), *Relational models theory: A contemporary overview* (pp. 197–220). Mahwah, NJ: Erlbaum.

Costa, P. T., & McCrae, R. R. (1992). *Revised NEO Personality Inventory (NEO-PI-R) and NEO Five-Factor Inventory (NEO-FFI) professional manual.* Odessa, FL: Psychological Assessment Resources.

Douglas, M. (1978). *Cultural bias* (Occasional Paper 35). London: Royal Anthropological Institute of Great Britain and Ireland.

Durkheim, E. (1933). *The division of labour in society* (George Simpson, Trans.). New York: Free Press. (Original work published 1893)

Durkheim, E. (1965). *The elementary forms of the religious life* (J. W. Swain, Trans.). New York: Free Press. (Original work published 1912)

Fiske, A. P. (1991). *Structures of social life: The four elementary forms of human relations.* New York: Free Press.

Fiske, A. P. (1992). The four elementary forms of sociality: Framework for a unified theory of social relations. *Psychological Review, 99*, 689–723.

Fiske, A. P. (1993). Social errors in four cultures: Evidence about universal forms of social relations. *Journal of Cross-Cultural Psychology, 24*, 463–494.

Fiske, A. P. (1995). Social schemata for remembering people: Relationships and person attributes that affect clustering in free recall of acquaintances. *Journal of Quantitative Anthropology, 5*, 305–324.

Fiske, A. P. (2000). Complementarity theory: Why human social capacities evolved to require cultural complements. *Personality and Social Psychology Review, 4*, 76–94.

Fiske, A. P. (2002). Socio-moral emotions motivate action to sustain social relationships. *Self and Identity, 1*, 169–175.

Fiske, A. P. (2004a). Relational models theory 2.0. In N. Haslam (Ed.), *Relational models theory: A contemporary overview* (pp. 3–25). Mahwah, NJ: Erlbaum.

Fiske, A. P. (2004b). Four modes of constituting relationships: Consubstantial assimilation; space, magnitude, time and force; concrete procedures; abstract symbolism. In N. Haslam (Ed.), *Relational models theory: A contemporary overview* (pp. 61–146). Mahwah, NJ: Erlbaum.

Fiske, A. P., & Haslam, N. (1996). Social cognition is thinking about relationships. *Current Directions in Psychological Science, 5,* 143–148.

Fiske, A. P., & Haslam, N. (1997). The structure of social substitutions: A test of relational models theory. *European Journal of Social Psychology, 25,* 725–729.

Fiske, A. P., Haslam, N., & Fiske, S. (1991). Confusing one person with another: What errors reveal about the elementary forms of social relations. *Journal of Personality and Social Psychology, 60,* 656–674.

Fiske, A. P., & Tetlock, P. E. (1997). Taboo tradeoffs: Reactions to transactions that transgress spheres of exchange. *Political Psychology, 18,* 255–297.

Fiske, S. T. (2004). *Social beings: A core motives approach to social psychology.* Hoboken, NJ: Wiley.

Foa, U. G., & Foa, E. B. (1974). *Societal structures of the mind.* Springfield, IL: Thomas.

Goodnow, J. J. (2004). Fiske's model of orientations to social life: The domain of work in households. In N. Haslam (Ed.), *Relational models theory: A contemporary overview* (pp. 167–196). Mahwah, NJ: Erlbaum.

Greenfield, P., Pfeifer, J. H., Fiske, A. P., Lim, H. C., & Blajesko, A. (2004). *Development of children's understanding of social relationships depicted in videos and still cartoons.* Manuscript in preparation.

Gurtman, M. B. (1991). Evaluating the interpersonalness of personality scales. *Personality and Social Psychology Bulletin, 17,* 670–677.

Haslam, N. (1994a). Categories of social relationship. *Cognition, 53,* 59–90.

Haslam, N. (1994b). Mental representation of social relationships: Dimensions, laws, or categories? *Journal of Personality and Social Psychology, 67,* 575–584.

Haslam, N. (1995). Factor structure of social relationships. *Journal of Social and Personal Relationships, 12,* 217–227.

Haslam, N. (1997a). Four grammars for primate social relations. In J. Simpson & D. Kenrick (Eds.), *Evolutionary social psychology* (pp. 293–312). Hillsdale, NJ: Erlbaum.

Haslam, N. (1997b). Personality disorders as social categories. *Transcultural Psychiatry, 34,* 473–479.

Haslam, N. (1999). Taxometric and related methods in relationships research. *Personal Relationships, 6,* 519–534.

Haslam, N. (2004). Research on the relational models: An overview. In N. Haslam (Ed.), *Relational models theory: A contemporary overview* (pp. 27–57). Mahwah, NJ: Erlbaum.

Haslam, N., & Fiske, A. P. (1992). Implicit relational prototypes: Investigating five theories of the cognitive organization of social relationships. *Journal of Experimental Social Psychology, 28,* 441–474.

Haslam, N., & Fiske, A. P. (1999). Relational models theory: A confirmatory factor analysis. *Personal Relationships, 6,* 241–250.

Haslam, N., & Fiske, A. P. (2004). Social expertise: Theory of mind or theory of relationships? In N. Haslam (Ed.), *Relational models theory: A contemporary overview* (pp. 147–163). Mahwah, NJ: Erlbaum.

Haslam, N., Reichert, T., & Fiske, A. P. (2002). Aberrant social relations in the personality disorders. *Psychology and Psychotherapy: Theory, Research and Practice, 75*, 19–31.

Iacoboni, M., Lieberman, M. D., Knowlton, B. J., Molnar-Szakacs, I., Moritz, M., Throop, C. J., & Fiske, A. P. (2004). Watching social interactions produces dorsomedial prefrontal and medial parietal BOLD fMRI signal increases compared to a resting baseline. *NeuroImage, 21*, 1167–1173.

Joiner, T. E., & Schmidt, N. B. (1998). Excessive reassurance seeking predicts depressive but not anxious reactions to acute stress. *Journal of Abnormal Psychology, 107*, 533–537.

Kahneman, D., & Tversky, A. (1984). Choices, values, and frames. *American Psychologist, 39*, 341–350.

Kiesler, D. J. (1983). The 1982 interpersonal circle: A taxonomy for complementarity in human transactions. *Psychological Review, 80*, 185–214.

Lickel, B., Hamilton, D. L., & Sherman, S. J. (2001). Elements of the lay theory of groups: Types of groups, relational styles and the perception of group entitativity. *Personality and Social Psychology Review, 5*, 141–155.

MacCrimmon, K. R., & Messick, D. M. (1976). A framework for social motives. *Behavioral Science, 21*, 86–100.

McGraw, P. A., Tetlock, P. E., & Kristel, O. V. (2003). The limits of fungibility: Relational schemata and the value of things. *Journal of Consumer Research, 30*, 219–229.

Meehl, P. E. (1992). Factors and taxa, traits and types, differences of degree and differences in kind. *Journal of Personality, 60*, 117–174.

Mills, J., & Clark, M. S. (1984). Exchange and communal relationships. In L. Wheeler (Ed.), *Review of personality and social psychology* (Vol. 3, pp. 121–144). Beverly Hills, CA: Sage.

Olaveson, T. (2004). "Connectedness" and the rave experience: Rave as new religious movement? In G. St. John (Ed.), *Rave culture and religion* (pp. 85–106). London: Routledge.

Ouchi, W. G. (1980). Markets, bureaucracies, and clans. *Administrative Science Quarterly, 25*, 120–142.

Parsons, T., & Shils, E. A. (Eds.). (1951). *Toward a general theory of action*. Cambridge, MA: Harvard University Press.

Piaget, J. (1973). *Le jugement moral chez l'enfant*. Bibliothèque de Philosophie Contemporaine. Paris: Presses Universitaries de France. (Original work published 1932) Translated by M. Gabain (1965) as *The moral judgment of the child*. New York: Free Press.

Polanyi, K. (1968). *Primitive, archaic, and modern economies: Essays of Karl Polanyi* (G. Dalton, Ed.). Garden City, NY: Anchor Books.

Ricoeur, P. (1967). *The symbolism of evil* (Emerson Buchanan, Trans.). Boston: Beacon Press.

Sahlins, M. (1965). On the sociology of primitive exchange. In Michael Banton (Ed.), *The relevance of models for social anthropology*. Association of Social Anthropologists, Monograph 1. London: Tavistock (pp. 139–236). Reprinted in M. Sahlins (1972), *Stone age economics.* New York: Aldine (pp. 185–275).

Simmel, G. (1900). *The philosophy of money* (2nd ed., David Frisby, Ed., T. Bottomore & D. Frisby, Trans.). London: Routledge. (Original work published 1900)

Soldz, S., Budman, S., Demby, A., & Merry, J. (1993). Representation of personality disorders in circumplex and Five-Factor space: Explorations with a clinical sample. *Psychological Assessment, 5,* 41–52.

Tönnies, F. (1988). *Community and society* (C. P. Loomis, Trans.). New Brunswick, NJ, and Oxford, UK: Transaction Books. (Original work published 1887)

Udy, S. H. (1970). *Work in traditional and modern society.* Englewood Cliffs, NJ: Prentice-Hall.

Vodosek, M. (2003). *Finding the right chemistry: Relational models and relationship, process, and task conflict in culturally diverse research groups.* Unpublished doctoral dissertation, University of Michigan Business School.

Weber, M. (1978). *Economy and society* (G. Roth and C. Wittich, Trans.). Berkeley and Los Angeles: University of California Press. (Original work published 1922)

Whitehead, H. (1993). Morals, models, and motives in a different light: A rumination on Alan Fiske's *Structures of social life. Ethos, 21,* 319–356.

Whitehead, H. (2000). *Food rules: Hunting, sharing, and tabooing game in Papua New Guinea.* Ann Arbor: University of Michigan Press.

Wiggins, J. (1980). Circumplex models of interpersonal behavior. In L. Wheeler (Ed.), *Review of personality and social psychology* (Vol. 1, pp. 265–293). Beverly Hills, CA: Sage.

Williamson, O. E. (1975). *Markets and hierarchies: Analysis and antitrust implications.* New York: Free Press.

Wish, M., Deutsch, M., & Kaplan, S. B. (1976). Perceived dimensions of interpersonal relations. *Journal of Personality and Social Psychology, 33,* 409–420.

12

Social Mentalities

A Biopsychosocial and Evolutionary Approach to Social Relationships

PAUL GILBERT

Social relationships are a source of our greatest joys and deepest sorrows. They can inspire us to love and compassion but also to vengeance and tragic cruelties (Gilbert, in press-a). They have major effects on immune, cardiovascular, and neurotransmitter systems (Cacioppo, Berston, Sheridan, & McClintock, 2000; Hofer, 1994) and mental health (Brugha, 1995; Wearden, Tarrier, Barrowclough, Zastowny, & Rahil, 2000). Our early relationships shape the maturation of the brain (Schore, 1994, 2001), the emergence of self-awareness and self–other schemas (Baldwin, 1992, and Chapter 2, this volume), and subsequent relating styles (Mikulincer & Shaver, Chapter 10, this volume). The chapter explores the evolution of social roles as forms of self–other co-constructed patterns of social relationships. They can vary as to whether they are (say) sexual or nonsexual, caring and affectionate or neglectful, competitive or cooperative. For the most part, a social role requires that we co-construct interacting sequences into meaningful patterns—for example, when caring for "an-other," the carer is sensitive to cues of distress in the other and seeks to be helpful and supportive. The one "cared for" will signal distress, seek out the caring other, and be responsive to the care he or she receives. Together they create an affectionate caring interaction and role. In competing, however, a person will in some way show his or her intent and power, be relatively nonresponsive to distress in the other, and may even be pleasured by it as a sign that he or she is winning. The one who is the target of the person's competitive attempts may back down, run away, submit, or fight back. What emerges between them is a co-constructed, ranked, social relational episode where one dominates and the other submits. If this pattern is repeated, they may form a dominant–subordinate role relationship.

Clinicians are interested in how people seek to create social roles with others (and see themselves as having been allocated social roles—e.g., as worthy of care or as subordinate) and how these role-forming processes bear centrally on mental health (Gilbert, 1984, 1989, 1992). The 1980s was a time when cognitive behavioral approaches to psychotherapy focused on people's thoughts and beliefs about themselves and others as sources for distress (Beck, Rush, Shaw, & Emery, 1979; Beck, Emery, & Greenberg, 1985). Although cognitive behavioral therapy was to provide an array of insights and techniques for engaging with and helping distressed people, there was concern on a number of fronts (Gilbert, 1992, 2002a). First, was there lack of clarity concerning how motives for certain social outcomes (e.g., for love, admiration, or revenge) related to cognitions: Were they simply products of styles of thinking? Second, there was lack of clarity on nonconscious processes or what is now called "implicit processing" (Haidt, 2001). Cognitive therapists often refer to cognition and information processing as if they are interchangeable. However, while computers, DNA, and neural pathways are information-processing systems, they can hardly be regarded as having "cognitions" as such. This has lead to unhelpful debates about cognitive processing versus emotional processing (Gilbert, 1992). Third, there was a lack of clarity on *archetypal processes*, the way we are motivated to create certain types of social relationship—for example, for caring, attachment, sex, or winning out over others. People can feel and think very differently when they are in different social roles. When people are bullied they feel, behave, and are physiologically organized very differently from when they are loved and valued (Cacioppo et al., 2000). Fourth, the social context plays a major role in cognition and emotion. For example, bullying may arise (or not) because social groups allow or even endorse it, or have strong social sanctions against it. Thus, my own interest has been in biopsychosocial formulations of social roles and states of mind (Gilbert, 1984, 1989, 1995). Figure 12.1 outlines the kinds of interactions that form part of this approach. Stated simply, our thoughts and emotions, our physiologies and social relationships are in a constant state of mutual influence. These in turn are contextualized in physical and social ecologies that influence social values and resource sharing.

The 1980s and 1990s were also a time for the growth of evolutionary psychology (Buss, 2003). There were three strands to this approach. The first focused on the evolution of *threat and defensive systems* that gave rise to various defensive emotions such as anger, anxiety, and disgust (Nesse,

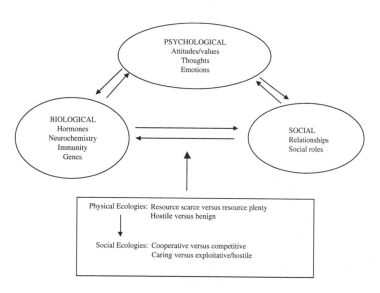

FIGURE 12.1. Biopsychosocial and ecological interactions.

1998) and to defensive behaviors such as fight, flight, submission, and expelling (e.g., noxious substances). These emotions and behaviors are common in a variety of mental health problems (Gilbert, 1993, 2001a). I also argued that there is a *safeness system* that is linked to a positive affect system and is sensitive to certain signals, such as affection and affiliation (Gilbert, 1989, 1993, in press-a). A second strand to evolutionary psychology was an interest in human *cognitive competencies* such as theory of mind, symbolization, and metarepresentation (Byrne, 1995; Suddendorf & Whitten, 2001). Recently Heyes (2003) has suggested that there are a number of evolved influences on cognitive mechanisms, including what they are attentive to, how they learn, and how they operate (e.g., through language). The third strand to evolutionary psychology was focused on *social roles*. Data showed that humans came into the world with basic needs and motives to create social roles. Evolutionary psychologists use the concept of social strategies rather than roles, and see social roles as phenotypes of strategies (Barrett, Dunbar, & Lycett, 2002; Buss, 2003; Smith, 2000). Evolved social strategies are shaped by experiences and social contexts into phenotypes that are expressed as social roles. Hence, for example, strategies for sexual role forming and investing in offspring may vary between the genders, with men being attracted to young, healthy females and wishing to avoid being cuckolded, while women may be attracted to men who control resources, and are more investing in their offspring (Buss, 1989, 2003). However, growing up in high care-investing versus low care-investing environments, or high resource versus low resource environments shapes the phenotypes of these strategies (Barrett et al., 2000), and thus social roles. For example, growing up in high investing environments may lead both men and women to being more altruistic, more orientated to long-term, stable pair bonds, and to more affectional investment in children, while growing up in low investing environments may orient individuals to an earlier age of reproduction, less stable pair bonds, and less investment in children (Belsky, Steinberg, & Draper, 1990). Many of the current key debates are on exactly how potential innate strategies become shaped into phenotypes (social roles and enactments), the flexibility of phenotypes, and the role of social learning (Li, 2003; Lickliter & Honeycutt, 2003; Malik, 2000).

Although there is a history of denial of the archetypal bedrock of human psychology (Pinker, 2002), there is also a long history in theories of psychopathology (Gilbert, 1989; McGuire & Troisi, 1989) and psychotherapy (Beck et al., 1985; Ellenberger, 1970; Ritvo, 1990) that suggest humans come into the world with a range of potentials and individual differences ready to unfold and be shaped by experiences. Running parallel to the evolutionary approaches, which focused on social strategies, were other approaches that also sought innate and evolved underpinnings for human psychology. Bowlby (1969, 1973) argued that we are born with innate potentials and needs to form attachments to caregivers; human infants die without them. Experiences with early caregivers shape internal working models of self and others, and later forms (phenotypes) of relating styles. Baumeister and Leary (1995) argued that with maturation we take an interest in peer relationships and belonging, and our evolved need to belong and form attachments to groups create contexts for social learning that will shape self-identities and values. Other approaches include Jung's archetype theory (Knox, 2003; Stevens, 2002), Guisinger and Blatt's (1994) suggestions of innate dispositions for individuality and relatedness; the circumplex model of social behavior that posits basic dispositions for dominance–submission and warmth–hate (Leary, 1957; Kiesler, 1983); social mentality theory (Gilbert, 1989, 1992, 2000a, in press-a); and many neurophysiological models (Panksepp, 1998). All these suggest *evolved* dispositions to human social behavior and cognition.

SOCIAL MENTALITY THEORY

Social mentality theory is a hybrid of many of these approaches (Gilbert, 1989, 1992). It seeks to integrate various stands of evolutionary psychology. First, it suggests that evolution has "designed into our brains'" systems for assessing threat and safeness and choreographing specific responses (Gilbert, 1993, 2001a, 2002a). All stimuli (both originating from outside a person and inside a person) will be assessed and tagged for how threatening (indicating injury, punishment, or loss) or safe they are. Second, it suggests that social roles (the phenotypes of strategies) can take various forms (e.g., sexual, caring, competing) and choreograph different specialized and nonspecialized processing systems for seeking out certain partners with whom to co-create a role (Gilbert, 1989). A social mentality, then, is not a specific module but is an organizing choreographer of various modules and subsystems needed for enactment of a role. Third, it suggests that information-processing systems, to evaluate and monitor interactions between self and other in the co-construction of roles (in humans), use specialized competencies (e.g., for facial expressions) and nonspecialized competencies (e.g., theory of mind, language, symbolic reasoning, and metarepresentations; see Chiappe, 2000).

This chapter focuses primarily on the evolution of social roles and whether we can "give form" to the various social roles we are motivated to co-create. Fiske and Haslam (Chapter 11, this volume) have approached the same question from a sociological and anthropological perspective focusing on the ecological influence of social roles. As noted, social mentality theory (Gilbert 1989, 1992, 2000a, in press-a) focuses on the evolution of *internal* processing systems, and the choreographies between social motives, threat and safeness, and cognitive competencies. It takes the standard evolutionary view that selective pressures on survival and reproduction lead to the evolution of psychological abilities to meet challenges (Buss, 2003). Social challenges include survival in the first phase of life, living in groups, attracting mates, care of the young, and competing for resources. All these challenges can only be meet in the co-construction of social roles between self and other. Evolution is a conservative process where "what works" is often maintained and modified to fit new challenges. Thus, for example, competing for resources, sexuality, and friend–foe recognition are strategies and competencies that have very early origins in the reptiles, while care providing, play, affection, affiliation, and cooperation emerge with the mammals (MacLean, 1990). Complex cognitive abilities that allow for new ways to create and enact social roles, such as symbolic self–other representations, metacognition, and theory of mind are late primate, and primarily human, abilities (Byrne, 1995).

In trying to identify an archetypal social role one needs to try to identify the challenges that it solves and the consequent psychological systems that have emerged to solve it. A rough classification, which, while not comprehensive captures some of the more important archetypal social roles, can be suggested (Gilbert 1989, 1992, in press-a).

1. *Care eliciting* involves relationship forming with another who can provide protection, needed investment for survival, and (in mammals) emotional regulation. It solves the problems of regulating (early) threat to self and having to provide for the self. Competencies include assessing

proximity to (an)other, distress calls, seeking the other, and being responsive to his or her (care) signals.

2. *Caregiving* involves relationship forming to another for providing investments of time, energy, and other resources (e.g., to an infant) that increase the chances of their survival, growth, and subsequent reproduction. It solves the problems of threat to young or "weakened" kin and allies. Competencies include responsiveness to distress, assessing (and providing for) the needs of another, and (in humans) empathy and sympathy.

3. *Formation of alliances* involves relationship forming for cooperation, with aggression inhibition, sharing-exchange, affiliation, friendships, group living, and reciprocal behavior. Competencies include judging who is similar to self, who is ingroup versus outgroup, and who is desirable as an ally. In humans this social mentality gives rise to thinking in terms of reciprocation, equity, fairness, and rights. It solves problems of constant infighting and allows for cooperative action to confront problems to survival (e.g., teamwork).

4. *Social ranking* involves relationship forming for direct competition for resources, gaining and maintaining rank/status (dominance/leader), accommodation to those of higher rank (submission/follower), and competing in ways that lead to being "chosen" by others for certain roles (e.g., as an ally, sexual partner, or leader). It solves the problem of constant infighting and offers social coherence. In humans what earns status can be socially constructed to fit an ecology.

5. *Sexuality* involves relationship forming for sexual behavior, involving attracting, being attracted to, courting, conception, and mate retention. Different strategies and blends of emotions and motives may operate for short-term mating verses forming long-term sexual bonds.

Each role requires both a signal-detecting system (e.g., of emotions and intents of others, to work out what role "the other" is trying to create with the self), and a signal-sending system (to send the appropriate signals to co-construct a role). From an evolutionary point of view, different role-forming mechanisms, or strategic orientations for a role, have been laid down at different times. Biosocial goals and role seeking evolved in various life forms because they were conductive to fitness—that is, animals that successfully enact these roles (e.g., for mating or caring for offspring) leave their genes behind in succeeding generations. Importantly, evolution is a process of gradual modification of what has gone before. It cannot go back to the drawing board and start again; adaptations must fit the system. Hence roles, with their appropriate motivating, searching, attracting, and signaling-to-others routines are retained if they work, but they are modified in their forms and the competencies needed to enact them. This implies that we can see evolution as a journey that is retaining some motives and competencies while also developing new ones, and modifying those retained. The way strategies and competencies become modified by evolution is subject to intense debate (Geary & Huffman, 2002).

Reptilian Roles

Many of the earliest forms of social behavior such as courting, sexual advertising, mating, threatening, harassing, defending territory, making ritual threat displays, and submitting can be observed in our early ancestors, the reptiles (MacLean, 1990). The hormone testosterone is an important hormone for these motives/behaviors and remains so in humans (Kemper, 1990; MacLean, 1990). Reptiles also need some kind of cognitive competency for *social comparison* and a recognition system of who can be challenged, who is dominant, and who should be avoided or submitted to, and when to flee rather than fight or submit. This cognitive competency is linked to what Maynard Smith (1982) called the *hawk–dove game/strategy*. Hawks always fight and doves always submit, but *social comparison*, aided by ritualistic displays to size up others, gives options to play either and thus becomes a flexible and stable part of the strategy. Because social comparison plays such a vital role in social interactions, it has (especially with humans) been subject to much modification in the motivational and cognitive competencies that support it and how and when it is used (Gilbert, Price, & Allan, 1995).

MacLean (1990) notes that threat displays, such as the goosestepping of soldiers on parade, involve muscular postures similar to those of reptiles issuing threats. Eye gaze can also be a threat signal in many species. Humans are capable of generating rich *fantasies*. It is interesting that the archetype of the devil and of evil (our thoughts and images about evil) typically involve both reptilian (visual) features and a mind that only has an interest in sex and power—that is, a mind completely devoid of a (mammalian) sense of kinship care, love, or compassion. In the real world too a mind without an interest in the welfare of others and who seeks to dominate and use others only for his or her own satisfaction is one to be feared.

Mammalian Roles

The motives for sex, control over reproductive opportunities, and abilities for social comparison (allowing animals to know who to challenge and who to submit to) did not disappear with the mammals but were retained and modified to track species-appropriate signals. This resulted in different forms of dominance hierarchies, styles of submissive behavior, group living, and competencies for such living (Gilbert, 2000b). Subordinates and dominants live close together and may forage as a group but with subordinates deferring and submitting to dominants. However, what was key to mammalian success was the evolution of live birth and postbirth care of offspring (Geary, 2000). Mammals brought a new set of motives, feelings, and competencies (ways of seeing and thinking about social relationships) into the world, which included kin recognition and kin care (fish may eat their own young if they don't disperse after birth; see MacLean, 1985; Bell, 2001). Thus caring behavior evolved with new motive systems (such as distress calling and answering), new signal detectors (e.g., to distress calls, and responding to physical, including body-to-body and skin-to-skin, closeness; Field, 2000), new cognitive competencies for assessing and seeking proximity to carers (in contrast to dispersion after birth) (Bowlby, 1969); new emotions (e.g., for affection, grief), and new hormone systems for caregiving and bonding (such as oxytocin; Bell, 2001; Carter, 1998; Panksepp, 1998; Wang, in press)—all needed to make possible attachment behavior as a reciprocal role relationship. The burden of care for young fell to females, and this influenced the sexual strategies of both males and females (Buss, 2003; MacDonald, 1992). These systems also provide a source for fantasies (e.g., for having children or being loved and cared for).

In addition to care and attachment, for certain species of predators (e.g., lions) and primates, cooperative behavior was a highly successful social role. Indeed, it was so successful that various forms of cooperation and alliance building gradually evolved with the motives and competencies to enact them (see below).

Social Environments

Importantly, the mammalian brain evolved with the assumption (expectations) that care would be available in the first days of life, and to search for and elicit it. Similarly, having motives for sex, or to form friendships and cooperate, would be useless if there were not others around who had (a mixed menu of) similar desires. Thus, as Caporael (1997) eloquently argues, types of social relationships (self–other roles) must also be replicated in succeeding generations to allow certain evolved motives and competencies to mature and be enacted. You can't have one without the other. Importantly, however, different human groups occupied different ecological niches (harsh, hostile, or benign) and so created different types of social niches that affected their strategies and role enactments (Barrett et al., 2002; Gilbert, in press-a). Maturation of brain systems, upon which mentalities depend, are highly influenced by early experiences of types of parental investment (care), degrees of threat in the social domain, and social values (Schore, 1994, 2002). Children mature to fit their social niche, and once matured for this niche will tend to develop certain types of role patterns and social-cognitive processes (e.g., men as tough and fearless, or loving and kind; Belsky et al., 1990; Gilmore, 1990), and thus re-create the social niche through reciprocal interactions and shared thoughts/values over the lifespan. To put this another way, social strategies seek to co-create roles with others. For example, if a person is hostile and aggressive to others, he or she is seeking to activate fear-based subordinate strategies in "the other" such that "the other" will defer to him or her. If a person is kind and altruistic, then these strategies can only work if they successfully activate altruism and liking of self in another. Gilbert and McGuire (1998) called this "role matching," or (in the circumplex model) "role complimentarity" (Leary, 1957; Kiesler, 1983).

Thus many theorists have argued that different motives and role-forming preferences have been laid down at different times in our evolution (Bailey, 1987). A combination of genes and learning harness our array of potential motives and competencies and pattern them during a person's life to fit a social niche and create a self-identity. In summary, then, archetypal desires and role-forming systems have been laid down over a long time. What is new for humans is not so much recent changes in desires, motives, and emotions, but the rapid change in cognitive competencies that give new meanings "to self in the world" and allow for integrated coregulating social interactions (Cacioppo et al., 2000; Mithen, 1996; Taylor, 1992). These self-identity and social systems, however, often have to regulate earlier evolved social motives (e.g., for sex, care, control over resources, and belonging) with their signal detectors.

Learning and Human Cognitive Competencies

Innate guides, for interpreting social signals, role seeking, signaling to others, and attracting, cannot provide all the information that animals need to achieve their goals. Learning provides the information that genes cannot. The more complex the environment (including the behavior of those to whom one will seek to relate to), the more complex this learning needs to be. From the simple laws of learning by association (which most species are capable of) to the highly sophisticated human capacity for symbolic thought, our abilities to learn, adapt, and coordinate component systems in our minds play a central role in social behavior (Heyes, 2003). There are a number of "self-and-other-focused" cognitive competencies that are key to *human* role formation and are relatively nonspecific—that is, they can be used in a variety of social roles (Chiappe, 2000; Mithen, 1996). These include symbolic self–other representations (Sedikides & Skowronski, 1997), theory of mind (Byrne, 1995; Nickerson, 1999), existential theory of mind (Bering, 2002), and metacognition (Wells, 2000). The frontal cortex seems especially important for these socially focused competencies and allows for our more basic role-forming motives and emotions to be organized, planned, or inhibited in new ways (Goldberg, 2002). Suddendorf and Whitten (2001) have pointed out that a mind with these types of abilities is a *collating mind*. This is a good term, for it describes well the ability to bring together (to assemble) different time periods to mind (e.g., past, present, and future) and run different simulations. It also allows role-forming mentalities to more flexibly bring together different attributes of mind in the service of role enactments, that is, motives, emotions, competencies, and evaluative abilities. These competencies give rise to abilities to form self-identities that are in turn patterned by social ecologies and social relationships (Gilbert, in press-a).

Different social mentalities that are role-focused will create different, sub- or mini-self-identities. One may have a self-identity when in the role of carer (e.g., father or psychotherapist) as a sexually attractive person, as a friend (e.g., as reliable), or as a competitor (e.g., as tough and assertive). We need to coordinate different aspects of our minds for different roles. Self-identities, then, are internally constructed models of a self with needs, desires, preferences, abilities, likes, and dislikes; a self that can be threatened in certain ways; a self as one wants to be (and does not want to be) in specific roles; a self that wants to be known/valued/respected (by self and others) via the roles one enacts. The ability to construct self-identities serves important role-regulating and -engaging functions (see Conway & Pleydell-Pearce, 2000, and McGregor & Marigold, 2003, for reviews).

Human cognitive flexibility also provides opportunities to *decouple* motives from actions. For example, the Dalia Lama once reported that even though he was a celibate Buddhist, this did not mean he did not have sexual feelings but rather that he learned to value them and control them in a different way from someone who wanted to form a sexual relationship. A person might be terrified but not run away and knowingly risk his or her life in a war. Or a person might be very hungry but not eat in order to lose weight to look more attractive to others or to stay healthy. One motive or felt need can come to override another through cognitive value systems. Although cognitive systems introduce powerful regulators on motives, emotions, and behaviors, they are not always accurate. Cognitive therapists, for example, have long argued that people can over- or underestimate the dangers of a particular event or social interaction (Beck et al., 1995). Cognitive therapists focus on beliefs, expectations, and attributional styles. However, these consciously available descriptions of our cognitive activity may be end products of highly complex processes in multiple component systems both conscious and nonconscious—a fact well articulated by Haidt, (2001), Teasdale (1999), and Lambie and Marcel (2002).

SOCIAL MENTALITIES

This section explores four of the five social mentalities outlined above. Sexual behavior is not explored here due to space limitations and to the large literature and debates that now exist for this form of relating.

Care Eliciting and Seeking

The first days of life can be a very threatening time for the young, many of whom will be eaten or come to harm in other ways. In some species only 1–2% will make it to adulthood to reproduce. For these species, it is the numbers produced that enables the species to continue. Things change rapidly with the advent of parental protection and care (Bell, 2001; MacLean, 1985; Wang, in press). Once a species has evolved kin recognition and provisioning (related to parental investment; see Geary, 2000), then infants will evolve to be highly motivated to seek parental care (Bowlby, 1969; MacLean, 1985). In mammals, the "need for others" in order to survive is active from the first days of life, and motives to be cared for, helped, and protected continue throughout life in increasingly complex ways. Different signals from a mother have different physiological effects on an infant (Hofer, 1994), with physical contact/affection being especially important for calming and sense of safeness (Field, 2000). Signals of protection, related to the accessibility and availability of (usually) the mother. Parental protecting functions were central to Bowlby's attachment theory. He theorized that disruptions to a child's access to his or her mother can result in anger, anxiety (Bowbly, 1973), or depression (Bowlby, 1980). Renewed and/or secure bonds result in joy and positive affect. As children's cognitive abilities unfold, they build internal working models of others as being available and helpful, or not. These internal models then influence a range of self–other relating styles (Mikulicner & Shaver, Chapter 10, this volume).

Protection is not the only signal that infants are responsive to; affection is also central to development. Recent work has shown that from the first days of life, infants are emotionally sensitive to a range of signals in their interactions with their caregivers. In particular, maternal facial expressions, holding and stroking, and the rhymes of voice tone have a major influence on the infant's internal state and physiological organization. This is called "intersubjectivity" (Trevarthen & Aitken, 2001). In addition to the protection-attachment system, MacDonald (1992) has suggested that infant–parent interactions operate through another system that he calls a "warmth system," which underpins affectional interactions. Thus, he argues that it is possible to have high warmth but low attachment in an interaction or high attachment but low warmth. Gilbert (1989, 1993) suggested that parental interactions not only regulate threat and stress, but also safeness. When individuals feel safe, they are psychobiologically organized in different ways from when they feel threatened. Safeness is not simply the absence of threat but requires specific signals to indicate safeness and warmth, and safeness may operate through opiate systems in the brain, giving rise to feelings of connectedness and contentment (Gilbert, in press-a). Providing signals of protection (Bowlby, 1969), warmth and affection (MacDonald, 1992), and empathic understanding (Koren-Karie, Oppenheim, Dolev, Sher, & Etzion-Carasso, 2002), enacted (in the first instance) via mutual intersubjectivity (Trevarthen & Aitken, 2001)—all influence brain development and social behavior (Schore, 1994), and in particular the degree of safeness children experience to external and internal signals. Thus, for example, a mother who is empathically attuned to her infant, and is understanding of and soothing to her infant's distress, anger, or anxiety will not only help to regulate her infant's distress, but that distress itself become relatively "nonthreatening." In contrast, a mother who withdraws or is aggressive in the face of her infant's distress can result in a child who is frightened of, or becomes disorganized by, his or her own distress (Steele, 2002; Liotti, 2000).

Later in life we attend to subtle cues of approval, care, and other people's empathic attunement to our feelings when working out if someone *really* cares about us. There can be a whole range of signals (or the absence of them) that we may take as indications of care. Moreover, we become increasingly discriminating on the type of care (investments) we seek. Thus, the care one seeks from a family doctor is different from what one seeks from a lover or parent, and the signals one will monitor will also vary. There will be some overlap, however, in that one may want both the family doctor and the lover to be accessible and understanding of one's needs and to have a positive and caring disposition toward self. People are often very attentive to the nonverbal signals of others and may track these using implicit processing systems (see Baldwin, Chapter 2, this volume). In psychotherapy the care-eliciting and -seeking mentality can come online and people will look for, and seek to elicit, certain types of "caring" signal(s) from their therapist. They want to know the quality of the relationship and if the therapist cares about them (Bailey, 2000, 2002). Some patients, especially those from difficult backgrounds, may feel they need easy and rapid access to a soothing, reassuring therapist. Others have closed down on this system and seek to be self-reliant, trusting no one to care for them, and fear feelings of vulnerability or needs for care; others oscillate between these two extremes (Liotti, 2000).

Care-eliciting roles thus arise from the co-construction of self with other. We may seek the protection of others and feel reassured by their signals that they will give it. Adult human care eliciting is often intended to seek practical help, regulate feelings of distress, and/or generate feelings of being valued or loved. Care eliciting can be about seeking signals from others so that they can sooth us, and to demonstrate to us that in their eyes we are someone to be valued and validated—we are worthy of their investment. When the desired signals from others are forthcoming (a role is matched in its co-construction), we may feel soothed, but if the other turns away, rejects us, or is aggressive, our care-eliciting efforts have failed (we are now role-mismatched), and we may become more distressed, more depressed, or close down this role-seeking system and look to our own efforts—or, as Bowlby (1980) noted, become compulsively self-reliant or avoidant. In the language of threat and safeness, care seeking becomes a threat, not an opportunity to feel soothed and reassured.

Caregiving

Caregiving evolved (in the first instance) from "kin caring." As MacDonald (1992) suggests, caring for others must evolve with *motivating* systems to provide care, and a sense of pleasure or threat from doing it, and *competencies* to detect signals from "the other" that indicate a need for care, with abilities to provide appropriate forms of care. Fogel, Melson, and Mistry (1986) define caregiving as "the provision of guidance, protection and care for the purpose of fostering developmental change congruent with the expected potential for change of the object of nurturance" (p. 55). The human desire (motivation) to care may be expressed to other humans, animals, inanimate objects (e.g., the family car), or the self. It takes in the concept of "looking after" and *concern* for the well-being of the other. Fogel et al. (1986) note four dimensions of caring: (1) choice of object, (2) expression of caring and nurturing feelings, (3) motivation to care and nurture, and (4) awareness of the role and need for caring. Emotions linked to caring can be positive—that is, pleasure from seeing the other prosper—or negative—triggered by distress in another—and the emotions of sympathy, distress and concern are central (Eisenberg, 2002).

Social caring behaviors may include providing needed resources (e.g., food), specific types of practical help, specific interpersonal stimuli (e.g., a cuddle), and protection. In addition, caring can be related to a preparedness to listen to and become empathically attuned with another and validating for him or her. We often express our mental state of being in a "caring state of mind" by our nonverbal communications. We monitor signals in others that might indicate that care is needed, would be beneficial, or would be valued by the other. The lack of *feeling* in caring can be very distressing to people—for example, if people think others are caring of them only out of their own self-interest, because they want something (e.g., "You are only nice to me because you want sex or something I have—not because you really care or have concern for me"; or a patient may say "You are only listening to me because you are paid to").

Serious problems arise in those who seem to lack the *motives* and feelings for caring. For example, psychopaths seem to lack feelings related to a desire and capacity to care and are not emotionally moved by the distress of others (Miller & Eisenberg, 1988). They can feel shame and humiliation—indeed these can ignite powerful defensive emotions of rage—but concern for others or guilt are not noted. They can, however, fake care (e.g., to impress desired sexual partners), but these feelings are superficial and only used to get what they want. Hence, competent caring behavior depends on certain evolved competencies for empathy and sympathy for others (Eisenberg, 2002). It is the care and concern system that makes possible guilt feelings (these are quite different from those of shame; see Gilbert, 2003). The caregiving mentality also underpins our abilities for compassion (Gilbert, in press-a).

The competencies for empathetic concern or sympathy are developed and socialized in family and social contexts (Eisenberg, 2002), and become built into a self-identity such that one values caring behavior (wants to see self as a caring person), recognizes its role in building and maintaining relationships, and accepts responsibility for the welfare of others (Staube, 2002). There may be gender differences in how we express care, with women being more focused on emotional forms of caring and more attentive to nonverbal communication, and males being more focused on instrumental and practical solutions to problems (Gilligan, 1982). These differences may relate to the fact that women carry the burden of investment in children, and thus these competencies and motives have been more "selected" in women (Taylor et al., 2000). The degree to which these differences are innate or the result of socialization remains a matter of debate and research, but the vast majority of people would like to see themselves (i.e., have a self-identity) as caring rather than uncaring, selfish, and egotistical. This does not mean that they *are* caring, of course. In regard to threat and safeness, it is known that if other people's distress becomes too threatening, costly, and/or distressing to self, then people may avoid or turn away from caring (Eisenberg, 2002).

However, care *is* an expensive resource to dispense and it is not given equally to any who seek it. We are more motivated to care for those with whom we are genetically related. For example, a mother who has just given birth wants to take home her own child, not just any newborn from the delivery room. Great distress is caused if there are mistakes in identification. Evolution theory predicts that caregiving will be greatest when it gains status, is likely to be repaid or reciprocated, and/or where it is directed to kin. However, much depends on the cost and nature of the threat that requires help. As both the threats and costs of caring increase, help provision may decrease (Burnstein, Crandall, & Kitayama, 1994).

Rescuing is an important quality of caring, often depends on courage, and does not always follow the genetic self-interest guides depicted by evolutionists. At times, it can override any personal concern with threat. People will die risking their lives to save strangers. As the morning of September the 11, 2001, unfolded, many people within the doomed buildings, and personnel from the emergency services, were to die in efforts to save others (knowing they were at risk), giving rise to the many stories of extraordinary heroism from ordinary people on that day. This does not mean that people would try to save other people's children before their own, or that they would try to save a trapped stranger on the floor below rather than a trapped friend on a floor above, or that many people weren't more concerned with their own safety than with that of others. What it does mean is that in extraordinary conditions our motives and emotions (in this case, to rescue and protect) can power us along and take us over. Clearly, these efforts have little to do with forming attachments as such, but seem to operate as a basic disposition to respond to distress and help others in danger, where lines of responsibility are clear.

It can also be noted that courageous rescuers are not necessarily "the warmest" of people in the sense of expressing affection. A patient of mine spoke of her three children. Peter was the most "difficult," not a very cuddly child or affectionate, and yet she said, "If there was ever any trouble in the family it was always Peter you could rely on to be there for you." It is also the case that some people put the needs of others first, partly because they want to earn other people's love and gratitude. Hence caring roles can take many forms and be inspired or enacted for many reasons. Nonetheless, without a caregiving mentality with its evolved motives and competencies for concern for the welfare of others, and with capacities for sympathy and empathy, it is unlikely that "caring" could exist in the way it now does in human relationships.

Cooperation and the Formation of Alliances

Large numbers in schools, herds, and other groups may attract more predators but also reduce an individual's chances of predation. Hence, preyed-on species tend to form larger groups than their predators—who operate either as individuals or in small groups. Some estimate the typical size of early human groups to have been around 100–150, although at times they could have been smaller or larger. There are many reasons why this size of group was adaptive—including the fact that more than this number and people would be unable to get to know everyone in the group and remember their transactions with them (Barett et al., 2002).

Baumeister and Leary (1995) have argued that the need to form into groups and derive a sense of belonging is an innate human need. Boehm (1999) argued that for humans (before agriculture), coalitions of subordinates, made possible by the ability to exchange information and jointly plan activities, shifted human social organization away from male-dominated groups to more egalitarian ones; people ganged up against aggressive and nonsharing others. Once within a group humans can work collectively to secure resources, defend them, and share them. For monkeys and humans alike, having alliances that reciprocate and share is a great advantage and is related to what has been called "reciprocal altruism" (Trivers, 1971). The social mentality to form alliances can involve aggression inhibition, sharing, affiliation, friendships, and reciprocal behavior. The motives to form alliances also evolved as a solution to threats (e.g., allies can remove parasites from each other or defend their interests more effectively than either alone). The *motive* to share is central to alliance formation. There are, of course, many types of alliance, such as pair-bonded sexual partners, family alliances, peer affiliative friendships, and cooperation within teams or larger groups such as armies.

Sharing and mutual helping is an important part of primate social life (de Waal, 1996). There are two aspects of human sharing that are significantly advanced by "theory of mind" competencies. These are sharing a goal (and an activity) and sharing contributions to a goal. Indeed, some argue that the benefits of sharing put pressure on humans to evolve some of their complex social-processing systems and use them in novel ways (Lock, 1999). Shared activity—such as playing in an orchestra or on a sports team or working as a member of the group that put a human on the Moon—is clearly highly rewarding and bonding. We are often highly motivated to be part of a team that has a goal or a shared activity. We gain a sense of "we-ness" (Plotkin, 2002), and at times we may lose our sense of individuality in the social activity (Gilbert, in press-a). When we share our values and goals, and the means to secure them, we feel in tune with others and positively disposed to them. However, a threat arises when we feel out of tune with those in our team/alliance. Then we become defensive and our emotions change. We are faced with the dilemma of conflict with them or of going along and changing ourselves. We may (often unconsciously) work out the cost of ostracism and becoming marginalized. One of the ways of avoiding this cost is to change our values and blend in. In cooperation there can thus also be a pressure (and a desire) to *conform*. The pressure to conform can be so strong that people may agree with things they know are wrong in order to be "like others" (Bond & Smith, 1996). Different cultures create different types of pressure to conform (Bond & Smith, 1996). People may also engage in very immoral behavior out of a need to conform and not be ostracized (Kelman & Hamilton, 1989; Straub, 2002).

Research has shown that one's feelings of belonging to a group (and being in conformity with it) also effects one's sense of personal identity and status (Abrams, 1996). Thus, for adolescents in particular, for whom building alliances outside the home and beginning their sexual adventures becomes a pressing issue, display behaviors (e.g., what kind of clothes or hairstyles one wears, or what type of music one is interested in) are all part of the social language of conformity. There can be a fear of stigma and exclusion by not having the right displays (i.e., looking right). One can feel personal pride or shame from the successes or failures of one's group or team—indeed, or one can feel it as a personal affront or attack if a member of one's group is threatened.

Different types of moral thinking emerge from the caregiving social mentality in contrast to the cooperative social mentality (Gilbert, 1989, in press-a; Gilligan, 1982). Caregiving focuses on the issue of need and wel-

fare of the other and uses sympathy. When Buddhists seek to tap our capacities for loving kindness and compassion, it is this caregiving mentality,
with its motives and emotions (e.g., sympathy), they are tapping into. Cooperation focuses on issues of justice, rights, and fairness, and is intended
to stop exploitation and intragroup conflicts (although dominant individuals often try to slant justice systems in their favor; see Scott, 1990). Thus
caring-based, and cooperative-based, moral systems require different types
of emotion-cognitive focus and processing (Gilbert, in press-a). Batson,
Klein, Highberger, and Shaw (1995) demonstrated that justice-focused versus care-focused motives (which they call "empathy-altruism") *are* different prosocial motives, which can produce different behaviors and at times
conflict.

Cooperation has sometimes been seen as a strategy: at times it is better
to be cooperative, to share, and to stay true, and at other times to defect
and to take the benefits (Axelrod, 1990). In a major review of this work,
Cohen (2001) discussed how cooperative strategies are related to the social
ecology and why poverty and resource inequalities may actually skew behavior to noncooperative and poor alliance-formation strategies (an "each
for him or herself" view of life). These are not necessarily conscious decisions (mostly they are not), but are part of a person's "strategic," social-
cognitive orientation to the social world, as they (nonconsciously) track
the type of social niche they are in. Cohen (2001) also points out that there
can be time lags. For example, if an ecology changes very quickly, then the
old values—rearing styles and so forth—may continue even though these
no longer fit the niche.

Threats to Cooperation and Alliance Building

Having our talents or attributes valued by others, such that they wish to
form an alliance with us, is good for our personal and genetic self-interests.
Our emotions respond to these signals of being valued and wanted or rejected (Gilbert, 2002a). A major threat is thus not having our contributions valued and/or we can't find people who want to share with us or will
not form the alliances and relationships we think we need. To be marginalized, rejected, or ostracized, and thereby fail to develop certain types of
alliance, have been major threats to many social animals, especially humans, for millions of years. Indeed, our survival and reproductive success
have long depended on forming alliances and being accepted into groups.
Baumeister and Tice (1990) have discussed how the fear of being left out of
social interactions or of being ostracized can be very easily triggered in humans. Williams, Cheung, and Choi (2000) suggest that ostracism can be
mild or severe, and encompasses a range of outcomes from not being
included in activities, to more severe forms of active social rejection, to
persecution. They set up a disc-throwing game on the Internet and then

manipulated how much each person (sitting miles away) got thrown the disc via his or her computer. They found that reducing the number of times participants were included in the game was aversive, and impacted on self-esteem and sense of belonging. This method is fascinating because participants did not know who was playing the game (unknown to them it was a computer), they were in their own home out of public view, and yet the effects were still robust. Ostracism is aversive even under these conditions of a cooperative participating game. It was not wining or losing that was the issue here but being included/excluded, suggesting a potent (and probably evolved) sensitivity for tracking inclusion/exclusion (Baumeister & Leary, 1995; Gilbert, 2001b).

Another threat to cooperation and alliance formation is cheating. Cheating has received much attention from evolutionists who believe we have attuned attention mechanisms and specialized ways of (modules for) reasoning to detect cheats (Cosmides & Tooby, 1992), although others disagree (Barrett et al., 2002). Cheating and detecting cheats involves many complex processes. We can cheat in a sexual relationship; we can fail to reciprocate with others such that we get more out of a relationship than we put in; we can feign illness and incapacity to make others care for us, or let us off our responsibilities; we can socially loaf on teams, and fake our talents, pretending we are better or more committed than we are; and we can simply lie about our true feelings and motives. There is also the issue of how conscious we are about our own social deceptions and manipulations (Nesse & Lloyd, 1992).

Different types of cheating may require different types of detection ability. Our sensitivity to being cheated probably relates to how trusting or gullible we are, theory of mind abilities (some people read deception into the most minor of things), history of being cheated, and social power (Scott, 1990). The ability to trust others is also the ability to feel safe with others. Cheating often ignites defensive emotions in us because to be cheated is a threat. Anger is a common reaction to being cheated, but so is anxiety, sadness (if it is by a loved other), disgust, and at times forgiveness. As for those doing the cheating, guilt (if someone is hurt), shame (when our reputations are damaged), and fear of retaliation can be regulators of cheating.

So our mentalities for cooperation and alliance formation will motivate us to seek alliances and join groups, compare ourselves with others to work out if we are "the same" as them and have the same values, conform to the norm, track who are the best allies to work with and how to secure relationships with them, monitor if we are being included or excluded, cheating or being cheated, and our emotions will be regulated according the "health" of these role relationships. However, forming alliances requires that others wish to form one with us, and for this we will usually have to be seen to be of some use to them (Tooby & Cosmides, 1996). Indeed, we may have to compete to prove ourselves worthy of the alliance.

This can give rise to conflict in how we wish to present ourselves and the degree to which we seek to "get ahead" or "fit in" (Wolfe, Lennox, & Cutler, 1986).

Social Ranking and Competing (for Status)

My clinics are regularly filled with people who seem in the grip of powerful feelings that are often focused on other people's relative power to hurt, control, or reject them. Over and over again one hears stories of (early) rejection, abuse, and the person's struggles to find a way to feel valued and wanted, to release him- or herself from the grip of feeling a failure, inferior, unworthy, depressed, and anxious. One can see these problems in cognitive terms, as related to core beliefs people hold about themselves and others. While useful and true (and it helps to explain attentional and evaluative biases), this can also be as much a description as an explanation (e.g., "You see yourself as inferior because you have an inferiority core belief/ schema"). Influenced by John Price's (1972) linkage of social rank to psychopathology, and many discussions with him, I have sought to explore the processes of "social power" from a biopsychosocial perspective (Gilbert, 1989, 1995) and how and why they are so saliently linked to various forms of mental health difficulties, including depression (Gilbert, 1984, 1992, 2004; Gilbert & Allan, 1998; Gilbert, Allan, Brough, Melley, & Miles, 2002), social anxiety (Trower & Gilbert, 1989; Gilbert, 2001b), shame (Gilbert, 1989, 1998, 2002b), and psychosis (Birchwood, Meaden, Trower, Gilbert, & Plaistow, 2000, Gilbert et al., 2001).

When people compete for material and social resources, and/or the pleasures or status linked to them, they create socially ranked relationships. Human competitive behavior still uses the old strategies of hawk-dove that reptiles use (Sprinkle, 2002), but obviously in far more complex ways because of our higher cognitive abilities, and because we compete to be attractive and chosen for roles—that is, we seek to stimulate various forms of positive affect in the minds of others such that they like and desire us (Etcoff, 1999; Gilbert, 1997; Gilbert & McGuire, 1998). There is now good evidence that social rank significantly affects the way we handle conflicts. We are more likely to be aggressive when dealing with subordinates but submissive when dealing with higher ranking others (Scott, 1990). Both the social contexts (bosses vs. workers) and the internal judgments of oneself as inferior, the same as, or superior to others affect how threatened we might feel in some contexts and how we deal with it. Fournier, Moskowitz, and Zuroff (2002) recently demonstrated this in an important study of the effect of rank on conflict and defensive behavior.

However, we should note three key human characteristics to human competition. First, human competition is marked by competing for reputations and symbolic representations of status. Any behavior can be turned into a competition. On our hospital's acute units, nurses are concerned that some patients compete to show they can be more self-harming, or take more drugs than others. Concern with how one is doing in comparison to others (i.e., social referencing) is key to social behavior. Stipek (1995) reported a study in which children were told that a tower-building game was competitive (to see who could build the fastest). Those below the age of 33 months who were slower (lost) carried on building their tower quite happily. After 33 months, however, children losing the contest often lost interest in their own tower. Hence, concern with social comparisons and awareness of the "meaning" of competition starts fairly early in life.

Second, humans can compete for respect or reputations (e.g., able to bear more pain, to do more self-harm, or to eat less than other patients on a ward) even if this is *not* socially approved of—it is a desire to be *noticed and respected*, or as one patient said to me of her eating disorder, "I want be a somebody rather than a nobody, to be good at something." In unsafe environments reputations for aggression may be one's best safety strategy (Pinker, 2002). However, by far the largest motivation underpinning human social competition is the desire for approval, to win a favored place in the minds of others, to stimulate positive emotions about us in the minds of others (Gilbert, 1997, 2002b). Thus, we compete so that our parents will love us, our friends want us as allies, our bosses admire and support our talents, our sexual partners desire us—we compete to belong and *to be participants* in roles/teams as much, if not more so, than for (high) rank as such. So we compete for the investments of others (Barkow, 1989; Etcoff, 1999), which Gilbert (1989, 1997) referred to as "social attention holding." Theory of mind plays a key role in helping us to work out what others will find attractive about us, and we often take our cues from how people attend to others—for example, higher status models. The cognitive competency for making social comparison (How am I doing compared to them?) can be used for, and in, a vast array of situations and on a vast number of different qualities. It can also be used to make judgments about the self and is linked to self-esteem (Gilbert et al., 1995).

Third, although animals may compete for the highest ranks they can get because rank is linked to control over resources, humans do not necessarily do so, in part because there are disadvantages from having too high a rank. The reasons for this are that pursuing and gaining rank is not cost-free, and rank is only useful insofar as it gives control over resources. People have to balance the costs and energies they put into gaining rank if it takes away from other goals, such as caring for one's children, or threatens helpful alliances with people who want to form a cooperative, sharing, and equalitarian relationship rather than let one person be top dog. Sometimes it is better not to be top dog. People who (perhaps to be accepted and liked) try to dominate conversations, grab the "the limelight," or lack modesty can be avoided, rejected, or shamed. Hence, what people compete for is control over their lives and sufficient resources (e.g., good enough al-lies, sexual partners) to balance threats and opportunities, have pleasures, and create a sense of safeness. In competing for approval from mates and alliances we must not engage in behavior that will result in ostracism for being too aggressive or selfish, or risk alliances forming against us, and sensitivity to self-presentation aids us in this (Baumeister, 1982). Generally, people will compete to be accepted, wanted, or popular and to avoid being unpopular or rejected—and shamed (Wolfe et al., 1986). They may be highly sensitive and overestimate how others view their (minor) mistakes (Savitsky, Epley, & Gilovich, 2001). Shame, unlike guilt, is organized through the social rank mentalities, that is, it is concerned with social standing, reputation, and relative attractiveness (Gilbert, 2002b). More-over, some people simply don't like having to do what it would take to gain top rank. A patient gave up a good position in a firm because it was down-sizing and he felt that to continue to get on he would have to become far too ruthless and put in too many hours at the office (against his self-identity as a caring man).

Like the other mentalities discussed above, there are individual differ-ences. For example, some people are far more ambitious and need to be higher ranking than others (Keltner, Gruenfeld, & Anderson, 2003). They can be very competitive in many aspects of their lives and "need to win." However, the psychology of pursuing high rank, and the psychology of *avoiding low rank*, while related, are also *quite different*. Just as there seem to be set points in the brain for deciding when one has had enough to eat, so with rank. And a lot depends on what one wants to do with one's rank if one gets it. For some people, gaining rank is a way to ensure that they have control over potential social harms and have allies who will obey them; for others, rank is about feeling secure and feeling valued; for still others, social power can be used to help others. In depression and some anxiety problems, avoiding inferiority (with the risk of rejection, loss of in-fluence, or being unable to participate in activities) is the issue. Indeed, it is usually cognitions about the self as inferior that are related to depression and social anxiety. The social rank theory of depression (Gilbert, 1992, 2000b, 2004) and social anxiety (Gilbert, 2001b) has thus always focused on *inferiority* and *loss* of control (not drives for superiority as such). In a recent study on reasoning tasks, Badcock and Allen (2003) found that in-ducing mild low mood made participants especially sensitivity and respon-sive to reasoning about social rank and social competition, somewhat more so than for tasks on attachment.

Going Up and the Dynamics of Power

In recent years much attention has been given to the idea that power cor-rupts. Keltner et al. (2003) have reviewed what is currently known about the psychology of social power. Social power, however, is not the same as social rank. For example, a figurehead monarch can have high social rank and status but little power; there are people who shun the limelight and status recognition but who have great power "in the backgound"; people can feel that they are low rank in a society but not that they are personally inferior or powerless to control their lives or achieve their goals; people can have high rank but still get depressed and feel powerless and inferior.

Hollander and Offerman (1990) suggest three types of power: *power over others*, the power to make or entice others to do things a person wants; *power to*, involving the degree of freedom to do as one wishes, also called "empowerment"; and *power from*, involving the ability/power to resist the wishes/demands of others. As they point out, high status often (but not always) involves all three forms of power, while subordinates have at best one or two and sometimes practically no such powers at all.

When it comes to considering the forms of power, psychologists have suggested five main forms (Podsakoff & Schriesheim, 1985). *Reward power* is the ability to provide something that others want and will work for (e.g., controlling access to wages, food, love, approval). *Coercive/ punishment power* is the ability to control others through actual or threatened aversive outcomes (e.g., to injure the other or to remove/withhold something of value to the other). Both of these forms of power are fairly direct, used by animals and humans. Another three types of power, however, require more complex psychologies. *Legitimate power* is linked to rights and obligations that require understanding and recognition of rights and obligations. It is used as a basis of law and socially defined roles (e.g., the power of the captain, teacher, or president). *Expert power* relates to an awareness of the superiority of another's knowledge or skill, and is linked with respect and at times admiration (e.g., for doctors, priests, scientists). *Referent power* refers more to attractiveness, liking, and a person's charm or charisma (Lindholm, 1993). Many forms of power and indeed leadership require that the dominant has access to, and can control, the *attention* of others. Whatever power one might think one has, if others don't recognize it and co-create the role, then the role (ranked relationships in that domain) cannot develop.

If one defines *social power* as the ability to influence others, some socially constructed roles come with a lot of power over others (e.g., teachers or doctors). How people perform in these roles is often related to personality and social expectations in a role. Our rank-aware psychology can and does take different forms in different cultures and social niches. Status on the back streets of London may come from carrying a gun, while at the stock market just a few miles away status comes for doing good deals and having certain business talents, and a few blocks away from the stock market, in the offices of (say) a woman's magazine, status comes from having a certain type of face and body.

Keltner et al. (2003), Gilbert (1995), and Scott (1990) point out that social power goes with different sensitivities to social threats and different social concerns. High power people can be less interested in the views and needs of lower ranking people and can exploit them for their own self-interests. High power people tend to be more positive in their feelings and moods and more risk taking. However, the dimension of affiliation is important to how power is used. For example, while some leaders are highly hostile and destructive (e.g., Hitler), others are highly prosocial and use their power to bring peace and to foster compassion (e.g., Nelson Mandala and Buddha). In the circumplex model this is the distinction between hostile and friendly dominance (Leary, 1957; Kiesler, 1983).

It may be a combination of genes, temperament, early experiences, social expectations (a number of patients have felt they have become less caring as work pressures have increased), and social role models that shape how one will strive for power and then use it if one gets it. Hitler was abused as a child while the Buddha was a high-ranking prince who did not have to compete for resources. Social environments may also select and advantage those who gain power and have relatively nonaffiliative traits. Some power-and social rank-focused people exhibit what has been called "the slime effect" or "upward licking, downward kicking" (Vonk, 1998). Vonk has shown that such individuals are more likely to express their anger and be bullies and exploitative with their subordinates, but submissive and compliant with their superiors. This was the typical style in the higher echelons of the Nazi Party. Some organizations in competitive environments may promote (thus select for rank/power positions) these people because they carry out orders no matter how ruthless they need to be. There is no doubt that the way people strive for social power and then use is has shaped human history. Hilter is an obvious example, but they are very many others.

Subordinates

The opposite side of the power coin is the appeasing and approval seeking of subordinates. Because building alliances with more powerful others can reduce the harm they pose and can be good for winning status (going up the ranks), people can subjugate their own genetic self-interests to win their approval—for example, by going on suicide missions. Jack Jones enticed nearly a thousand suicides, with parents killing their children and themselves, in the mass suicide of 1978 (Lindholm, 1993). Moreover, to win approval, subordinates can do some very immoral things (Kelman & Hamilton, 1989). Subordinates will also show what has been called "reverted escape" where they will return and try to appease a dominant who has just threatened or hurt them, a process that can be involved in some religious practices (Gilbert, 2000b). Subordinates may try to resist the power

of dominants, but as Scott (1990) points out, they may often do so in se-
cret or from "disengaged subcultures."

Subordinate voices are often excluded from social narratives. Those
who are "allowed" to reflect on themselves and pass their views on to the
wider group are the dominants. In the historical record the stories of the
experiences of the subjugated, be these of the life experiences of the de-
feated, slaves, women, children, or "lower" castes and classes are notable
for their absence. The social cognitions and values of those rendered
subordinate are poorly understood (are unrecognized) and instead psychologists sometimes prefer rarefied and individualistic concepts such as "self-
esteem." I have been interested in social power and social rank and it
relationships to psychopathology because the social rank mentality may be
the best mentality to organize self–other roles when one is faced with the
hostility and low care of others. I have been wary of the self-esteem
concept in part because it now carries negative connotations as if there is
something "wrong" with a person or even he or she has the "disease" of
low self-esteem. Although low self-esteem goes with increased risk of a
variety of emotional problems, in social mentality theory low self-esteem is
a defensive strategy of the social rank mentality, where people focus on
threat (from more powerful or rejecting others) and damage limitation.
Those with low self-esteem may be operating in the best way they can, and
low self-esteem is a nonconscious strategy for coping with a threatening social world (Gilbert, 2002a).

Group and Social Mentalities

So far the focus has been primarily on how an individual relates to others
and the various social mentalities that underpin the co-construction of social roles. However, social mentalities can become organizing frameworks
for the co-constructions for intra- and intergroup interactions (see Fiske &
Haslam, Chapter 11, this volume). For example, groups/societies that
value caring and the *welfare* of others and seek equity have lower rates of
crime and various forms of illness than groups that focus on self-interest
and self-promotion (Arrindell, Steptoe, & Wardle, 2003). Indeed, there is
increasing concern that competitive economic systems, while good for
business and the creation of material comforts, can create many contexts
for crime and poor mental health, in part because they create highly segre-
gated communities of haves, have nots, and have lots (Kasser, 2002;
Wilkinson, 1996). Social ecologies, economic systems, and social values re-
cruit social mentalities that become enacted between people and groups
and shape self-identities (Gilbert, in press-a).

Subgroups often seek to dominate other groups, defend their own interests, attempt to limit subordinate groups' access to resources, and at
times attack them. Indeed, groups can engage in a range of narratives that

can even cultivate hatred of other groups (Gay, 1995). In a different paradigm, Pratto, Sidanius, Stallworth, and Malle (1994) have explored the social rank mentality at the group level and referred to it as "social dominance orientation." They consider how people take their self-identities from their own group and set about subordinating other groups. Hence, even between groups subordinate positions can be aversive. They point out that

> ideologies that promote or maintain group inequality are the tools that legitimize discrimination. To work smoothly, these ideologies must be widely accepted within a society, appearing as self-apparent truths; hence we call them *hierarchy-legitimizing myths*. By contributing to consensual or normalized group-based inequality, legitimizing myths help to stabilize oppression. That is, they minimize conflict among groups by indicating how individuals and institutions should allocate things of positive or negative social value, such as jobs, gold, blankets, government appointments, prison terms, and disease. For example, the ideology of anti-black racism has been instantiated in personal acts of discrimination, but also in institutional discrimination against African-Americans by banks, public transit authorities, schools, churches, marriage laws, and the penal system. Social Darwinism and meritocracy are examples of other ideologies that imply that some people are not as "good" as others and therefore should be allocated less positive social values than others. (p. 741)

The boundaries that define and separate ingroup from outgroup or high from low status (sub)groups can therefore be various. They may be made on the basis of race, gender, age, profession, economics, locality, or religion. Since the aim of superiority is to exert control over things that bring resources and pleasures, and reduce harms, *group practices must discriminate to avoid a collapse into equality*. Equality would put severe limits on the pleasures and comforts some can claim access to at the expense of others. Hence, dominant groups that are privileged need to see others as less deserving and inferior in order to protect their own self-identities of being honorable people. Slavery was excused in exactly this way (Gay, 1995). The importance of laws and values that support fairness and sharing cannot be overstated. It would be incorrect to say that all groups act like this, for it is clear that some groups will form precisely to fight against discrimination and injustice (e.g., Amnesty International) and many religions seek to generate more compassionate ways of being in the world (Davidson & Harrington, 2002).

Self-to-Self Relating

If the sense of self emerges out of our evolved strategic dispositions for creating social roles, shaped by experiences, then social mentality theory can also be used to explore internal self-to-self relationships. It can be suggested that self-evaluation and self-identity formation competencies evolved because they gave advantage to the enactment of social roles. In particular, self-evaluation and self-identity help us keep track of the social niche we are operating in. Learning to be confident, friendly, and trusting may be advantageous in a socially caring and mutually supportive environment but far less so in a neglectful and hostile one. In hostile and competitive environments it might be better to adopt either social roles of fear and submissiveness or go for a higher risk, high-gain strategy of aggressive self-promotion and lack of caring interest in others (Gilbert, 2002a, in press-a). As Baldwin (1992) has eloquently argued, self-evaluations are rooted in interpersonal schema. Thus, for example, if you show people a subliminal picture of a hostile, disapproving face they are more likely to rate their own ideas as less worthy than if they are primed with an approving face (see Baldwin, Chapter 2, this volume; Baldwin & Fergusson, 2001). Self-evaluations are not therefore autonomous systems of cognition but are linked to models of others and in particular to how others have related to, and are likely to relate in the future to the self. Moreover, we copy their behavior into simulations and metacognitive processing (what will others think about me) via recourse to memory. Thus, if a child is constantly labeled as stupid and inadequate, this may be copied into both implicit (fear of others) and explicit self-referent systems. These can then act as sources of information for how others are likely to treat her if she tries to assert herself (Gilbert & Irons, in press). This is precisely how shame works (Gilbert, 2002b). Over time the social behavior of others comes to regulate self and is coded into self-regulation and self-evaluation.

There is another aspect to the process of incorporating others evaluation of self into self-evaluation. Self-to-self experience is inherently relational too (Gilbert, 2000a). We can thus speak of having a 'relationship' with ourselves as objects for our own self-evaluations. Thus I can enact a caring nurturing and supportive role to myself, or (say) a hostile and contemptuous one. The later is more likely if self has been subjected to other's people criticisms and put down's (Gilbert & Irons, in press). When some people are self-critical it is not just that they have critical thoughts, but that they *feel* angry with or contemptuous of the self. They may want to punish or hurt the self, order the self to act differently ("You must try harder, you lazy person"), and can feel beaten down and harassed by their own self-attacks (Gilbert, Clarke, Kempel, Miles, & Irons, 2004). In extreme cases (e.g., auditory hallucinations in psychosis), these internal attacks can be experienced as external voices of condemnation and commands (Gilbert et al., 2001).

Recent evidence also suggests that high self-critics are relatively poor at being able to generate warm and compassionate images of and to themselves (Gilbert et al., 2004). This "warm" self-to-self role appears underdeveloped and its development can be a focus for psychotherapy (Gilbert, 2000a; Gilbert & Irons, in press). Hence in the last 10 years or so, I have focused on how one might activate more caring mentalities, and in particular compassion, toward the self and to others. We are thus currently investigating psychotherapy methods to do this. This work is still preliminary, but social mentality theory suggests that the development of compassion can have major reorganizing effects on physiological systems (Wang, in press), psychological systems (Gilbert & Irons, in press), social values, and relationships (Davidson & Harrington, 2002). It is not just attacks (in both inter- and intrapersonal relationships) that can lead to distress but also the lack of warmth.

CONCLUSION

Many of our social roles and desires for types of social relationships have evolved over many millions of years—traceable back to the reptiles, the emergence of the mammals, and then to the success of the primates. For humans, social roles are built from both innate dispositions and competencies to recognize and enact roles. But they are also built from complex cognitive abilities that mature in social contexts and shape how we think about our roles and our self-identities. Social mentalities are a way of thinking about how various components of our minds are organized to co-create social roles. Hence social mentalities are not like "modules" but are organizing systems that choreograph motives, emotions, thoughts, and behaviors both in and outside consciousness. From the reptiles through to us, evolution has fashioned a range of desires and competencies for relating, and in the process we have become self-aware. Studies in evolutionary, developmental, and social psychology all point to the extraordinary way we have evolved, such that social relationships shape the essence of who we are, and regulate our identities, values, feeling, and moods.

REFERENCES

Abrams, D. (1996). Social identity, self as structure and self as process. In W. P. Robinson (Ed.), *Social groups and identities: Developing the legacy of Henri Tajfel* (pp. 143–162). Oxford, UK: Butterworth-Heinemann.

Arrindell, W. A., Steptoe, A., & Wardle, J. (2003). Higher levels of depression in masculine than in feminine nations. *Behaviour Research and Therapy, 41*, 809–817.

Axelrod, R. (1990). *The evolution of cooperation*. London: Penguin Books.

Badcock, B. T., & Allen, N. B. (2003). Adaptive social reasoning in depressed mood and depressive vulnerability. *Cognition and Emotion, 17*, 647–670.

Bailey, K. (1987). *Human paleopsychology: Applications to aggression and pathological processes*. Hillsdale, NJ: Erlbaum.

Bailey, K. (2000). Evolution, kinship and psychotherapy: Promoting psychological health through human relationships. In P. Gilbert & K. G. Bailey (Eds.), *Genes on the couch: Explorations in evolutionary psychotherapy* (pp. 71–92). London: Brenner-Routledge Press.

Bailey, K. (2002). Recognizing, assessing and classifying others: Cognitive bases of evolutionary kinship therapy. In P. Gilbert (Ed.), *Cognitive psychotherapy: An international quarterly* (Special issue: Evolutionary psychology and cognitive therapy), *16*, 367–366.

Baldwin, M. W. (1992). Relational schemas and the processing of social information. *Psychological Bulletin, 112*, 461–484.

Baldwin, M. W., & Fergusson, P. (2001). Relational schemas: The activation of interpersonal knowledge structures in social anxiety. In W. R. Crozier & L. E. Alden (Eds.), *International handbook of social anxiety: Concepts, research and interventions relating to the self and shyness* (pp. 235–257) Chichester, UK: Wiley.

Barkow, J. H. (1989). *Darwin, sex and status: Biological approaches to mind and culture*. Toronto: University of Toronto Press.

Barrett, L., Dunbar, R., & Lycett, J. (2002). *Human evolutionary psychology*. London: Palgrave.

Batson, C. D., Klein, T. R., Highberger, L., & Shaw, L. L. (1995). Immorality from empathy-induced altruism: When compassion and justice conflict. *Journal of Personality and Social Psychology, 68*, 1042–1054.

Baumeister, R. F. (1982). A self-presentational view of social phenomena. *Psychological Bulletin, 91*, 3–26.

Baumeister, R. F., & Leary, M. R. (1995). The need to belong: Desire for interpersonal attachments as a fundamental human motivation. *Psychological Bulletin, 117*, 497–529.

Baumeister, R. F., & Tice, D. M. (1990). Anxiety and social exclusion. *Journal of Social and Clinical Psychology, 9*, 165–195.

Beck, A. T., Emery, G., & Greenberg, R. L. (1985). *Anxiety disorders and phobias: A cognitive approach*. New York: Basic Books.

Beck, A. T., Rush, A. J., Shaw, B. F., & Emery, G. (1979). *Cognitive therapy of depression*. New York: Wiley.

Bell, D. C. (2001). Evolution of care giving behavior. *Personality and Social Psychology Review, 5*, 216–229.

Belsky, J., Steinberg, L., & Draper, P. (1990). Childhood experiences, interpersonal development, and reproductive strategy: An evolutionary theory of socialization. *Child Development, 62*, 647–670.

Bering, J. M. (2002). The existential theory of mind. *Review of General Psychology, 6*, 3–34.

Birchwood, M., Meaden, A., Trower, P., Gilbert, P., & Plaistow, J. (2000). The power and omnipotence of voices: Subordination and entrapment by voices and significant others. *Psychological Medicine, 30*, 337–344.

Boehm, C. (1999). *Hierarchy in the forest: The evolution of egalitarian behavior*. Cambridge, MA: Harvard University Press.

Bond, R., & Smith, P. D. (1996). Culture and conformity: A meta-analysis of studies using Asch's (1952b, 1956) line judgement. *Psychological Bulletin, 119*, 111–137.

Bowlby, J. (1969). *Attachment and loss: Vol. 1. Attachment*. London: Hogarth Press.

Bowlby, J. (1973). *Attachment and loss: Vol. 2. Separation: Anxiety and anger.* London: Hogarth Press.

Bowlby, J. (1980). *Attachment and loss: Vol. 3. Loss: Sadness and depression.* London: Hogarth Press.

Brugha, T. (Ed.). (1995). *Social support and psychiatric disorder. research findings and guidelines for clinical practice.* Cambridge, UK: Cambridge University Press.

Burnstein, E., Crandall, C., & Kitayama, S. (1994). Some neo-Darwinian rules for altruism: Weighing cues for inclusive fitness as a function of biological importance of the decision. *Journal of Personality and Social Psychology, 67,* 773–807.

Buss, D. M. (1989). Sex differences in human mate preference: Evolutionary hypotheses tested in 37 cultures. *Brain and Behavioral Sciences, 12,* 1–49.

Buss, D. M. (2003). *Evolutionary psychology: The new science of mind* (2nd ed.). Boston: Allyn & Bacon.

Byrne, R. W. (1995). *The thinking ape.* Oxford, UK: Oxford University Press.

Cacioppo, J. T., Berston, G. G., Sheridan, J. F., & McClintock, M. K. (2000). Multilevel integrative analysis of human behavior: Social neuroscience and the complementing nature of social and biological approaches. *Psychological Bulletin, 126,* 829–843.

Caporael, L. R. (1997). The evolution of truly social cognition: The core configuration model. *Personality and Social Psychology Review, 1,* 276–298.

Carter, C. S. (1998). Neuroendocrine perspectives on social attachment and love. *Psychoneuroendocrinology, 23,* 779–818.

Chiappe, D. L. (2000). Metaphor, modularity and the evolution of conceptual integration. *Metaphor and Symbol, 15,* 137–158.

Cohen, D. (2001). Cultural variation: Considerations and implications. *Psychological Bulletin, 127,* 451–471.

Conway, M. A., & Pleydell-Pearce, C. W. (2000). The construction of autobiographical memories in the self-memory systems. *Psychological Review, 107,* 261–288.

Cosmides, L., & Tooby, J. (1992). Cognitive adaptations for social exchange. In J. H. Barkow, L. Cosmides, & J. Tooby (Eds.), *The adapted mind: Evolutionary psychology and the generation of culture* (pp. 193–228). New York: Oxford University Press.

Davidson, R., & Harrington, A. (Eds.). (2002). *Visions of compassion: Western scientists and Tibetan Buddhists examine human nature.* New York: Oxford University Press.

de Waal, F. (1996). *Good natured: The origins of right and wrong in humans and other animals.* Cambridge, MA: Harvard University Press.

Dixon, A. K. (1998). Ethological strategies for defence in animals and humans: Their role in some psychiatric disorders. *British Journal of Medical Psychology, 71,* 417–445.

Eisenberg, N. (2002). Empathy-related emotional responses, altruism, and their socialization. In R. Davidson & A. Harrington (Eds.), *Visions of compassion: Western scientists and Tibetan Buddhists examine human nature* (pp. 131–164). New York: Oxford University Press.

Ellenberger, H. F. (1970). *The discovery of the unconscious: The history and evolution of dynamic psychiatry.* New York: Basic Books.

Etcoff, N. (1999). *Survival of the prettiest: The science of beauty.* New York: Doubleday.

Field, T. (2000). *Touch therapy.* New York: Churchill Livingston.

Fogel, A., Melson, G. F., & Mistry, J. (1986). Conceptualising the determinants of nurturance: A reassessment of sex differences. In A. Fogel & G. F. Melson (Eds.), *Origins of nurturance: Developmental, biological and cultural perspectives on caregiving* (pp. 53–67). Hillsdale, NJ: Erlbaum.

Fournier, M. A., Moskowitz, D. S., & Zuroff D. C. (2002) Social rank strategies in hierarchical relationships. *Journal of Personality and Social Psychology, 83,* 425–433.

Gay, P. (1995). *The cultivation of hatred.* London: Fontana Press.

Geary, D. C. (2000). Evolution and proximate expression of human parental investment. *Psychological Bulletin, 126,* 55–77.

Geary, D. C., & Huffman, K. J. (2002). Brain and cognitive evolution: Forms of modularity and functions of the mind. *Psychological Bulletin, 128,* 667–698.

Gilbert, P. (1984). *Depression: From psychology to brain state.* Hove, UK: Erlbaum.

Gilbert, P. (1989). *Human nature and suffering.* Hove, UK: Erlbaum.

Gilbert, P. (1992). *Depression: The evolution of powerlessness.* Hove, UK, and New York: Erlbaum and Guilford Press.

Gilbert, P. (1993). Defence and safety: Their function in social behaviour and psychopathology. *British Journal of Clinical Psychology, 32,* 131–153.

Gilbert, P. (1995). Biopsychosocial approaches and evolutionary theory as aids to integration in clinical psychology and psychotherapy. *Clinical Psychology and Psychotherapy, 2,* 135–156.

Gilbert, P. (1997). The evolution of social attractiveness and its role in shame, humiliation, guilt and therapy. *British Journal of Medical Psychology, 70,* 113–147.

Gilbert, P. (1998). The evolved basis and adaptive functions of cognitive distortions. *British Journal of Medical Psychology, 71,* 447–463.

Gilbert, P. (2000a). Social mentalities: Internal "social" conflicts and the role of inner warmth and compassion in cognitive therapy. In P. Gilbert & K. G. Bailey (Eds.), *Genes on the couch: Explorations in evolutionary psychotherapy* (pp. 118–150). Hove, UK: Psychology Press.

Gilbert, P. (2000b). Varieties of submissive behaviour: Their evolution and role in depression. In L. Sloman & P. Gilbert (Eds.), *Subordination and defeat: An evolutionary approach to mood disorders* (pp. 3–46). Hillsdale, NJ: Erlbaum.

Gilbert, P. (2001a). Evolutionary approaches to psychopathology: The role of natural defences. *Australian and New Zealand Journal of Psychiatry, 35,* 17–27.

Gilbert, P. (2001b). Evolution and social anxiety: The role of social competition and social hierarchies. In F. Schnieder (Eds.), *Psychiatric clinics of North America* (Special issue: Social anxiety), *24,* 723–751.

Gilbert, P. (2002a). Evolutionary approaches to psychopathology and cognitive therapy. In P. Gilbert (Eds.), *Cognitive Psychotherapy: An International Quarterly* (Special issue: Evolutionary psychology and cognitive therapy), *16,* 263–294.

Gilbert, P. (2002b). Body shame: A biopsychosocial conceptualisation and overview, with treatment implications. In P. Gilbert & J. Miles (Eds.), *Body shame: Conceptualisation, research and treatment* (pp. 3–54). London: Brunner-Routledge.

Gilbert, P. (2003). Evolution, social roles and the differences in shame and guilt. *Social Research, 70,* 401–426.

Gilbert, P. (2004). Depression: A biopsychosocial, integrative and evolutionary approach. In M. Power (Ed.), *Mood disorders: A handbook of science and practice* (pp. 99–142). Chichester, UK: Wiley.

Gilbert, P. (in press-a). Compassion and cruelty: A biopsychosocial approach. In P. Gilbert (Ed.), *Compassion: Conceptualisations, research and use in psychotherapy.* London: Brunner-Routledge.

Gilbert, P. (Ed.). (in press-b). *Compassion: Conceptualisations, research and use in psychotherapy.* London: Brunner-Routledge.

Gilbert, P., & Allan, S. (1998). The role of defeat and entrapment (arrested flight) in depression: An exploration of an evolutionary view. *Psychological Medicine, 28,* 584–597.

Gilbert, P., Allan, S., Brough, S., Melley, S., & Miles, J. (2002). Anhedonia and positive affect: Relationship to social rank, defeat and entrapment. *Journal of Affective Disorders, 71,* 141–151.

Gilbert, P., Baldwin, M., Irons, C., Baccus, J., & Clark, M. (2004). *Self-criticism and self-warmth: An imagery study exploring their relaion to depression.* Manuscript submitted for publication.

Gilbert, P., Birchwood, M., Gilbert, J., Trower, P., Hay, J., Murray, B., Meaden, A., Olsen, K., & Miles, J. N. V. (2001). An exploration of evolved mental mechanisms for dominant and subordinate behaviour in relation to auditory hallucinations in schizophrenia and critical thoughts in depression. *Psychological Medicine, 31,* 1117–1127.

Gilbert, P., Clarke, M., Kempel, S., Miles, J. N. V., & Irons, C. (2004). Forms and functions of self-criticisms and self-attacking: An exploration of differences in female students. *British Journal of Clinical Psychology, 43,* 31–50.

Gilbert, P., & Irons, C. (in press). Focused therapies and compassionate mind training for shame and self-attacking In P. Gilbert (Ed.), *Compassion: Conceptualisations, research and use in psychotherapy.* London: Brunner-Routledge.

Gilbert, P., & McGuire, M. (1998). Shame status and social roles: The psychobiological continuum from monkeys to humans. In P. Gilbert & B. Andrews (Eds.), *Shame: Interpersonal behavior, psychopathology and culture* (pp. 99–125). New York: Oxford University Press.

Gilbert, P., Price, J. S., & Allan, S. (1995). Social comparison, social attractiveness and evolution: How might they be related? *New Ideas in Psychology, 13,* 149–165.

Gilligan, C. (1982). *In a different voice: Psychological theory and women's development.* Cambridge, MA: Harvard University Press.

Gilmore, D. D. (1990). *Manhood in the making: Cultural concepts of masculinity.* New Haven, CT: Yale University Press.

Goldberg, E. (2002). *The executive brain: Frontal lobes and the civilized mind.* New York: Oxford University Press.

Guisinger, S., & Blatt, S. (1994). Individuality and relatedness: Evolution of a fundamental dialectic. *American Psychologist, 49,* 104–111.

Haidt, J. (2001). The emotional dog and its rational tail: A social intuitionist approach to moral judgment. *Psychological Review, 108,* 814–834.

Heyes, C. (2003). Four routes of cognitive evolution. *Psychological Review, 110,* 713–727.

Hofer, M. A. (1994). Early relationships as regulators of infant physiology and behavior. *Acta Paediatiricia, 397*(Suppl.), 9–18.

Hollander, E. P., & Offerman, L. R. (1990). Power and leadership in organizations: Relationships in transition. *American Psychologist, 45,* 179–189.

Kasser, T. (2002). *The high price of materialism.* Cambridge, MA: MIT Press.

Kelman, H. C., & Hamilton, V. L. (1989). *Crimes of obedience*: New Haven, CT: Yale University Press.

Keltner, D., Gruenfeld, D. H., & Anderson, C. (2003). Power, approach and inhibition. *Psychological Review, 110,* 265–284.

Kemper, T. D. (1990). *Social structure and testosterone: Explorations of the socio-bio-social chain*: New Brunswick, NJ: Rutgers University Press.

Kiesler, D. J. (1983). The 1982 interpersonal circle: A taxonomy for complementarity in human transactions. *Psychological Review, 90,* 185–214.

Knox, J. (2003). *Archetype, attachment, analysis: Jungian psychology and the emergence of mind.* London: Brunner-Routledge.

Koren-Karie, N., Oppenheim, D., Dolev, S., Sher, S., & Etzion-Carasso, A. (2002). Mothers' insightfulness regarding their infants' internal experience: Relations with maternal sensitivity and infant attachment. *Developmental Psychology, 38,* 534–542.

Lambie, J. A., & Marcel, A. J. (2002). Consciousness and the varieties of emotion experience: A theoretical framework. *Psychological Review, 109,* 219–259.

Leary, T. (1957). *The interpersonal diagnosis of personality.* New York: Ronald Press.

Li, S. C. (2003). Biocultural orchestration of developmental plasticity across levels: The impact of biology and culture in shaping the mind and behavior across the life span. *Psychological Bulletin, 129,* 171–194.

Lickliter, R., & Honeycutt, H. (2003). Developmental dynamics: Toward a biologically plausible evolutionary psychology. *Psychological Bulletin, 129,* 819–835 (plus peer commentary, 836–872).

Lindholm, C. (1993). *Charisma.* Oxford, UK: Blackwell.

Liotti, G. (2000). Disorganised attachment, models of borderline states and evolutionary psychotherapy. In P. Gilbert & B. Bailey (Eds.), *Genes on the couch: Explorations in evolutionary psychotherapy* (pp. 232–256). Hove, UK: Brunner-Routledge.

Lock, A. (1999). On the recent origin of symbolically-mediated language and its implications for psychological science. In M. C. Coballis & M. E. G. Lea (Eds.), *The descent of mind: Psychological perspectives on humanoid evolution* (pp. 324–355). New York: Oxford University Press.

MacDonald, K. (1992). Warmth as a developmental construct: An evolutionary analysis. *Child Development, 63,* 753–773.

MacLean, P. D. (1985). Brain evolution relating to family, play and the separation call. *Archives of General Psychiatry, 42,* 405–417.

MacLean, P. D. (1990). *The triune brain in evolution.* New York: Plenum Press.

Malik, K. (2000). *Man, beast and zombie: What science can and cannot tell us about human nature.* London: Weidenfeld & Nicolson.

Maynard Smith, J. (1982). *Evolution and the theory of games.* Cambridge, UK: Cambridge University Press.

McGregor, I., & Marigold, D. C. (2003). Defensive zeal and the uncertain self: What makes you so sure? *Journal of Personality and Social Psychology, 85,* 838–852.

McGuire, M. T., & Troisi, A. (1998). *Darwinian psychiatry.* New York: Oxford University Press.

Miller, P. A., & Eisenberg, N. (1988). The relation of empathy to aggressive behaviour and externalising/antisocial behavior. *Psychological Bulletin, 103,* 324–344.

Mithen, S. (1996). *The prehistory of the mind: A search for the origins of art and religion.* London: Thames & Hudson.

Nesse, R. M. (1998). Emotional disorders in evolutionary perspective. *British Journal of Medical Psychology, 71,* 397–416.

Nesse, R. M., & Lloyd, A. T. (1992). The evolution of psychodynamic mechanisms. In J. H. Barkow, L. Cosmides, & J. Tooby (Eds.), *The adapted mind: Evolutionary psychology and the generation of culture* (pp. 601–624). Oxford, UK: Oxford University Press.

Nickerson, R. S. (1999). How we know—and sometimes misjudge—what others know: Inputting one's own knowledge to others. *Psychological Bulletin, 125,* 737–759.

Panksepp, J. (1998). *Affective neuroscience.* New York: Oxford University Press.

Pinker, S. (2002). *The blank slate: The modern denial of human nature.* New York: Alan Lane.

Plotkin, H. (2002, July 5–7). *Evolution of culture.* Paper presented at the Evolutionary Psychology Conference, Open University, University of Nottingham, UK.

Podsakoff, P. M., & Schriesheim, C. A. (1985). Field studies of French and Raven's bases of power: Critique, reanalysis and suggestions for future research. *Psychological Bulletin, 97,* 387–411.

Pratto, F., Sidanius, J., Stallworth, L. M., & Malle, B. (1994). Social dominance orientation: A personality variable predicting social and political attitudes. *Journal of Personality and Social Psychology, 67,* 741–763.

Price, J. S. (1972). Genetic and phylogenetic aspects of mood variations. *International Journal of Mental Health, 1,* 124–144.

Ritvo, L. B. (1990). *Darwin's influence on Freud: A tale of two sciences.* New Haven, CT: Yale University Press.

Savitsky, K., Epley, N., & Gilovich, T. (2001). Do others judge us as harshly as we think?: Overestimating the impact of our failures, shortcomings, and mishaps. *Journal of Personality and Social Psychology, 81,* 44–56.

Schore, A. N. (1994). *Affect regulation and the origin of the self: The neurobiology of emotional development.* Hillsdale, NJ: Erlbaum.

Schore, A. N. (2001). The effects of early relational trauma on right brain development, affect regulation, and infant mental health. *Infant Mental Health Journal, 22,* 201–269.

Schore, A. N. (2002). Dysregulation of the right brain: A fundamental mechanism of traumatic attachment and the psychopathologies of posttraumatic stress disorder. *Australian and New Zealand Journal of Psychiatry, 36,* 9–30.

Scott, J. C. (1990). *Domination and the arts of resistance:* New Haven, CT: Yale University Press.

Sedikides, C., & Skowronski, J. J. (1997). The symbolic self in evolutionary context, *Personality and Social Psychology Review, 1,* 80–102.

Smith, E. A. (2000). Three styles in the evolutionary analysis of human behavior. In L. Cook, N. Chagnon, & W. Irons (Eds.), *Adaptation and human behavior: An anthropological perspective* (pp. 23–46). New York: Aldine de Gruyter.

Smith E. O. (2002). *When culture and biology collide: Why we are stressed, depressed and self-obsessed.* New Brunswick, NJ: Rutgers University Press.

Sprinkle, R. H. (2002). Hawks, doves and birds of paradise. *Politics and the Life Sciences, 21,* 1–12.

Steele, H. (2002). State of the art: Attachment theory. *The Psychologist, 15,* 518–522.

Stevens, A. (2002). *Archetype revisited: An update on the natural history of the self.* London: Brunner-Routledge.

Stipek, D. (1995). The development of pride and shame in toddlers. In J. P. Tangney & K. W. Fischer (Eds.), *Self-conscious emotions: The psychology of shame, guilt, embarrassment and pride* (pp. 237–252). New York: Guilford Press.

Straub, E. (2002). Emergency helping, genocidal violence, and the evolution of responsibility and altruism in children. In R. Davidson & A. Harrington (Eds.), *Visions of compassion: Western scientists and Tibetan Buddhists examine human nature* (pp. 165–181). New York: Oxford University Press.

Suddendorf, T., & Whitten, A. (2001). Mental evolutions and development: Evidence for secondary representation in children, great apes and other animals. *Psychological Bulletin, 127,* 629–650.

Taylor, C. (1992). *Sources of the self: The making of the modern identity.* Cambridge, UK: Cambridge University Press.

Taylor, S. E., Klein, L. B., Lewis B. P., Gruenwald, T. L., Gurung, R. A. R., & Updegaff, J. A. (2000). Biobehavioral responses to stress in females: Tend and befriend, not fight and flight. *Psychological Review, 107,* 411–429.

Teasdale, J. D. (1999). Emotional processing: Three modes of mind and the prevention of relapse in depression. *Behaviour Research and Therapy, 37,* 29–52.

Tooby, J., & Cosmides, L. (1996). Friendship formation and the bankers paradox: Other pathways to the evolution of adaptations for altruism. *Proceedings of the British Academy, 88,* 119–143.

Trevarthen, C., & Aitken, K. (2001). Infant intersubjectivity: Research, theory, and clinical applications. *Journal of Child Psychology and Psychiatry, 42,* 3–48.

Trivers, R. L. (1971). The evolution of reciprocal altruism. *Quarterly Review of Biology, 46,* 35–57.

Trower, P., & Gilbert, P. (1989). New theoretical conceptions of social anxiety and social phobia. *Clinical Psychology Review, 9,* 19–35.

Vonk, R. (1998). The slime effect: Suspicion and dislike of likeable behavior toward superiors. *Journal of Personality and Social Psychology, 74,* 849–864.

Wang, S. (in press). A conceptual framework for integrating research related to the physiology of compassion and the wisdom of Buddhist teachings. In P. Gilbert (Ed.), *Compassion: Conceptualisations, research and use in psychotherapy.* London: Brunner-Routledge.

Wearden, A. J., Tarrier, N., Barrowclough, C., Zastowny, T. R., & Rahil, A. A. (2000). A review of expressed emotion research in health care. *Clinical Psychology Review, 5,* 633–666.

Wells, A. (2000). *Emotional disorders and metacognition: Innovative cognitive therapy.* Chichester, UK: Wiley.

Whitten, A. (1999). The evolution of deep social mind in humans. In M. C. Corballis and S. E. G. Lea (Eds.), *The descent of mind: Psychological perspectives on humanoid evolution* (pp. 173–193). New York: Oxford University Press.

Wilkinson, R. G. (1996). *Unhealthy societies: The afflictions of inequality.* London: Routledge.

Williams, K.,D., Cheung, C.,K.,T., & Choi, W. (2000). Cyberostracism: Effects of being ignored over the Internet. *Journal of Personality and Social Psychology, 79,* 748–762.

Wolfe, R. N., Lennox, R. D., & Cutler, B. L. (1986). Getting along and getting ahead: Empirical support for a theory of protective and acquisitive self-presentation. *Journal of Social and Personality Psychology, 50,* 356–361.

13

Role-Relationship Models

Addressing Maladaptive Interpersonal Patterns and Emotional Distress

JODENE R. BACCUS *and* MARDI J. HOROWITZ

"No man is an island."
—JOHN DONNE, *Devotions upon*
Emergent Occasions, no. 17 (1624)

Humans cannot exist independent of others; social interactions are important and necessary facets of human life. For some people, close relationships are characterized by comfort, security, and happiness. For others, relationships are a chore characterized by anxiety, ambivalence, and unhappiness. In this chapter we explore the idea that people's states of mind—their emotions, motivations, and thought processes—can be directly linked to cognitive representations of relationships. We use the concept of role-relationship models to outline the cognitive representations of self and other, and to explore how conflict within and between these self–other representations can lead to maladaptive patterns and contribute to personal distress. Later in the chapter, we look at what happens to representations of self and other when a relationship ceases to exist—specifically, through the death of a spouse. The aim of this chapter is to provide the reader with a working knowledge of role-relationship models, and to make the case that they provide a framework for addressing maladaptive interpersonal patterns and emotional distress both during everyday life and during times of interpersonal change.

THE EVOLUTION OF PSYCHOANALYTIC VIEWS OF THE SELF-CONCEPT

It is widely accepted that the concept of the self involves multiple self-representations that are associated in some way with conceptualizations of others. However, early research into the self instead began with the typical image of the self being that of a single, independent unit, corresponding with the body as a single unit. The common notion was "one body, one mind" (Horowitz, 1988). In 1928 the American Psychological Association created a committee to address the issue of the self-concept in psychoanalytic and general psychology (Horowitz, 1988). This committee came up with the definition of the self as "a special complex or integration of content in which the body as object of consciousness is fundamental" (Viney, 1969, p. 355). This definition reaffirmed the belief that the self was a single unit (Horowitz, 1979).

However, at the same time there were theorists, such as Freud, who challenged the notion of a unitary self-construct. Because we draw heavily on Freud's theorizing, it is worth reviewing some of his central ideas. He saw the mind as consisting of the *id*, the *ego*, and the *superego* (Freud, 1900/1953). The *id* refers to our motivation, or inner drives and wishes that press toward specific impulses and intentions to act (Horowitz, 1988). Inner drives tend to focus on meeting biological needs (e.g., satisfying hunger, finding shelter, engaging in reproductive behavior), while wishes tend to focus on self-growth and self-satisfaction (e.g., social recognition and appreciation, gaining social status or power). The *superego* refers to our value system, or what we believe to be "bad" thoughts and actions versus "good" thoughts and actions. Finally, while Freud often used the term *ego* to refer to a central processor of information with many functions, he also used the term to represent a sense of self. In some work, he looked beyond the self in isolation and developed the idea that self-experience varied with interpersonal relationships (Horowitz, 1979). While Freud acknowledged the influence of social factors on the self-concept, it was, however, not a main focus of his theory.

Another important facet of Freud's work involved his examination of cognitive self-organization. Freud (1900/1953) created zones of thinking and feeling; from most accessible to least so, these zones were called *conscious*, *preconscious*, and *unconscious*. These zones were separate from each other, and information passing from one zone to another could be either facilitated or inhibited. Freud theorized that certain unconscious desires, deemed immoral by the *superego*, might never become consciously accessible to the mind. He believed these unconscious desires were often sexual or hostile in nature, and were repressed to avoid fear, guilt, or shame. The threat of these desires arriving at consciousness created feelings of anxiety, which was reduced by maintaining the inhibition of these desires. Freud viewed inhibited repressed desires as disowned aspects of the self, but argued that repressed wishes exerted dynamic force from the unconscious, manifested as neurotic symptoms (Horowitz, 1988). An important implication of Freud's theory of the unconscious, preconscious, and conscious mind is the notion that unconscious cognitive representations can influence conscious experience and behavior, while the conscious recognition of the motives and meanings involved might simultaneously be prevented (Horowitz, 1988). In other words, the self is not a single, conscious unit; some facets of the self exist at an unconscious level.

If one attempts to map the aspects of the self that are not consciously accessible onto the two unconscious domains of the self-concept postulated by Freud (the *id* and the *superego*), one sees that, theoretically, they do not align perfectly (Horowitz, 1988). In the 1970s and early 1980s, many critiqued Freud's classic structural model of the *id*, *ego*, and *superego*. Among other objections, they noted that it did not adequately account for all of the mental processes involved in conflict (Gedo & Goldberg, 1973; Klein, 1976; Peterfreund, 1971; Slap & Saykin, 1983; Thickstun & Rosenblatt, 1977). One aspect of these critiques was a call for a better theory of self and object depiction in the mind, including a model of conflict between the main body of integrated ideas (schematized as self) and sets of repressed, active, unconscious urges and beliefs (schematized as alternative selves, dissociated selves, or warded-off components of self-organization) (Jacobson, 1964; Kernberg, 1975, 1980; Kohut, 1972; Slap & Saykin, 1983).

ROLE-RELATIONSHIP MODELS

We now turn to describing a theoretical framework that outlines the cognitive representation of self and other interactions, and the influence these representations have on people's states of mind.

States of Mind

At the core of our approach is the phenomenon we term *state of mind*. It is important to note that from our perspective a state denotes more than an expression of emotion. Rather, a state refers to a pattern of many features that includes both verbal (e.g., vocal inflection, pace, tone) and nonverbal patterns (e.g., facial expression, posture, gesture, action, style) (Horowitz, 1991). It is similar to mood but, unlike mood, refers to accompanying cognition, behaviors, and affect (Horowitz & Eells, 1997). Importantly, states give clues to underlying motives. For example, incongruence between verbal and nonverbal patterns suggests underlying conflict (Horowitz, 1979).

States can be given descriptive and customized names in order to facilitate their explanation. For example, if a person has a racing heartbeat, light-headedness, thoughts of impending harm, and confusion about what to do next, a label of *distraught fear* might be used. This would be more effective than simply using the word *anxiety* (Horowitz, 2001a). Formulating states of mind introduces concepts about wishes for desired states, fear of dreaded states, and defenses (Horowitz, 2001a), as we shall discuss shortly.

States are defined by examining both mood and self-regulation. There are four types of states of mind: well-modulated, undermodulated, overmodulated, and shimmering (Horowitz, 1979, 1988). A *well-modulated state of mind* is one in which a person appears to be in self-command, expressions are appropriate to the situation, and impulses are adequately controlled. In an *undermodulated state*, a person exhibits poor control and displays impulsive expressions (e.g., intense sobbing, uncontrolled outburst of anger). A person in an *overmodulated state* displays restricted expressions with a lack of spontaneous affect to the extent that the expression appears feigned or false. Finally, a *shimmering state* is one where a rapid shifting between undermodulated and overmodulated states of mind is displayed.

Anatomy of a Role-Relationship Model

We maintain that a person's state of mind at any moment is closely tied to his or her cognitive representations of self and other. This is most obvious in the context of an actual interaction. Our social interactions include various people, both familiar to us and not. How we act with another obviously depends, in part, on whether or not we have previously interacted with the person in question. When we are communicating with people who are familiar to us, such as family and close friends, we likely have an idea of which behaviors are acceptable (e.g., hugging Uncle Joe when he says he's had a bad day) and unacceptable (e.g., slapping Aunt Flo on the back and saying "What's up, Flo?"). Just as we have expectations regarding how we will interact with others, people who are familiar to us likely have expectations of how we will behave. These expectations are developed and represented in enduring schemas we term *role-relationship models*.

Role-relationship models are combinations of a self-schema, a schema for at least one other person, and a script of transactions between them (Horowitz, 1991). The script is a sequence of actions, including communications of ideas and feelings, and appraisals of goodness or badness (Horowitz, 1991). This sequence typically involves the self expressing feelings or acting in a specific way in relation to another person, the expected response of the other, and the subsequent reactions of the self. Reference to a self-schema therefore does not imply the self in isolation, but rather accommodates our contention that self-schemas contain self-with-other relationship patterns. They are internalized views of the self in relation to another.

All role-relationship models focus on a theme, which could concern a specific relationship or a particular type of relationship (Horowitz et al., 1991). In general, role-relationship models are focused on attaining a desired state (e.g., comfortable companionship) or avoiding a dreaded state (e.g., lonely guilt). They include motivational information summarizing several steps that are organized and used like a step-by-step script for how to proceed from wish to satisfaction. Freud (1905/1953, 1920/1950) originally focused on the sexual drive (*libido*) as a primary motive for thought and action but later added aggressive drives. Some theorists found this binary model too limiting, and added self-development and integration as basic strivings (Colarusso & Nemiroff, 1981; Erikson, 1950, 1956, 1959; Jung, 1959; Kagan & Moss, 1983; Klein, 1976; Kohut, 1972, 1977; Levinson, 1978; Murray, 1937; Stevens, 1982; Weiss & Sampson, 1986). A common theme among these theories is the notion that people are motivated to increase pleasure and to avoid displeasure. Pleasure can be found in many forms of self-development, such as learning to do something well (competency) and being liked by others (affiliation) (Horowitz, 1988). Displeasure can be characterized by incompetence and rejection.

Role-Relationship Models, Working Models, and States of Mind

Role-relationship models develop in the context of interpersonal behavioral patterns and then serve as enduring schemas to guide such behavior in the future (Horowitz, 1991). They help us sort out the social information presented to us in an organized and predictable fashion. As we perceive the social world, our existing schema fills in missing information with what we have come to expect in similar situations. The role-relationship model contains information about past, present, and future interpersonal relationships; it prepares the self for what is likely to happen next (Horowitz, 1991).

However, information the schema provides may not always be correct. To help control for this vulnerability to error, people use multiple schemas at a time, relying on a type of "best-fit" process. A *working model* is a temporary concept of the interaction with a person derived from both observations and inner schemas (Bowlby, 1973). A working model operates "in the moment," allows us to interpret what others are intending, and organizes our decisions about how to respond. As we interact with a specific person more and more, we unconsciously tweak the working model, and occasionally make conscious decisions regarding our responses. Over time, the working model becomes an enduring *role-relationship model*, a mental schematization of the characteristics of self and other, and a script for how each responds to the other (Horowitz, 1988). In some literatures, the terms "working model" and "enduring schema" are used synonymously. It is important to note that here, the term "working model" refers to temporary, dynamic models, and the term "enduring schema" refers to static role-relationship models.

At any moment, then, working models and enduring schemas interact with each other. A working model of an interaction integrates information from the external social world, that is, actual perceptions of the current situation, and internal information, or information gathered from enduring schemas such as previously established role-relationship models (Horowitz, 1991). In some cases, as we shall discuss momentarily, the strength of an internal model can override the information from the actual social event, leading to an error in the working model.

Role-relationship models and working models are directly related to the state of mind a person is in, and can be seen as organizers of state of mind (Horowitz, 1988, 1989). A person's state of mind and a person's self-schema are mirrors of each other. A healthy self-schema will include adaptive patterns of interpersonal relationships and positive representations of self and other, while a negative self-schema will include maladaptive interpersonal patterns of behavior and negative or ambivalent representations of self and other. A positive self-schema will be reflected in a positive state of mind, whereas a maladaptive self-schema will be reflected in an inappropriate and unhealthy state of mind. A well-developed and effective self-organization results in a successful and coherent ego mediation of the often conflicting demands of reality, id, and superego. In a less mature or abnormal self-organization, id or superego attributes might dominate, producing under- or overmodulated states of mind and resulting in maladaptive behavior such as excessive impulsivity or conformity (Horowitz, 1988).

States of mind clarify how the "role of the self pertains to internalized views of relationships with others" (Horowitz, 1991, p. 69). For example, if Paul is in a friendly state, Chris might be likely to respond in a similar manner. However, if Paul is in an irritable state, Chris may know that he can respond in several ways, depending in part on his own preexisting state. He could respond in a sensitive manner and try to calm Paul down, he could become irritated and verbally attack Paul, or he could ignore him. Chris's responses will lead to further reactions from Paul, such as becoming calmer if Chris is supportive or becoming hostile if Chris attacks him. What we see here is that our present state of mind is not only influenced by our own schemas, but also by the way other people react to us based on their perception of our schema and their own state of mind.

People are not consciously aware of their role-relationship models, unless they are brought to their attention. However, the feelings surrounding the interaction, as well as calculations about past, present, and future interactions, are conscious (Horowitz, 2001a). Because role-relationship models operate without conscious awareness, emotional reactions to situations may be experienced without the person having conscious recognition of how and why the feeling has been evoked (Horowitz, 1991).

INTERPERSONAL AND INTRAPSYCHIC CONFLICT

The notion of role-relationship models is a useful tool in trying to interpret various phenomena of interest to social and clinical psychologists. We now briefly discuss interpersonal conflict, and two forms of intrapsychic conflict.

Interpersonal Conflict Arising from Maladaptive Role-Relationship Models

In well-coordinated interactions, two people adjust their responses to each other according to their perceptions of the other's state of mind. They base their responses on what they have learned from observing past patterns of behavior, which leads to a sense of understanding between the two people. However, an inaccurate working model can lead to misunderstandings and inappropriate responses within the situation. In extreme situations, maladaptive working models can be repeated, and patterns of negative interactions and incorrect expectations can occur.

Take, for example, the following scenario involving two sisters, Kelly and Cheryl. Cheryl is 10 years older than Kelly, and has always had a slightly maternal feel toward her. They have a close relationship and talk to each other several times a week. Kelly has just bought a new home, and Cheryl is helping her to move in. Cheryl thinks about when she moved into her own house, and remembers what a hassle it was to unwrap all the dishes and glasses and put them away in the kitchen. While Kelly is out shopping, Cheryl unpacks all of Kelly's kitchenware and arranges them in the cupboards and drawers. She imagines how happy and relieved Kelly will be when she sees all work that Cheryl has done for her. However, when Kelly arrives home she rudely tells Cheryl that things aren't set up the way she wants them. Cheryl feels hurt and offended, and tells Kelly that she won't be able to go out for dinner as they had planned.

Cheryl and Kelly had this falling out because they both approached the situation with a different set of expectations and a different model of their respective roles in the relationship. Prior to Kelly arriving home, Cheryl saw herself as the helpful older sibling, lending support to her sister and lightening her workload. She imagined that Kelly would be grateful for her actions, and would look up to her as a big sister. Kelly, on the other hand, saw her new home as a step toward independence. She perceived Cheryl's gesture as bossy and condescending, and interpreted it as Cheryl failing to respect her capabilities as a grown woman. Cheryl's fantasy of Kelly as an appreciative little sister rather than an adult woman led to the sharp discrepancy between Cheryl's expectation and Kelly's actual behavior.

This scenario illustrates how discord, or mismatch between schemas, can evoke sharp emotional arousal (Horowitz, 1991). The fundamental outline of this type of role-relationship model can be seen in Figure 13.1. As mentioned previously, the basic components are a self-schema, schema of other, and a relationship script. The script includes the following: (1) an anticipated action, emotion, wish, or motivation of the self; (2) the expected response of the other; (3) the reaction of the self to the response of the other; (4) a self-appraisal of these reaction; and (5) the expected other's appraisal of these reactions.

Once a role-relationship model is set in motion, one tends to act according to the sequences contained within its script and to expect responses from the other accordingly. Even in new relationships, the unconscious mind tends to repeat past schemas (Horowitz, 2001a). Recurrent use of inappropriate role-relationship models can lead to repetitive maladaptive interpersonal behavioral patterns in social situations. Thus, a person might operate from a working model that is quite irrational in regard to the actual present situation (Horowitz, 1991). This is called a *transference reaction*. Recent empirical support for this effect has been described by Andersen and colleagues (Andersen & Berk, 1998; Andersen & Miranda, 2000; Chen & Andersen, 1999). Furthermore, because people have varied self-schemas and varied role-relationship models within their overall self-organization, they may behave differently at different times with the same significant other (Horowitz, 2001a). For example, a husband may be very affectionate toward his wife when his goal is to receive affection from her. However, he may behave in an aloof manner when his goal is to avoid an argument with his wife. Thus, certain shifts between

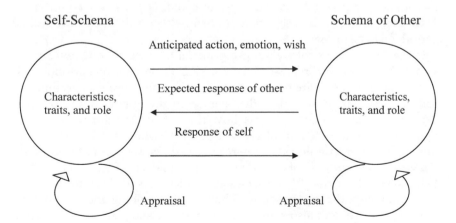

FIGURE 13.1. A basic role-relationship model of self and other.

models may become predictable, such as behavior expressing a desired wish or defensive reactions to threat.

In general, then, role-relationship models are helpful cognitive tools when functioning in a variety of social situations. However, these schemas can become problematic when they are used too rigidly, or when they do not match the situation and the expectations of others.

Conflict within a Role-Relationship Model as a Source of Intrapsychic Conflict

Recognizing the importance of role-relationship models provides a novel view of intrapsychic, as well as interpersonal, conflict. Simply put, intrapsychic conflict is hypothesized to result from internally inconsistent and incompatible scripts within the individual's representation of a relationship. First, recall that, as a rule, the outcome of a completed script is the fulfillment of a goal, usually in the form of a desire (e.g., "When I visit my mother-in-law we talk about cooking, I ask for one of her recipes, she feels complimented, and I feel satisfied."). In general, role-relationship models are based on the attainment of wishes and the avoidance of fears. However, as we shall see, conflict can occur in role-relationship models, leading to distressed states of mind. Furthermore, because the state of mind of one person is likely to influence the response of the other, a vicious circle is easily formed that helps to maintain a sense of validity regarding the maladaptive state of mind. States of mind are commonly used in clinical therapy to help people recognize and identify patterns of behavior. When used in therapy, defining a state introduces concepts about wishes for desired states, fears of dreaded states, and defenses (Horowitz, 1988). *Desired states* are those that a person would like to enter, while *dreaded states* are those that a person fears and hopes to avoid. *Defenses* are compromise states used to avoid risks that may occur in either a dreaded or a desired state (Horowitz, 1988).

The first level of role-relationship model conflict we now examine is within the interaction represented by a single role-relationship model. It occurs between the desire to act a certain way or to express a certain emotion and the fear of how the other person might respond and how that response, in turn, might influence how the self reacts (Horowitz, 1988). Figure 13.2 outlines a typical type of conflict within a role-relationship model. This conflict follows a wish–response–threat sequence. As an example, we will use the case of a graduate student and supervisor relationship. As expressed by arrow #1, the graduate student has a desire to be strong and to challenge the supervisor, who has been controlling and dominating. However, this student also respects his supervisor and does not feel hatred or animosity toward the supervisor. Arrow #2 expresses the student's belief that his supervisor would feel embarrassed at his loss of status should the

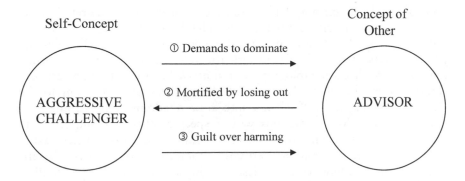

FIGURE 13.2. A typical wish–response–threat sequence within a role-relationship model.

student's desire for power be fulfilled. An expectation of this kind leads to another imagined consequence, as outlined by arrow #3: the self (i.e., the student) will feel guilt in harming the other (i.e., the supervisor). In this example, the wish or desire of the student will have directly caused harm to the esteem of the supervisor. As seen in Figure 13.2, the conflict is portrayed sequentially, from the initial wish to dominate the supervisor, to the expected shame of the supervisor. This expected response of the other leads to the next step of inferred guilt over harming the mentor. The guilt is a schematized composite of self-criticism, retaliatory rage from the supervisor, and criticism by others (Horowitz, 1989). Because of the expected outcome of guilt, this role-relationship model becomes a *dreaded* one, even though the first step in the sequence is a wish-like motive. Instead of representing a fulfilling satisfaction of a wish, therefore, the role relationship model represents a dysfunctional, conflicted pattern transforming a wish into a feared, dreaded outcome.

Conflict among Models: Role-Relationship Model Configuration

A second level of conflict occurs between different perspectives of the same interpersonal situation, or conflict between two or more role-relationship models. Here, a person experiences conflict when unconsciously trying to decide which of several possible role-relationship models to engage for the present situation.

Role-relationship model configuration (RRMC) was created to examine conflict between role-relationship models. Initially created for and still used in psychotherapy, RRMC was designed to be a systematic way of recording inferred conflicts at the schematic level (Horowitz et al., 1991). An RRMC is an organization of role-relationship models. It draws on the assumption that self-schemas include models of the self in relation to others, and that each person may have a repertoire of multiple role-relationship models relating to a single other person. That is, a person may have several schematized scripts of different ways to behave with another. The roles and potential acts of the self placed into the role-relationship model format may be those that are habitually desired as well as those that are dreaded (Horowitz et al., 1991). Figure 13.3 shows the typical diagram for an RRMC, dividing the self-schema into four quadrants representing four possible models for interactions with a specific other. It is important to note that the self-schema outlined in the configuration is not necessarily the most powerful, or identified with, component of the overall self-organization. In a more complex design addressing the third level of conflict, which is not discussed here, several configurations might be constructed classifying role-relationship models into sets according to relationship or type of self-schema (see Horowitz, 1988).

Within the four quadrants, the bottom right quadrant represents a desired role-relationship model; it organizes states of satisfaction, and includes wishes for relationship pleasures or relief from distress (Horowitz et al., 1991). This model does not necessarily contain only positive desires—it might also contain neurotic patterns stemming from an expected negative response from the other should the wish be fulfilled (Horowitz & Eells, 1997). The bottom left quadrant is the dreaded role-relationship model; it organizes states of suffering and loss of control. The top half of the configuration makes up the compromise role-relationship models, which organize states of greater control. They are divided into more or less adaptive versions. The adaptive compromise, in the top right of the model, takes into consideration the strongest wishes and fears of both the desired and

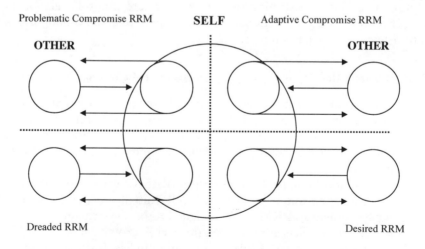

FIGURE 13.3. A basic diagram of a role-relationship model configuration.

the dreaded models, and works to organize a situation where dreaded outcomes are lessened and harmful desires are stifled (Horowitz et al., 1991). The problematic compromise also takes into consideration the strongest wishes and fears; however, it is more maladaptive than the compromising role-relationship model as it tends to emphasize a "problematic" state, such as a "blind rage" or the tendency to manipulate others. The problematic role-relationship model might be used when the adaptive compromise cannot be maintained. It is better than the dreaded model, but still contains some maladaptive patterns.

To clarify the mapping of an RRMC, we return to the case of the graduate student and his supervisor. As detailed in Figure 13.4, we can see the dreaded role-relationship model in the bottom left quadrant. This is the exact model that was used to describe the conflict within a role-relationship model, where the student has a wish to dominate over the supervisor, yet ultimately expects to feel guilt for causing the supervisor to feel shame. In the bottom right quadrant, the *desired* quadrant, we see a wish similar to that of the dreaded script, except it is formulated as a desire to develop original, independent research. In this model, the student expects the supervisor to respond in a supportive way, encouraging the student and providing positive feedback. As noted above, a desired model does not necessarily contain only positive desires. In this example, we see that the expected support of the supervisor actually leads to anxiety over dominating the supervisor. Thus, while the end result is a state of competency, there is also anxiety associated with it.

Moving to the top portion of the configuration, we consider the two remaining models. In the top right corner of the quadrant, we see a compromise role-relationship model. In this case, the student can draw away from the supervisor, reducing closeness and declaring self–sufficiency. While this compromise might work for a while, the student will ultimately realize that he needs contact with others, including the supervisor. Furthermore, the relationship with the supervisor cannot be severed. This leads us to the final model in the upper left quadrant, the problematic role-relationship model. Here, the tendency for the student to act in a manipulative fashion is activated. For example, the student may use an unrelated issue, such as a minor illness, as a weapon against the supervisor. The student might claim that his illness has made him unable to meet the demands of the supervisor, and ask for freedom to focus on research projects he is more capable of handling at this time. In turn, the supervisor might concede that he has been placing considerable demands on the student, bearing his illness in mind, and give the student more autonomy. Consequently, the student feels anxious about "winning" the interpersonal battle in this fashion.

Overall, RRMCs allow for several different interpersonal scenarios with one other person. By mapping out the various self-schemas repre-

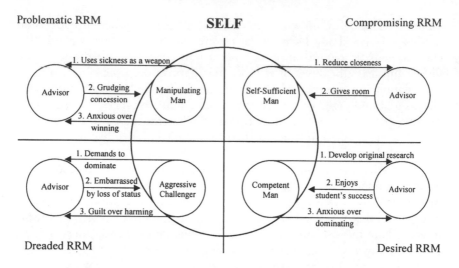

FIGURE 13.4. An example of a role-relationship model configuration.

sented within the configuration, the influence of wishes and fears becomes clearer and maladaptive interpersonal patterns can be identified.

Role-Relationship Model Configuration and Psychotherapy

In a clinical framework, psychotherapists can use RRMC as a part of a configurational analysis. As outlined in Horowitz and Eells (1997), configurational analysis is an approach to psychotherapy case formulation that considers the patient's clinically salient states of mind, his or her concept of self and other, and his or her habitual ways of coping with and responding to emotional information. Once maladaptive emotional themes and defensive patterns have been identified, psychotherapy can help alter role-relationship models. The psychotherapist assists the patient in identifying maladaptive states and patterns, which leads to greater self-awareness and an increased sense of control. The therapist then helps the patient develop healthier role-relationship models. New forms of experience can lead not only to new role-relationship models but also to the development of supraordinate integrations of previously contradictory attitudes. These larger systems of person schematization can soften prior tendencies to extreme ambivalence, as positive attitudes are recallable, and thus can ameliorate hate upon immediate frustrations of wants or perceived failure to meet personal needs. In other words, people can go from extreme conflict and relatively dissociated organization of states by diverse role-relationship models to a more harmonious balance and so a less explosive change from one state to another when under stress or strain. As the person uses more appropriate role-relationship models from a personal repertoire the result will be a reduction of the impact of prior unconscious fantasies about relationship, and improved ability to act on real opportunities for cooperation, friendship, and the experience of the compassion of others.

GRIEF AND THE PERSISTING EFFECTS OF ROLE-RELATIONSHIP MODELS AFTER THE DEATH OF A SIGNIFICANT OTHER

Undeniably, the death of a spouse is one of the most devastating and stressful life events, especially if the relationship had existed for an extended period of time. Grief has been a special situation for the study of schema change (Bowlby, 1969; Horowtiz, 1988). During mourning, one must abandon certain schemas and learn new ones (Horowitz, 1988). Because schemas endure and tend to change relatively slowly, the role-relationship model may remain relatively unchanged in the mind even after the external social aspects of the relationship are no longer there, and even when the mind consciously recognizes that the relationship is over. Recall that role-relationship models are enduring schemas made up of generalizations from previous relationships, while a working model draws on both internal schema information and external information from the actual current social events. With the death of a spouse comes the necessary process of developing a new enduring schema. This involves, in a sense, reconstructing the identity in accord with the new reality of oneself as single. During the period of developing new enduring schemas, self-organization becomes somewhat unclear and chaotic. The internal role-relationship models do not fit with reality, which contributes to the intense feelings of grief and depression following death. To explore these issues, we turn to recent empirical work on spousal bereavement.

The Hypothesized Role of Ambivalence in Bereavement

Freud (1917/1957) hypothesized that pathological grief following the death of a spouse might be preceded by a relationship that was characterized as ambivalent. He theorized that ambivalence in a relationship could produce guilt and self-hate, which could subsequently increase the depressive aspects of grief following the death of the significant other. In the attachment literature, "ambivalence" refers to a strong desire for intimacy together with insecurity about others' responses to this desire and a high fear of rejection (Mikulincer, 1995). It represents the simultaneous existence of opposing tendencies, such as the desire to approach and avoid another person at the same time, or coexisting feelings of love and disgust toward another person (Horowitz, 1988). However, recent studies have suggested that the type of grief reaction typically associated with ambiva-

lence (e.g., self-blame, hatred, disgust) and hypothesized by early researchers to be pathological is, in fact, not uncommon in people who are otherwise mentally healthy (Raphael, 1983; Parkes, 1972; Horowitz, 1986).

In 1998, a group of researchers set out to empirically test how interpersonal ambivalence affects the grief responses of recently bereaved individuals (Bonanno, Notarius, Gunzerath, Keltner, & Horowitz, 1998).
Conjugally bereaved participants who had sustained the death of their
spouse between 3 and 6 months earlier were recruited for this study, along
with a control group of nonbereaved adults. Bereaved participants were
between the ages of 21 and 55, and had either been married to or living
with their partner for at least 3 years. Participants completed several questionnaires including the Dyadic Adjustment Scale (DAS; a measure of relationship adjustment), measures of perceived health and distress, and the
Semantic Representation of Others Scale (SROS), which was developed
specifically for this study and measures interpersonal ambivalence through
perceptions of the spouse and a current important other. Grief was assessed
through an interview measure that assessed grief-related cognitive intrusions, behaviors that delayed or minimized the finality of the loss, and difficulties adapting to the loss. Participants completed the SROS once for
their deceased partner, and once for an additional person, other than a parent, whom they considered to be currently important in their lives. They
rated separately the positive aspects of the specified person while ignoring
the person's negative qualities, and, on a separate page, rated the negative
aspects of the person while ignoring the positive aspects. To calculate an
ambivalence score, positive and negative adjectives were matched according to inverse correlation and conceptual opposition, then compared following a complex mathematical method (developed by Scott, 1966; see
Bonanno et al., 1998, for a full description of the scoring).

Results found that ambivalence toward the partner, as measured by
the SROS, was generally associated with distress and poor perceived
health, regardless of bereaved/nonbereaved status and, in the bereaved
sample, was associated with grief. However, ambivalence did not prolong
grief. Participants who exhibited high ambivalence in their relationship
with their deceased spouse did not differ in rating of distress and poor
health at 25 months of bereavement compared to those who scored low in
ambivalence. On the other hand, early grief was related to increased later
ambivalence. That is, initial grief (as measured through interviews and self-
reports of distress) at 6 months predicted subsequent ambivalence and
poorer recollections of the quality of the lost relationship and of current relationships. One of the explanations the authors provide for the link between grief and increasingly negative views of the ended relationship is that
the intense change in emotional expression caused by the loss leads to a
form of state-dependent memory, similar to that observed in depression
(Blaney, 1986). Because the bereaved individual is in a grief state of mind,

memories of times in which similar states were experienced (i.e., painful or undesirable features of the relationship) become more and more accessible to recall. Over time, this would result in a more negative reconstruction of the relationship overall. This research demonstrates, then, that ambivalence in a relationship prior to the death of a spouse is not necessarily related to pathological or prolonged grief reactions after the death. Rather, this study provides insight into how role-relationship models continue to affect the bereaved individual's state of mind following the death of his or her spouse.

Phases of Grief

Extreme emotional reactions can occur following the death of a spouse, sometimes without any conscious awareness of what has triggered the response. These reactions tend to follow a series of phases. These phases of grief are a variant on the states of mind that are common following other stressors or major life events (e.g., unemployment or divorce). These emotional reactions can be classified as either normal or pathological. What distinguishes between the two depends on, to a large extent, how much the loss has affected the self-schema and existing role-relationship models, the likelihood of previously dormant role-relationship models (e.g., an anxious model from childhood) becoming activated in reaction to the loss, and the amount of social support following the loss (Horowitz, 1988). As people move through the phases of grief, changes to their self-schema and role-relationship models are being made to accommodate for the absence of the loved one in the script (Horowitz, 1990). In each stage, the person must deal with the conflict between his or her working model (i.e., other as deceased) and his or her enduring schema (i.e., other as alive).

Phase 1: Outcry

The outcry phase is a response to first hearing the news of the death. It involves intense expression of emotion. In this phase a person can enter into various states of mind: panic (e.g., erratic behavior, uncontrollable fear, and grief), dissociation (e.g., withdrawal, loss of a sense of connection), or even a reactive psychotic state (e.g., highly irrational and bizarre beliefs about why the death happened). These strong emotional reactions are directly activated by the discrepancy between the enduring schema and the current working model of the immediate situation. At first, the working model might inaccurately reflect the external reality, that is, the working model may depict the loved one not as dead, but rather as under a great threat of harm (e.g., the threat of being "torn away" from life). The intense emotional arousal is, in part, a reaction to the threat.

Donnelly, Field, and Horowitz (2000–2001) hypothesized that a greater discrepancy between the working model and the enduring schema will exist when the death of a spouse is unexpected (e.g., due to an accident). Their study examined the impact of expectancy of death on adjustment to subsequent grief following the death of a partner. The influence of this factor can be examined using a cognitive framework, using the schemas perspective outlined throughout this chapter. In an unexpected death, the bereaved spouse has not had time prior to the death to reevaluate and reconfigure the role-relationship model. Conversely, if the death is expected, there will be time for the current schema to undergo revisions. Thus the death will be less discrepant with schemas and less distressful for the bereaved person. Since past empirical research has produced mixed findings regarding the impact of expectancy of death, the researchers conducting this study took care to improve on methodology and to operationally define "expectancy of death." Both objective and subjective expectancy measures were included. Participants were adults who had lost their spouse through death in the past 3–6 months. They completed several questionnaires, were given a structured grief interview, and were asked to complete follow-up questionnaires at 13 and 25 months postbereavement. Subjective expectancy was measured by each participant's response to the question "How expected was the loss of your spouse?" Objective expectancy was measured by the length of each participant's forewarning of spousal death, defined as participants' reports of the interval between receiving the first news of the spouse's terminal condition and the spouse's death. Results showed that objective expectancy was a significant predictor of both depressive and grief-specific symptoms at 6, 13, and 25 months postbereavement. That is, cases with the least forewarning tended to involve the greatest symptoms. However, subjective expectancy showed no relationship to depression or grief. On the whole, bereaved individuals are probably more aware of the duration between the spouse's terminal condition and death than they are aware of how they experienced or processed the information. Thus, their response to the objective question was likely more accurate than their response to the subjective question. These findings suggest that long terminal illnesses allow time for the spouse to address the inevitable schema change, thus leading to a more prepared schema once the death occurs. The smaller discrepancy between the enduring schema and the working model in turn leads to less distress and grief.

Phase 2: Denial

Following the outcry phase comes the denial phase, characterized by increased efforts at cognitive control. In this phase, the person tends to avoid thoughts and reminders of his or her partner as deceased. The person enters into states such as emotional blunting or numbness. Pathological states such as risk taking or drug and alcohol abuse can also potentially occur at this time. During this phase, the person may preserve the enduring role-re-lationship model of the deceased as alive, with the potential to interact with the self. Working models of the other as deceased may develop, but are not always used. For example, a person may continue to refer to the deceased partner in the present tense (e.g., "John loves it when I bake these cookies.").

As discussed above, the first stage of grief is the most intense, due in part to the sharp contrast between the enduring schema and the working model. Over time, and as the bereaved individual creates a new enduring schema that involves accepting the end of the relationship, and including the other as deceased, the grief emotions become less intense. For many individuals, focusing on the implications of the loss during the grief stage can evoke powerful emotions. During the denial phase they may engage in cognitive and instrumental efforts to maintain a sense of continuing attachment to the spouse to help counteract the pain of separation (Shuchter & Zisook, 1988). These cognitive experiences may include experiencing a sense of their spouse's presence (Conant, 1996), or gaining comfort through fond memories (Moss & Moss, 1996). An example of an instrumental effort would be placing high value on the deceased's possessions, such as clothes or books, as a vehicle for maintaining a sense of connection with the deceased (Gentry, Kennedy, Paul, & Hill, 1995). There has been conflicting research regarding whether or not a continued bond with the deceased helps or hinders the mourning process. However, most recently the view seems to be that expressions of continuing attachment are adaptive by providing the bereaved with a sense of continuity in the context of the loss. Expressions of continuing attachment allow for overlap between old enduring schemas and new working models.

A recent study examined the role of continuing attachment following the death of a spouse (Field, Nichols, Holen, & Horowitz, 1999). The researchers used the empty-chair monologue paradigm to assess levels of distress when discussing the bereaved, and to examine the relationship between expressions of continuing attachment and levels of distress. The empty-chair monologue is a methodology used to study internal dialogue with a deceased person (Field & Horowitz, 1988). The bereaved spouse is told that he or she will be given the opportunity to speak to his or her deceased spouse "one last time." Several instructions are given in order to elicit an emotionally engaging response. In this study, four types of expressions of continuing attachment were coded from the empty-chair monologue session: (1) recurrent sense of the deceased's presence, (2) maintaining the deceased's possessions, (3) seeking comfort through contact with belongings, and (4) gaining comfort through memories.

Results showed that the relationship between continuing attachment and bereavement is quite complex. Different expressions of continuing attachment created different levels of emotional grief. Those who reported using belongings of the deceased to gain comfort and security were more likely to express and experience greater distress. However, those who reported using memories of the deceased to gain comfort and security were more likely to express and experience less distress. This suggests that expressing continuing attachment through the use of belongings might represent an avoidance of reality, or an unwillingness to cope with the loss of the spouse. Alternatively, gaining comfort through recalling memories of the deceased appears to be a more adaptive way of coping, and represents greater acknowledgment and acceptance of the death.

Phase 3: Intrusion

Following the denial phase, a bereaved individual may enter into the next phase of grief. Here, intrusive thoughts about the deceased increase. The content of these thoughts are often negative, such as the recollection of negative relationship incidents, bad dreams during sleep, and daytime preoccupation. At a pathological level, these intrusions could intensify to the point where the person feels fear at his or her lack of control over the thoughts, and the phase may subsequently last for months or years. During this time the individual may become preoccupied with evaluating the state of the relationship prior to the death of his or her partner.

A recent study by Field, Hart, and Horowitz (1999) examined the perceived quality of the past relationship with the spouse (i.e., the positivity vs. negativity of the enduring role-relationship model) in relation to adjustment following the death of a partner. It obviously cannot be assumed that at the time of the death of one spouse all husbands and wives have mutually positive enduring schemas of the relationship. According to past research in the bereavement literature, a prior highly conflictual relationship with the deceased (as opposed to an ambivalent relationship, as discussed earlier) is believed to result in greater difficulty adjusting to the loss (Horowitz, Bonanno, & Holen, 1993). In the case where a conflict existed between the couple, the death of one spouse may evoke guilt over lack of efforts to resolve the conflict or for not working harder at making the relationship work, or anger at having wasted years in an unhappy marriage. These types of emotions can be referred to as *blame-related* emotions, and can have a negative effect on adjustment following loss.

This study drew on the work on self-discrepancies by Higgins (1987). In his work, Higgins has shown that a low proximity (or a "discrepancy," in his terms) between the actual and the ideal self—conveying nonattainment of one's hopes or wishes—is associated with dejection-related emotions (e.g., sadness), whereas a low proximity between the actual and ought self—conveying violation of prescribed duties or obligations—is related to greater agitation-related emotions (e.g., anxiety).

This study examined two proximities believed to capture important aspects of the perceived quality of the past relationship with the spouse. The first represents the proximity of the representation of the spouse to the representation of what the self expected of the spouse (i.e., the person the spouse ought to have been), which is referred to as the *Deceased-Expected of Deceased* proximity. The second term represents the proximity of the representation of the self in relation to the spouse to the representation of what the spouse expected of the self (i.e., the person the self thought the bereaved person expected him or her to be in the relationship), which is referred to as the *Self-Expected of Self* proximity. It was hypothesized that the Deceased-Expected of Deceased proximity would be more strongly associated with expressed anger toward the deceased. A lower proximity score here would reflects an appraisal of the spouse as not having lived up to what the bereaved individual expected of him or her. It was also hypothesized that the Self-Expected of Self proximity would be more strongly related to guilt. A lower proximity score here would reflect an opposite appraisal, that is, the bereaved spouse would believe that he or she did not live up to the expectations of the spouse.

To assess the emotions expressed by the bereaved individual toward the deceased spouse, the empty-chair monologue procedure described above was used. Transcripts of these sessions were then rated for blame toward the deceased and self-blame. A large amount of deceased blame indicated that the bereaved individual held the deceased person accountable for the negative consequences of the loss. Self-blame indicated that the bereaved individual felt personal responsibility for the loss. Participants also completed several questionnaires that elicited representations of self and other, including the Persons and Their Attributes Questionnaire (PTAQ), and the Symptom Checklist (to measure distress). They also completed the Self and Other Matrix Approach (SOMA), which is a computer-rating task that provides calculations for the proximity scores.

The results supported both hypotheses. A low level of Deceased-Expected of Deceased proximity was related to high levels of anger toward the deceased. A low level of Self-Expected of Self proximity was related to high levels of guilt. These results demonstrate how bereaved people can experience different types of grief-related emotions (e.g., anger vs. guilt) depending on the way in which they construe the relationship. It is important to consider this when examining the impact of relationship conflict on bereavement, as it leads to a clearer picture of the type of unresolved emotions that are likely to be evoked when focusing on the loss.

Phases 4 and 5: Working Through and Completion

There is a lack of empirical research addressing the final two stages in the process of mourning: *working through* and *completion*. In the working-though stage, the bereaved individual may experience oscillations of denial and intrusion themes (Horowitz, 1988). The state here is one of increased rational acceptance and a deep emotional realization that the death is actual. As time progresses and new enduring schemas are formed during the completion stage, there is less of a discrepancy between working models and enduring schemas, leading to more positive states of mind such as a sense of self-coherence and a readiness for new relationships.

Summary of Role-Relationship Models and Spousal Bereavement

In his *Mourning and Melancholia* (1917/1957, pp. 126–127), Freud discussed the loss of a significant other through death, and stated that "all the time the existence of the lost object is continued in the mind . . . when the work of mourning is completed the ego becomes free and uninhibited again." As modern research has shown, Freud was not far off in his conceptualization of how it "feels" when a significant other dies. The loss of a person in real life does not automatically remove that person from existing role-relationship models. The death of a significant other causes considerable disruption in self-organization and only schema change can help the individual regain a sense of self-coherence. As outlined above, these changes or shifts that occur in schemas happen in unconscious mental processing and are reflected throughout the phases of grief as various states of mind. The ability to map out thoughts about a significant other through the use of role-relationship models contributes to our understanding of reactions to spousal death, and highlights the cognitive processes that are necessary for a healthy journey through the phases of grief.

SUMMARY AND CONCLUSION

No man is an island, indeed. Identity is supported in part by working models of current relationships with others, their reflectance of who the self is, and which self-schema from a repertoire of several is emphasized. Role-relationship models organize current interactions of self with others and give rise to the current state of mind, representative of how identity is experienced at that moment.

Role-relationship models represent and structure the interaction of roles, traits, characteristics, emotional potentials, and intended or expected action sequences. They allow mental calculation of the motives of others and the consequences of various possible engagements. Because each person has multiple role relationships, these also can be organized into configurations of what is desired and dreaded, and how defensive compromises can avoid feared consequences of relationship dilemmas. Finally, considering the enduring nature of self-with-other representations allows us to understand some of the cognitive mechanisms underlying expressions of grief in spousal bereavement.

In psychotherapy, as we have discussed briefly (see Horowitz, 2001b, 2003, for a more detailed review), a patient's maladaptive states of mind can be assessed and a configural analysis can be conducted to identify problematic and, in some cases, no longer accurate representations. Psychotherapy can then be used to reconfigure maladaptive role-relationship models into healthier ones, leading to more effective self-organization and more accurate responses to interpersonal situations, reflected in better modulated states of mind.

In grief, especially in complicated grief, identity reorganization is almost always required to complete, or nearly complete, the mourning process. This process often includes a containment of ambivalences beyond that achieved before the loss. Understanding person schemas theory helps us understand posttraumatic growth processes, and how to facilitate them.

REFERENCES

Andersen, S. M., & Berk, M. S. (1998). The social-cognitive model of transference: Experiencing past relationships in the present. *Current Directions in Psychological Science, 7*, 109–115.

Andersen, S. M., & Miranda, R. (2000). Transference: How past relationships emerge in the present. *Psychologist, 13*, 608–609.

Blaney, P. J. (1986). Affect and memory: A review. *Psychological Bulletin, 99*, 229–246.

Bonanno, G. A., Notarius, C. I., Gunzerath, L., Keltner, D., & Horowitz, M. J. (1998). Interpersonal ambivalence, perceived relationship adjustment, and conjugal loss. *Journal of Consulting and Clinical Psychology, 66*, 1012–1022.

Bowlby, J. (1969). *Attachment and Loss. Vol. 1: Attachment.* New York: Basic Books.

Bowlby, J. (1973). *Attachment and Loss. Vol. 2: Separation: Anxiety and anger.* New York: Basic Books.

Chen, S. & Andersen, S. M. (1999). Relationships from the past in the present: Significant-other representations and transference in interpersonal life. In M. P. Zanna (Ed.), *Advances in experimental social psychology* (Vol. 31, pp. 123–190). San Diego, CA: Academic Press.

Colarusso, C. A., & Nemiroff, R. A. (1981). *Adult development.* New York: Plenum Press.

Conant, R. D. (1996). Memories of the death and life of a spouse: The role of images and sense of presence in grief. In D. Klass, P. Silverman, & S. Nickman (Eds.), *Continuing bonds: New understandings of grief* (pp. 179–198). Washington, DC: Taylor & Francis.

Donnelly, E. F., Field, N. P., & Horowitz, M. J. (2000–2001). Expectancy of spousal death and adjustment to conjugal bereavement. *Omega—Journal of Death and Dying, 42*, 195–208.

Erikson, E. H. (1950). *Childhood and society.* New York: Norton.

Erikson, E. H. (1956). The problem of ego identity. *Journal of the American Psychoanalytic Association, 4,* 56–121.

Erikson, E. H. (1959). Identity and the life cycle. In *Psychological Issues* [Monograph 1, pp. 50–100]. New York: International Universities Press.

Field, N. P., & Horowitz, M. J. (1998). Applying an empty-chair monologue paradigm to examine unresolved grief. *Psychiatry, 61,* 279–287.

Field, N. P., Hart, D., & Horowitz, M. J. (1999). Representations of self and other in conjugal bereavement. *Journal of Social and Personal Relationships, 16,* 407–414.

Field, N. P., Nichols, C., Holen, A., & Horowitz, M. J. (1999). The relation of continuing attachment to adjustment in conjugal bereavement. *Journal of Consulting and Clinical Psychology, 67,* 212–218.

Freud, S. (1953). The interpretation of dreams. In J. Strachey (Ed. and Trans.), *The standard edition of the complete psychological works of Sigmund Freud* (Vol. 4–5, pp. 281–392). London: Hogarth Press. (Original work published 1900)

Freud, S. (1953). Three essays on the theory of sexuality. In J. Strachey (Ed. and Trans.), *The standard edition of the complete work of Sigmund Freud* (Vol. 7, pp. 125–245). London: Hogarth Press. (Original work published 1905)

Freud, S. (1957). Mourning and melancholia. In J. Strachey (Ed. and Trans.), *The standard edition of the complete works of Sigmund Freud* (Vol. 14, pp. 239–258). London: Hogarth Press. (Original work published 1917)

Freud, S. (1950). Beyond the pleasure principle. In J. Strachey (Ed. and Trans.), *The standard edition of the complete works of Sigmund Freud* (Vol. 18, pp. 7–64). London: Hogarth Press. (Original work published 1920)

Gedo, J., & Goldberg, A. (1973). *Models of them mind.* Chicago: University of Chicago Press.

Gentry, J. W., Kennedy, P., Paul, D., & Hill, R. (1995). Family transitions during grief: Discontinuities in household consumption patterns. *Journal of Business Research, 34,* 67–79.

Higgins, E. T. (1987). Self-concept discrepancy: A theory relating self and affect. *Psychological Review, 94,* 319–340.

Horowitz, M. J. (1979). *States of mind.* New York: Plenum Press.

Horowitz, M. J. (1986). Stress–response syndromes: A review of posttraumatic and adjustment disorders. *Hospital and Community Psychiatry, 3,* 241–249.

Horowitz, M. J. (1988). *Introduction to psychodynamics: A new synthesis.* New York: Basic Books.

Horowitz, M. J. (1989). Relationship schema formulation: Role-relationship models and intrapsychic conflict. *Psychiatry: Journal for the Study of Interpersonal Processes, 52,* 260–274.

Horowitz, M. J. (1990). A model of mourning: Change in schemas of self and other. *Journal of the American Psychoanalytic Association, 38,* 297–324.

Horowitz, M. J. (1991). Person schemas. In J. J. Horowitz. (Ed.), *Person schemas and maladaptive interpersonal patterns* (pp. 13–31). Chicago: University of Chicago Press.

Horowitz, M. J. (2001a). Configurational analysis of the self: A states-of-mind approach. In J. C. Muran (Ed.), *Self-relations in the psychotherapy process* (pp. 67–81). Washington, DC: American Psychological Association.

Horowitz, M. J. (2001b). *Stress response syndromes: Personality styles and intervention* (4th ed.). Northvale, NJ: Jason Aronson.

Horowitz, M. J. (2003). *Treatment of stress response syndromes*. Washington, DC: American Psychiatric Press.

Horowitz, M. J., Bonanno, G. A., & Holen, A. (1993). Pathological grief: Diagnosis and explanation. *Psychosomatic Medicine, 55*, 260–273.

Horowitz, M. J., & Eells, T. D. (1997). Configurational analysis: States of mind, person schemas, and the control of ideas and affect. In T. D. Eells (Ed.), *Handbook of psychotherapy formulation* (pp. 166–191). New York: Guilford Press.

Horowitz, M. J., Merluzzi, T. V., Ewert, M., Ghannam, J. H., Hartley, D., & Stinson, C. (1991). Role-relationship models configuration. In M. J. Horowitz (Ed.), *Person schemas and maladaptive interpersonal patterns* (pp. 115–154). Chicago: University of Chicago Press.

Jacobson, E. (1964). *The self in the object world*. New York: International Universities Press.

Jung, C. G. (1959). The archetypes and the collective unconscious. In R. F. C. Hull (Trans.), *The collected works of C. G. Jung* (Vol. 9, Part I, pp. 3–41). Princeton, NJ: Princeton University Press. (Original work published 1954)

Kagan, J., & Moss, A. (1983). *Birth to maturity*. New Haven, CT: Yale University Press.

Kernberg, O. (1975). *Borderline conditions and pathological narcissism*. New York: Jason Aronson.

Kernberg, O. (1980). *Internal world and external reality: Object relations theory applied*. New York: Jason Aronson.

Klein, G. S. (1976). *Psychoanalytical theory*. New York: International Universities Press.

Kohut, H. (1972). Thoughts on narcissism and narcissistic rage. *Psychoanalytic Study of the Child, 27*, 360–400.

Kohut, H. (1977). *Restoration of the self*. New York: International Universities Press.

Levinson, D. (1978). *The seasons of a man's life*. New York: Ballantine Books.

Mikulincer, M. (1995). Attachment style and the mental representation of self. *Journal of Personality and Social Psychology, 69*, 1203–1215.

Moss, M., & Moss, S. (1996). Remarriage of widowed persons: A triadic relationship. In D. Klass, P. Silverman, & S. Nickman (Eds.), *Continuing bonds: New understandings of grief* (pp. 163–178). Washington, DC: Taylor & Francis.

Murray, E. (1937). *Explorations in personality*. Cambridge, UK: Cambridge University Press.

Parkes, C. M. (1972). *Bereavement: Studies of grief in adult life*. New York: International University Press.

Peterfreund, E. (1971). Information, systems, and psychoanalysis. *Psychological Issues, 7*, 25–26.

Raphael, B. (1983). *The anatomy of bereavement*. New York: Basic Books.

Scott, W. A. (1966). Measure of cognitive structure. *Multivariate Behavior Research, 1*, 391–395.

Shuchter, S. R., & Zisook, S. (1988). Widowhood: The continuing relationship with the dead spouse. *Bulletin of the Menninger Clinic, 52*, 269–279.

Slap, J. W., & Saykin, A. J. (1983). The schema: Basic concept in a nonmetapsychological model of the mind. *Psychoanalysis and Contemporary Thought, 6,* 305–325.

Stevens, A. (1982). *Archetypes: A natural history of the self.* New York: William Morrow.

Thickstun, J. T., & Rosenblatt, A. D. (1977). Monograph on information processing and PSA theory. *Psychological Issues, 11,* 42–43.

Viney, L. (1969). Self: The history of a concept. *Journal of the History of the Behavioral Sciences, 5,* 349–359.

Weiss, J., & Sampson, H. (1986). *The psychoanalytic process: Theory, clinical observation, and empirical research.* New York: Guilford Press.

14

Interpersonal Schemas
Clinical Theory, Research, and Implications

POLLY SCARVALONE, MELANIE FOX, and JEREMY D. SAFRAN

Schema theory has provided common ground for scientist-practitioners and cognitive researchers alike to explore representational structures, study their roots and development, and understand how schemas direct psychological functioning (Stein, 1992; Anderson & Cole, 1990; Bartlett, 1932). Cognitive constructivists may use the theory to frame psychotherapy through a scientific lens—for example, as a process of formulating and testing personal hypotheses, of reconstructing and revising early maladaptive schemas, or as a communicative action and conversational elaboration between therapist and patient (Martin & Sugarman, 1997). Similarly, the schema concept helps clinical researchers assess and explain the development of psychopathology as well as key aspects of psychotherapeutic process and outcome (Beck, 1967; Beck & Freeman, 1990; Horowitz, 1991; Eagle, 1984; Mitchell, 1988; Wachtel, 1997).

Since social-cognitive researchers have begun to investigate *relational schemas*, or how individuals represent their beliefs and expectations about interaction in significant relationships (for a review, see Baldwin, 1992), schema theory has allowed for even greater interplay between cognitive science and clinical research and theory. Such an integrative construct affords the opportunity to predict and explain psychological change from divergent perspectives and assessment methods. This chapter locates the historical foundations of relational schemas in the psychoanalytic theories of Sullivan and Bowlby—namely, in the dynamics of interpersonal behavior and the primacy of attachment needs. We also describe the development and utility of a measure, the Interpersonal Schema Questionnaire (ISQ; Hill & Safran, 1994), which is particularly relevant to assessing how people represent interactions with significant others across various clinical theories and models. A summary of key findings culled from studies using the ISQ leads to the description of a clinical research program that proposes a more fine-grained and theoretically based investigation of the influence and ubiquity of interpersonal schemas.

SULLIVAN'S INTERPERSONAL THEORY

Harry Stack Sullivan, the father of interpersonal psychoanalysis, significantly enhanced our understanding of the relational self. He shifted focus from the traditional Freudian conception of the individual as self-contained and the mind as intrapsychically structured to the notion that the individual is embedded in a web of emotionally laden relationships. In Sullivan's view, the individual cannot be understood outside of an interpersonal context. This interpersonal web shapes one's perceptions of self at the same time it influences one's perceptions of others.

Many authors have acknowledged the ease with which Sullivan's basic concepts can be assimilated into social cognition theory, from schemas of self and of others to schematic processing (Carson, 1969, 1982; Kiesler, 1982; Safran, 1998; Baldwin, 1992). In fact, Sullivan's (1940, 1953) *personifications* are what may now be called self- and other schemas. Acquired in childhood through actual interactions with caregivers, these representational structures develop, differentiate, and help guide perceptions of oneself and the social world. In self-personifications, people experience and understand themselves in terms of characteristics that belong to a "good-me," a "bad-me," or a "not-me." Sullivan suggested that the good-me results from childhood experiences and personal qualities that were highly regarded and rewarded by caretakers, while aspects of the bad-me and the not-me consist of characteristics that were either not accepted or were punished by caretakers.

The nature of the personification that evolves depends on the level of anxiety that the child experiences in response to interactions with caregivers. Positive, predictable, and satisfying interactions result in representations of self as good. If early experiences are negative but only moderately anxiety-producing, they become associated with bad self-schemas or personifications. When the anxiety provoked is extreme or severe, overwhelming the child's capacity to tolerate and assimilate it—even as a representation of a bad self—such early experiences are then dissociated from the self. Personifications that are not-me remain unacknowledged or disowned; in fact, they are barely personified or are represented at a rudimentary level.

In this way, one's sense of security is yoked to experience of the good-me or to self-esteem, whereas anxiety-provoking situations and anxiety-laden personifications are inversely related to self-esteem (reflecting the bad-me or disowned self). Sullivan (1953) proposed that individuals attempt to reduce anxiety and thus maintain and protect their sense of self through what he called *security operations*. For example, one might selectively ignore self-discrepant information, via selective inattention. This operation is consistent with findings in the early social cognition literature demonstrating that people process and recall adjectives relevant to their self-schemas faster and more accurately than characteristics that do not match their self-schemas (Markus, 1977; Rogers, Rogers, & Kuiper, 1979). Similarly, people actively seek social feedback that confirms their self-concept in preference to information that does not (Swann & Reade, 1981). Thus, personifications, like schemas, can be viewed as cognitive-affective mental structures that are developed and maintained through dynamic processes.

Sullivan suggested that anxiety not only resides in the individual, as when a child is punished by a caregiver, but can be transmitted directly. If a mother feels anxious in the process of breast feeding, the infant would also feel anxious and could represent the interaction as a bad- me or, in cases of overwhelming anxiety, a not-me personification. Conversely, if the mother feels calm, confident, and loving, the infant would be more likely to internalize feelings of goodness and safety in relation to others.

For Sullivan, interpersonal expectations arise in early childhood, evolve over time, and provide a structure to guide and facilitate processing of new social information. While experiences of security and satisfaction with others as a child form a basis for expectations of positive interactions in adulthood, negative and anxious early experiences can result in biased or rigid ways of interpreting new information, particularly regarding perceptions of others. In this way, a person with a cold and rejecting mother may come to expect and therefore view all women as rejecting. Sullivan (1954/1970) referred to this commonly occurring phenomenon as *parataxic distortion*. It is a feature of all relationships that individuals elaborate on and distort reality, including "the *real* characteristics of the other fellow" (p. 25). These distortions and misconceptions are especially germane to therapeutic process:

> In other words, parataxic distortion may actually be an obscure attempt to communicate something that really needs to be grasped by the therapist, and perhaps finally to be grasped by the patient. Needless to say, if such distortions go unnoted, if they are not expected, if the possibility of their existence is ignored, some of the most important things about the psychiatric interview may go by default. (1954/1970, p. 25)

Sullivan (1940) believed that one's self-understanding and self-esteem are inherently interpersonal. The infant constructs a sense of self out of what Sullivan called *reflected appraisals*, knowledge about the self derived from feedback from another, based on how the caretaker communicates and responds to the infant's needs. These appraisals result in self-worth contingencies, or rules for how one should behave in interactions in order to maximize the possibility of human relatedness, and therefore self-esteem.

More specifically, Sullivan theorized that people, in an effort to remain securely related to others, acquire "me–you" patterns of representations that consist of the self and the other interacting in a complementary fashion. For example, a positive personification may include a belief that informs the person to act submissively in social situations. At the same time, he or she may perceive or personify the other person in the interaction as controlling or dominant. These representations of submissive self and dominant other serve to provide a sense of security in the world, as they help the person predict and guide future interactions in ways that the individual believes will preserve key relationships. Clearly, in Sullivan's view, self and other personifications were not two different concepts; rather, they were intertwined in a dynamic interpersonal representation of self with other.

BOWLBY'S ATTACHMENT THEORY AND INTERNAL WORKING MODELS

Both Sullivan and John Bowlby believed that humans are relational by nature, and that the self is defined and shaped through interactions with others. They both emphasized the importance of connection and proximity to others, and they both suggest that anything that poses a potential threat to key attachment relationships will cause intense anxiety for an individual. Bowlby's (1969, 1973) attachment theory, however, by employing an ethological perspective, provides a greater elaboration of why such a need for connection exists.

The link between anxiety and the loss, or threat of loss, of key relationships is given primary status in attachment theory. Bowlby argued that humans are genetically predisposed to a wired-in or biological feedback system that triggers anxiety in the face of danger. Considering the essential role that maintaining closeness to others plays in the continuation of the human species, as particularly evident in the profound dependency needs of human infants, it makes sense that people would feel anxious when faced with cues signaling a potential threat to their interpersonal relationships.

He further proposed the concept of *internal working model* to explain how the individual attempts to maintain proximity to key attachment figures (Bowlby, 1969). An internal working model is a cognitively based strategy for facilitating attachment; it provides information about the conditions under which attachment to the caregiver, who is the source of safety and sustenance, are likely to occur. Similar to Sullivan's personifications, internal working models are templates of relational patterns that are formed through early experiences with caregivers. Such encoding of representations of early interpersonal experiences is critical to human adaptation, in that they help guide and plan interpersonal encounters. As Bowlby wrote,

> Each individual builds working models of the world and of himself in it, with the aid of which he perceives events, forecasts the future, and constructs his plans. In the working model of the world that anyone builds, a key feature is his notion of who his attachment figures are, where they may be found, and how they may be expected to respond. Similarly, in the working model of the self that anyone builds a key feature is his notion of how acceptable or unacceptable he himself is in the eyes of his attachment figures. (1973, p. 203)

These internal working models can be evoked in the therapeutic setting, just as Sullivan's parataxic distortions could extend to the therapist. Bowlby believed that the patient's perceptions of the analyst and his forecasts of the analyst's behavior were particularly valuable in revealing the nature of the working models that exert a dominant influence in the patient's life. In Bowlby's view, the analyst should invite the patient to consider the validity of his working models and, perhaps, revise them.

Since Bowlby's attachment theory emphasizes the importance of close relationships in reducing stress and anxiety, observational research has focused on supporting the link between early interactions with caregivers and later behavior in stressful situations (Ainsworth, Blehar, Waters, & Wall, 1978; Main, Kaplan, & Cassidy, 1985). Other writers have been concerned with how relational knowledge can be active in shaping the construal of knowledge and yet be out of awareness (Bretherton, 1987; Crittenden, 1988). Stern (1985) offers a representational bridge to actual social events in infancy in an extension of Bowlby's internal working models.

Stern (1985) suggested that after a series of similar events with caregivers, infants develop a prototype, or template, about the likely course of events. Over time, different interpersonal events, such as feeding at the mother's breast, become organized into *representations of interactions that have been generalized* or RIGs, which contain images, episodic memories, and whatever expressive motor and autonomic responses were evoked. In this view, an internal working model is an aggregate of RIGs, averaged together and forming an even more abstract representation of interpersonal interactions (Safran, Segal, Hill, & Whiffen, 1990). Thus, the gist of numerous episodes at the mother's breast becomes a generalized representation of the self-and-mother relationship.

Theoretically, people would develop several working models for different types of people in their lives—one prototype for mother, another for lover, and so on. In turn, such relational prototypes would be averaged again, forming an even more abstract schema—for example, a representation of oneself with a dominant other or with a submissive other. It is these high-level generalized representations that contain the elaborated and implicit rules, beliefs, goals, action plans, and "if–then" strategies related to the self in interaction, and form part of what we consider procedural versus declarative knowledge.

Stern (1985) also points out that mothers' affect attunement plays a central role in helping the child interpret and articulate emotional experiences. As the mother attends to and responds to her child's affective states, the infant develops a sense of selfhood or agency as well as security, out of which evolve flexible, adaptive relational schemas. If she fails to recognize and attune to her child's emotional states, anxiety and insecurity along with mistrust of caregivers are likely to ensue. In cases of misattunement, the child may learn to avoid risks or new situations with others, and consequently constrict his or her range and type of behaviors. Without intervention, that individual may lack the flexibility and range of behaviors necessary to adapt to the variety of social interactions presented throughout life (Safran, 1998).

INTERPERSONAL SCHEMA THEORY

Interpersonal schema theory (Safran, 1990) emerges from Sullivan's interpersonal approach as well as Bowlby's attachment theory, in particular from the notion of an internal working model. The *interpersonal schema* contains generalized representations of self–other interactions, as opposed to isolated representations of self and others, and is therefore relational in nature (Safran, 1990, 1998). It evolves out of actual experiences with caregivers, and employs a level of abstraction that allows for the prediction of patterns and interactions that will ensure continuing relatedness. While interpersonal schemas are initially formed in the context of attachment relationships, they are also later applied to more general interpersonal situations, and thus play a central role in shaping thoughts, feelings, and behaviors in the interpersonal domain (Main et al., 1985).

Interpersonal schemas contain survival-relevant information regarding the self in interaction with the environment (Bowlby, 1969; Greenberg & Safran, 1987). As emotions are critical to survival, schematic information contains an affective component that is at least partially coded in expressive motor form and/or preverbally (Bucci, 1985; Greenberg & Safran, 1987; Zajonc & Markus, 1984). Through conceptual appraisals, integration of emotional experiences and motoric expression, and the subsequent abstraction of important details in the environment, the goals, beliefs, and rules that concern how to behave in interpersonal relationships become encoded and represented in implicit, procedural memory structures (Leventhal, 1984). Moreover, when new interpersonal encounters occur and a schema is triggered, experienced, and appraised, any new information becomes assimilated into the already existing structure. As a result, these cognitive–affective schemas are continuously elaborated upon and adapted to the environment.

Typically, attachment is forged under conditions of mutual and positive reciprocity between the child and the caretaker, where the child's expression of needs elicits complementary efforts from the caretaker to attune to and satisfy those needs (Bowlby, 1969; Tronick, 1989). However, in a maladaptive early environment, the typical pattern of mutual reciprocity is disrupted and the child learns that to be interpersonally engaged means to be neglected, controlled, or somehow mistreated, and that such mistreatment offers a way to be connected. Since schemas are templates for future behaviors, and they are automatically activated, such attachment patterns can easily guide the adult toward repeating activities that are maladaptive in adulthood.

For example, a young woman from an abusive family who has developed the understanding that interpersonal relatedness is contingent on being exploited may offer or allow sex as a way of emotionally connecting to others, whether or not she is interested in a sexual interaction. This attitude or rigid belief structure may lead to multiple sexual partners, and thus to a higher risk of sexual assault. It can also close off opportunities to engage in nonsexualized or nonabusive relationships. This woman may selectively ignore discrepant information, or distort it in an automatic attempt to maintain relatedness and avoid anxiety. Alternately, she may not recognize a nonabusing person as having characteristics with which an attachment can be negotiated (Cloitre, Cohen, & Scarvalone, 2002).

In this way, negativity and rigidity of interpersonal schemas along with their impenetrability to feedback result in distorted and inflexible responding. Such responding makes individuals more likely to evoke from the environment what is maladaptively expected. In other words, interpersonal schemas pull for behaviors that result in a perpetuating vicious cycle or *cognitive-interpersonal cycle* (Safran, 1990). For example, a man who expects a controlling response from a significant other may act in a suspicious and unfriendly way, thereby evoking the expected response and confirming his preexisting expectation. Moreover, his partner, who has now been treated with mistrust and hostility, will react in a way compatible with his *own* interpersonal schema, and thus behave in an even more controlling manner. The more anxiety-laden early attachment relationships are, the more the individual will fail to process relevant emotions, and will feel the need to manipulate the situation in an effort to keep the significant other at close proximity. This may result in an inflexible interpersonal schema that inhibits the individual from expressing and experiencing feelings of vulnerability when relating to others.

THE INTERPERSONAL CIRCUMPLEX

The question then arises, How can we best assess interpersonal schemas and measure their processes and impact? Safran and colleagues looked to interpersonal theory, and particularly the interpersonal circle, as an empirical foundation for this purpose. Leary (1957) created the interpersonal circle or circumplex in an attempt to capture what he saw as predictable, reciprocal patterns in relationship functioning. Influenced by Sullivan's theory on the effect of relationships on one's experience and even identity, Leary proposed that interpersonal acts could best be conceptualized as falling somewhere on a circle. The horizontal axis of the interpersonal circle depicts a continuum of affiliative behaviors, whereas the vertical axis depicts a continuum of controlling behaviors, as interpersonal behavior was conceptualized as the essential, overarching interaction between affiliation and dominance (Kiesler, 1983; Carson, 1969; Leary, 1957). Therefore, any social act can be plotted on the interpersonal circle according to its degree of affiliation and control, which allows for measurement and predictions according to what Leary (1957) called the "principle of reciprocal interpersonal relations" (p. 123).

Since the 1950s, studies based on the interpersonal circumplex model have burgeoned, from investigations of personality and psychopathology to psychotherapy process and outcome (Benjamin, 1974; Coady & Marziali, 1994; Henry, Schacht, & Strupp, 1986; Najavits & Strupp, 1994). One influential development in the interpersonal circle literature was Benjamin's Structural Analysis of Social Behavior (SASB; Benjamin, 1974, 1996). The SASB is the only circumplex model to incorporate interdependence and autonomy into its structure, by redefining the vertical (control) axis. Instead of control as the polar opposite of submission, in the SASB model both control and submission are on the opposite side of autonomy and emancipation in relationships. Also unique is the SASB's three-dimensionality, as all other circles are constructed in two dimensions. Of its three surfaces, the first and second are both interpersonal, describing actions directed by another person ("He rejects me") as well as reactions to another person's (perceived) initiations ("I withdraw from him"). The third surface is intrapersonal, to reflect Sullivan's principle of introjection and portray the expected impact of a caregiver's behavior on the self-concept ("I attack and blame myself").

Kiesler (1979, 1983), another key figure in interpersonal theory, came to the circumplex model through earlier work concerning communication in psychopathology and in the psychotherapy relationship. In an interpersonal transaction, a person (the encoder) sends an "evoking message" comprised of verbal and nonverbal meanings. When the message is received and decoded by the other person in the transaction, it has an "impact message." The impact message consists of cognitive, affective, and behavioral reactions triggered by the other's communication, and unless specifically attended to they will remain outside of the receiver's awareness. Kiesler argued that impact messages lead to automatic overt responses that are reciprocal and that confirm the encoder's initial expectations of social interactions. If an individual smiles while greeting another, he or she may automatically elicit a friendly response in return, without awareness of the smile's contribution. In the same vein, a depressed person may half-heartedly greet another and send an impact message of disinterest or dislike, thus leading to an unhappy interaction or one that reinforces a pessimistic outlook.

Kiesler (1983) turned to the theory and empirical utility of the interpersonal circle in order to research the impact message, and formulated his own version (see Figure 14.1.). The new version was significant in two ways. First, in order to clarify definitions of each circumplex segment and to provide more interactional and observable anchors versus simple notations of personality styles, Kiesler described overt behaviors, using transitive verbs and unambiguous adjectives as much as possible. In effect, he created an action-based circumplex model that was conducive to evaluating behavioral transactions in relationships, as opposed to evaluating interpersonal styles outside the relational context.

Second, Kiesler developed a version of the interpersonal circle that more fully integrates complementarity theory with Leary's methodology and the circle's roots in interpersonal theory (Carson, 1969; Foa, 1961; Leary, 1957; Wiggins, 1982). In general, *complementarity* refers to the ways in which an individual's particular type of behavior elicits a particular behavioral response from another individual. There are two types of behavior that can be mapped onto the interpersonal circle according to the laws of complementarity (Leary, 1957; Carson, 1969). The first is *correspondence*, which is represented on the affiliation axis, in which hostile behavior begets others' responding in a hostile way, and friendly behavior elicits friendliness in return. The second is termed *reciprocity*, depicted on the control axis, in which dominance elicits the opposite response, submission, and submissive behavior pulls for its opposite, dominance. According to Kiesler (1992), any interpersonal act is designed to elicit from another

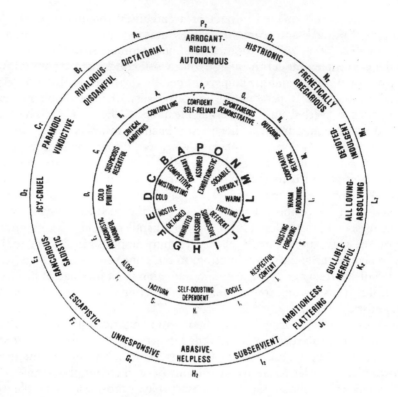

FIGURE 14.1. Kiesler's (1982) interpersonal circle. From Kiesler (1983, p. 189). Copyright 1983 by American Psychological Association. Reprinted by permission.

person complementary responses "that confirm, reinforce or validate a person's self-representation, and cause that person to repeat similar interpersonal acts" (p. 78).

Kiesler advanced the notion of complementarity by articulating semantic opposites for each interpersonal transaction style. In other words, he located each behavior around the circumplex in a bipolar fashion, creating 16 segments or eight axes, with the complementary behavior at either the other end of the pole. In doing so, he provided an empirical foundation for the theoretical notion that each relational acts pulls for a corresponding and/or reciprocal reaction. Thus, one can more precisely map out how a person who is controlling and hostile will evoke a submissive hostile response from the other person.

In these refinements of the interpersonal circle, Kiesler advanced the circumplex model into an even more relational realm. He gave it the potential to systematically assess interactive processes taking place, to define and measure myriad relational acts, and to predict behavior according to theoretically coherent laws. Such a revision lends itself to empirical study and validation across many different versions, and to application in a variety of interpersonal contexts and from divergent perspectives. In addition to the Interpersonal Schema Questionnaire (described below) other well-validated examples include the Checklist of Interpersonal Transactions (CLOIT; Kiesler, 1987a), a behavioral measure of interpersonal interaction, and the Impact Message Inventory (IMI; Kiesler, 1987b), which assesses the therapist's subjective or covert reactions in response to a patient's overt interpersonal behavior.

THE INTERPERSONAL SCHEMA QUESTIONNAIRE

Hill and Safran (1994) developed the ISQ to assess individuals' prototypic ways of construing interactions with important others. Using Kiesler's 1982 interpersonal circle, the authors generated a series of 16 scenarios of socially based actions, each anchored along the interpersonal circle, and asked respondents to imagine themselves in the interaction, and then to indicate the kinds of responses they might expect from the other person. Thus, responses would elicit memories and expectations that are associated with specific close relationships, namely, with mother, father, and romantic partner or close friend. Ratings would represent the generalized rules, goals, contingencies, or strategies comprising the respondent's interpersonal schema. The authors selected Kiesler's 1982 version of the circumplex as the basis for the ISQ for three reasons. Kiesler's descriptions of interpersonal behaviors improve adherence to circumplex terminology; his model systematizes complementarity, thus allowing the operationalization of dynamic interactions; and it samples the full range of interpersonal behaviors in a rigorous and theoretically guided fashion (Hill & Safran, 1994).

Both imagined behaviors and anticipated responses are grounded in scenarios that represent hostile or friendly and dominant or submissive interpersonal situations. These situations allow for indices of the level of affiliation and control in the anticipated responses to be mapped onto the circumplex, reflecting different degrees of affiliative and control behaviors on the part of the participant, and creating a sampling of behaviors around the circumplex (see Figure 14.2.). There are eight choices of expected responses by the other, following the octant version of the interpersonal circle. The octant version is created by collapsing adjacent segments of the circumplex together to form the following subscales: controlling, mistrustful, hostile, distant, submissive, trusting, friendly, and interested. Each of these choices represents some blend of affiliation and control characteristics derived from a location within the two axes of the circle. It is important to note that by collapsing segments together, perfect complementarity

Situations *(1982 Interpersonal Circle letters in parentheses)*

1 (A) Imagine that you and your _____ are collaborating on something. You have more knowledge and expertise in this area than your _____, so you take the lead in making decisions.
2 (E) Imagine yourself feeling angry and argumentative towards your _____.
3 (I) Imagine yourself feeling weak or passive and wanting your _____ to take the lead.
4 (M) Imagine yourself being friendly and helpful with your _____.
5 (B) Imagine yourself in a game (tennis, scrabble, etc.) with your _____. You act very competitive and work hard to win the game.
6 (F) Imagine yourself being preoccupied with your own thoughts and detached with your _____.
7 (J) Imagine yourself in an unmotivated or lazy mood where you feel like just going along with whatever your _____ is doing.
8 (N) Imagine yourself expressing genuine interest and concern for your _____.
9 (C) Imagine a situation where you feel that your _____ has disappointed you.
10 (G) Imagine yourself in a serious mood where you are reserved and not sociable with your _____.
11 (K) Imagine yourself confiding in your _____ something that is important to you.
12 (O) Imagine feeling uninhibited and spontaneous with your _____.
13 (D) Imagine that you have had a terrible day and are feeling peeved off with the whole world. You are definitely not feeling affectionate or cordial toward anyone.
14 (H) Imagine feeling not very confident or sure of yourself and feeling dependent on your _____.
15 (L) Imagine yourself feeling warm and affectionate towards your _____.
16 (P) Imagine yourself acting independently and confidently about something you have never done before, and not feeling that you need assistance from _____.

Responses *(1982 Interpersonal Circle letters in parentheses)*

A (PA) Would take charge, or try to influence me.
B (BC) Would be disappointed, resentful, or critical.
C (DE) Would be impatient, or quarrelsome.
D (FG) Would be distant, or unresponsive.
E (HI) Would go along with me, or act unsure.
F (JK) Would respect me, or trust me.
G (LM) Would be warm, or friendly.
H (NO) Would show interest, or let me know what he/she thinks.

CODING OF THE ISQ

Responses are recoded to reflect the amount of control and affiliation each represents.

ISQ Response	Octant	Control	Affiliation
A	Controlling	.875	.125
B	Mistrustful	.625	−.375
C	Hostile	.125	−.875
D	Distant	−.375	−.625
E	Submissive	−.875	−.125
F	Trusting	−.625	.375
G	Friendly	−.125	.875
H	Interested	.375	.625

FIGURE 14.2. Content and coding of the Interpersonal Schema Questionnaire (ISQ).

is not possible; however, subjects found choosing among 16 different responses too unwieldy in pilot studies of the ISQ (Hill & Safran, 1994).

The ISQ yields three key indices: affiliation and control (with mean scores ranging from −1 to +1) and desirability. Scores on the affiliation index (the horizontal axis) begin with 0 and are represented at the center of the circle. Positive scores indicate greater affiliation and movement toward the right of the circle (the friendly pole of the axis). Negative scores indicate greater hostility and movement toward the left of the circle (the hostile pole of the axis). Scoring for the control index is similar, with a 0 score represented in the center of the circle. Positive scores indicate dominance responses and movement toward the top of the circle, while negative scores indicate submissive responses and movement toward the bottom of the circle. To illustrate, the anticipated response from the other person of "Would take charge, or try to influence me" is very controlling but neutral in relation to affiliation, and thus would be scored +1 for control and 0 for affiliation. On the other hand, the response "Would respect me, or trust me" is relatively submissive as well as friendly, and thus would be scored −.5 for control and +.5 for affiliation.

Following the scoring of individual responses, two sets of indices are created to represent overall affiliation and dominance of expected responses. Each index is the mean of the participant's scores across the four behavioral domains (dominant, submissive, friendly, or hostile), across the three significant others (mother, father, and close friend), and across the three behaviors representing that context (individual items pertaining to each axis on the ISQ). There is also a desirability index that represents subjects' perception of the desirability of each expected response from the other. Desirability scores range from 1 (least desirable) to 7 (most desirable).

EMPIRICAL STUDIES USING THE INTERPERSONAL SCHEMA QUESTIONNAIRE

Development and Validation of the ISQ

In their seminal paper on the development of the ISQ, Hill and Safran (1994) assessed the validity and reliability of the measure with 344 university students. As expected, due to the inherent properties of the interpersonal circle, affiliation and control axes were orthogonal or uncorrelated ($r = .07$). Thus, knowledge of whether a person expects a friendly or a hostile response from others does not predict the same person's tendency to expect dominant or submissive responding. Internal consistency was high for affiliation and desirability, but not for the control dimension (alphas = .81, .90, .62, respectively). Similarly, test–retest correlation coefficients for the 34 students who rerated the ISQ over a 4-week interval were high for affiliation and desirability, but not for control (r's = .88, .87, .44, respectively).

These findings of overall good validity with a relative lack of consistency in the control index were replicated in cross-cultural validation studies of the ISQ in Turkey. In Boyacioglu and Savasir's (1995) study of 93 university students rating the Turkish version of the ISQ, independent judges gave high ratings in suitability for each dimension and in congruence of its situational categories. The measure's content validity was further supported by factor analysis, which demonstrated that the interpersonal situations have theoretically consistent and strong factorial patterns. Test–retest reliability was also evidenced by correlations ranging from .66 to .88 for situational and desirability subscales. However, alpha coefficients in a follow-up study of 378 Turkish students (Soygut & Savasir, 2001) demonstrated lower internal consistency for each subscale, especially in the control situation (alphas = .62, .61, .40, and .63 for friendly, hostile, dominant, and submissive situations, respectively), while desirability across all situations was highly consistent (alpha = .90).

Desirability ratings will likely always be more internally consistent for statistical reasons, in that the desirability scale comprises 48 items versus nine items for each situational subscale. However, the finding that the control situation showed less consistency led the authors to suggest that consistency may be context-specific—it may make sense in some domains (e.g., affiliation) and yet not as much in others (e.g., control) or it may be dependent on the specific individuals and populations studied. For example, perhaps psychologically healthy individuals expect consistency to their friendly behavior, whereas those expecting consistency in dominant or submissive situations are likely to have interpersonal difficulties (Hill & Safran, 1994; Soygut & Savasir, 2001).

Additional support of the measure's construct validity stems from the ISQ's ability to detect the presence of complementarity as well as to differentiate populations in predictable ways. In the original pilot and test-construction studies, Hill and Safran (1994) found a significant relationship between interpersonal expectations and psychiatric symptomatology on all three indices represented on the questionnaire (affiliation, control, and desirability). With the affiliation index, the high symptomatic students, as measured by the SCL-90 (Derogatis, 1977), were significantly less likely than low symptomatic students to expect friendly, sociable, and trusting responses from significant others. They were also more likely to expect hostility to their own lack of friendliness to others.

Interpersonal Schemas and Depression

Evidence for differing interpersonal expectations is consistent with various theoretical models hypothesizing that impaired cognitive structures and negative early attachment relationships play a role in the development of symptomatology, particularly depression (Blatt & Maroudas, 1992; Bartholomew & Horowitz, 1991; Carnelley, Peitromonoco & Jaffe, 1994), as well as research suggesting that depressed people evoke more negative feelings and aversive reactions from others (Coyne, Burchill, & Stiles, 1991; Marcus & Nardone, 1992; Segrin & Abramson, 1994; Burns, Sayers, & Moras, 1994).

On the control index, Hill and Safran found that depressed students, as measured by the Beck Depression Inventory (Beck, 1978), tended to expect dominance from others when they were acting in a controlling fashion, and submissive responses when they were behaving submissively. Notably, these expected responses are *anticomplementary* because the control axis typically pulls for opposite responses (dominance should beget submission and vice versa). Thus, this finding suggests an interpersonal schema that predicts failure in attempts to dominate social interactions, as well as failure to elicit controlling responses from others when needed. One can interpret these responses as evidence of the depressive's working model of helplessness concerning his or her role in negotiating relationships (Seligman, 1980). In another finding consistent with interpersonal theory, high symptomatic and/or depressed individuals were more likely than psychologically healthy individuals to expect undesirable responses. Thus, people who are psychologically healthy expect more positive responses in social interactions, whereas those who are psychologically unhealthy expect more negative responses from others (Hill & Safran, 1994; Safran & Segal, 1990).

In cross-cultural follow-up studies, researchers replicated these findings (Boyacioglu & Savasir, 1995; Soygut & Savasir, 2001). They found that depressed Turkish students expected less complementary responses than those who were not depressed. In fact, the depressed individuals were more likely than nondepressed subjects to expect complementary responses to their own hostile behavior or, in other words, for their lack of warmth or friendliness to elicit hostility from others. The depressed Turkish students also tended to expect less desirable responding from others overall.

If vulnerability to depression is related to internalization of early representations of neglect and rejection on the part of caregivers (Bowlby, 1973; Blatt & Zuroff, 1992), then parent–child interactions should be related to a depressed individual's expectations and behaviors in new social encounters in adulthood. Mongrain (1998) pursued this question in studies of how parental representations influence interpersonal behavior. In a sample of 102 undergraduate students rating the ISQ and the Depressive Experiences Questionnaire (DEQ; Blatt, D'Afflitti, & Quinlan, 1976), she found that the ISQ successfully discriminates parental representations related to dependent versus self-critical personality styles in individuals at risk for depression. Dependent participants anticipated a more positive and accepting response from their mothers when they behaved in a warm, friendly way; they also expected their fathers to be warmer and friendlier when they behaved submissively, and to be more impatient and quarrelsome when they behaved in an angry or argumentative way. A self-critical personality style predicted more negative, pervasive responses from both parents. These results suggest that in depression-prone individuals, a dependent personality style is associated with greater expectations of interpersonal support, greater submissiveness, and less expression of anger (Mongrain, 1998).

Interpersonal Schemas and Self-Esteem

Investigation into the interpersonal roots of self-esteem using the ISQ has also yielded theoretically interesting results. Baldwin and Keelan (1999) hypothesized that feelings of insecurity would negatively affect relationship functioning. They asked 182 college students to fill out a self-esteem inventory and to rate their interpersonal schemas via the ISQ. Results showed strong evidence for complementarity, both in terms of correspondence in affiliation and reciprocity in dominance. As predicted, all participants expected affiliative responses to their own corresponding friendly behavior and less affiliative responses to their hostile behavior. Furthermore, the students expected minimal dominance from others in response to their own dominant behaviors; at the same time, they did expect greater control from others when they were submissive. More important, Baldwin and Keelan found that self-esteem, gender, and affiliative interpersonal expectations interacted in a significant way:

> Contrary to the most straightforward interpretation of the interpersonal roots of self-esteem, high self-esteem individuals in this study were not blithely secure in an expectation that others would respond to them in a positive, affiliative manner equally across all situations. Rather, interpersonal expectations showed clear if–then, behavior-outcome patterns. (p. 830)

Individuals with high self-esteem had more confidence in their ability to bring about affiliation from others and expected more friendly responses to their own friendliness than those with low self-esteem. With less positive expectations, insecure individuals may be consequently less likely to seek out social interactions and thus engage in self-fulfilling prophecy. The results also showed that women were more likely than men to expect affiliation in response to their friendliness and submissiveness. Consistent with the literature on gender roles in interactional contexts (Eagly, 1987; Wiggins, 1991), women with high self-esteem marginally expected that their submissiveness would evoke more desirable outcomes, whereas men with high self-esteem expected somewhat less desirable outcomes when being submissive. As Baldwin and Keelan (1999) suggest, "even minor differences between people in their if–then social expectations can influence both information processing and social behavior, and ultimately lead to important differences in self-esteem and security in significant relationships" (p. 832).

Effects of Disability on Interpersonal Schemas

The question then arises as to how these relational schemas affect individuals' expectancies and behavior in a quasi-clinical arena. In investigating interpersonal characteristics of the physically disabled and of the counselors training to work with them, Heubler and colleagues first asked whether students in rehabilitation counseling differed from other students. They used the ISQ as a measure of expectations of affection, consistency, and satisfaction in primary relationships, as well as two measures of capacities and impediments in interpersonal behavior (Battery of Interpersonal Capabilities [BIC]; Martin & Paulhus, 1984) and of desire for and expression of interpersonal interaction (Fundamental Interpersonal Orientation Scale—Behavior [FIRO—B]; Schutz, 1978). The results revealed significant gender differences on the latter two measures: women were more likely to expect and express more affection and reported more difficulty in exhibiting a wide range of behaviors than male students. In addition, all three measures showed that counselors-to-be, regardless of gender, were more likely to anticipate affection from others, to be affectionate and accepting of others, and to express satisfaction with their relationships than noncounselors. Thus, in this study interpersonal expectations were not only related to gender role but to the assumption of a counseling role.

Of particular interest to interpersonal schema researchers, students with disabilities had different expectations of control and submission depending on whether their disability was acquired or was congenital. Those with acquired disabilities expected the most control from others, yet desired the least amount of dominance by them. Those who were disabled from birth expressed conflicting needs: for structure and control from others, while at the same time for others to respond submissively to them. Such patterns of interpersonal expectations are likely to stem from actual experiences of becoming and being disabled, losing a measure of autonomy and independence, as well as from subsequent risks of increased interference from others. The clinical implications of these results include counselors' accommodation to these interpersonal expectations in order to facilitate their clients' engagement in and benefit from treatment. In effect, the counselor would assume a more submissive style to counteract the expectation that others will be overcontrolling, or the therapist might use a slightly more dominant stance to help a disabled person's ability to tolerate being submissive. Notably, a large number of rehabilitation counselors-in-training in the study (40%) expressed a low capability to be submissive, even when the situation would require it. If the clients with disabilities they plan to treat generally expect others to respond with submission, then these counselors could unwittingly reinforce expectations of overcontrol in the disabled and a power struggle could ensue (Heubner & Thomas, 1996).

Subsequently, Heubner and colleagues explored the interpersonal consequences of physical disability in a sample of 178 undergraduates, again using the ISQ, the BIC, and the FIRO—B (Heubner, Thomas, & Berven, 1999). Factor analysis yielded three different and exclusive factors, suggesting that each of these measures represented an independent, unidimensional construct. While they found no difference in interpersonal schemas or attachment behaviors between college students who were disabled and those without physical disabilities, the students with disabilities were five times more likely to use mental health services. In fact, those students who used services more actively also demonstrated on the ISQ that they expected increased hostility and inconsistency in their relationships and less satisfaction in attachment relationships than students with disabilities who did not seek therapy. In the "best case scenario," the therapeutic relationship would provide an alternative model for relating that would disconfirm the negative expectations of students with disabilities.

Maladaptive Interpersonal Schemas and Personality

Clinical populations can also provide rich resources for examining the nature and implications of rigid interpersonal schemas. In a study of problematic personality styles, Soygut, Nelson, and Safran (2001a) assessed relationship expectations via the ISQ of 92 patients in cognitive behavioral treatment, and correlated them by domain with personality characteristics, as measured by the Millon Clinical Multiaxial Inventory (MCMI; Millon, 1983). Results showed that histrionic patients tended to expect submissiveness to their own submissive behavior, instead of others' dominance, whereas schizotypal individuals tended to expect coldness and hostility in response to their friendliness, instead of friendly responses. The authors suggest that such anticomplementary expectations reflect maladaptive personality styles, in that individuals with rigid personalities may be more likely to ignore environmental feedback and pull for the responses similar to their own, regardless of the actual situation. In contrast, subjects with healthier personality types may adapt more easily to the individual situation, thereby exhibiting a more flexible interpersonal style that pulls for an appropriate complementary response.

Maladaptive Interpersonal Schemas and Abuse History

A further implication is that it is not just schematic content that can be maladaptive, but aspects of the schema's formal properties as well. Cloitre et al. (2002) explored the relationship between key aspects of maladaptive interpersonal schemas—negative content, rigidity in range of schemas, and their inappropriate or excessive generalization—and abuse history and its consequences. They administered the ISQ to 67 women with and without early abuse experiences in order to see how various attachment experiences in childhood linked with interpersonal schemas in adulthood. Interestingly, the psychometric properties of the ISQ were solid in this clinical population. Internal consistencies of expected responses for each of the significant others were excellent: alphas = .91 for mother, .89 for father, and .86 for current significant other, and .96 for overall desirability. In addition, there was no correlation between the control and affiliation indices as predicted by the circumplex model.

Following the trauma literature, the authors expected to find specific characteristics of abuse-related interpersonal schemas: that a limited range of negative schemas would be uniformly and inappropriately applied to different contexts, and that generalization of these schemas in adulthood would be associated with the experience of revictimization. Since abused individuals typically are raised with highly rigid family roles and a great degree of social insularity, abused children may have limited opportunities to develop additional or alternative interpersonal schemas, beyond those emerging in the context of the family.

As expected according to interpersonal schema theory, the researchers found that women who had never been sexually abused tended to report warm and submissive expectations of their parents and of significant others. On the other extreme, women who were sexually abused as children and again in adulthood expected hostile and controlling responses from their parents and significant others, even in social interactions in which they imagined themselves acting in a warm and friendly manner. However, women who were sexually abused in childhood, but not later in life, reported hostile-submissive interpersonal schemas of their parents. Moreover, unlike those who had never been abused and those who had been revictimized, this group did not generalize their expectations of their parents to significant others. Rather, their interpersonal schemas for romantic partners or close friends consisted of warmth and submissiveness. As the authors suggest, this discrepancy may be related to the submissive element within the submissive-hostile parental schemas reported by these women. In other words, the low level of parental control, or childhood neglect, may have paradoxically provided them with an opportunity to seek out and establish alternative relationships (e.g., with schoolteachers, neighbors, or therapists) that provided warm, supportive, and accepting interpersonal experiences when they were children.

Interpersonal schema theory assumes that all individuals tend to "repeat" their history through the automatic application of relationship schemas. This tendency applies across people with a variety of childhood experiences, but it elicits attention only when the interpersonal outcome is negative and repeated. For those whose lives have been filled with positive experiences and loving interpersonal relationships, the automatic activation of interpersonal schemas does no harm, and, in fact, may enhance the likelihood of long-lasting, satisfying relationships. It is a pattern of repetition that goes unnoticed. In contrast, those who have been abused by caregivers are likely to activate schemas that put them at risk for continued abuse and assault. These results suggest that the problem of revictimization is not the tendency to repeat one's history but rather is the misfortune of having a particular history. By identifying and changing maladaptive schemas, abused individuals may reduce their risk of repeating the past (Cloitre et al., 2002).

Interpersonal Schemas and the Therapeutic Relationship

Thus, the cognitive-interpersonal cycle has powerful implications for treatment, in that psychotherapy is an arena in which maladaptive interpersonal schemas can be elicited, explained, and possibly changed. These schemas may especially give rise to problems in the therapeutic relationship. A patient who finds the therapist's occasional silence as excessive and withholding may betray a deep-seated expectation that others are emotionally unavailable, whereas another person who experiences a therapist's active style as hindering may believe others are excessively controlling (Safran, 1998). Thus, more general beliefs regarding social interactions, particularly with intimate others, may inform the way a patient construes a therapist's interventions.

Among the many reactions a patient can have to a therapist, there is often a collaborative attitude toward helping professionals in general, as well as realistic, positive appraisals of the therapist's person, behaviors, or interpersonal style. These components are typically referred to as the "working alliance," in which the patient bonds with the therapist and together they develop consensus regarding the tasks and goals of treatment (Bordin, 1979). Problematic therapeutic reactions, on the other hand, are viewed as the unconscious displacement onto the therapist of unresolved and conflictual patterns of relating, formed with early caregivers in childhood (Freud, 1912/1958; Greenson, 1967). Typically intense, inappropriate, and persistent, such responses are called "transference" reactions, and they can impinge on the treatment process whether they are overly positive and idealizing or critical and devaluing of the therapist. At the same time, transference is a crucial part of therapy, and can serve to enhance understanding of the patient's relational patterns and encourage resolution or reduction of their negative impact (Wachtel, 1997).

Since perceptions of interactions with parents are theoretically related to transference reactions, the ISQ was used to predict the quality and extent of transference in psychoanalytic counseling sessions (Multon, Patton, & Kivlighan, 1996). Sixteen counseling clients rated the parent versions of the ISQ prior to treatment, which yielded high internal consistency ratings for both mother and father (alphas = .91 and .87, respectively) across situational domains. The 16 counselors completed the Multon et al.'s measure, the Missouri Identifying Transference Scale (MITS) as well as three single-item ratings of transference (overall amount, amount of positive, and amount of negative reactions) after each session. The researchers cross-validated the MITS using 24 treatment dyads nationwide who were in the middle of treatment; in this sample, clients rated a therapist version of the ISQ (alpha = .84), whereas their therapists rated the clients' transference reactions with the MITS after the same session.

Multon and colleagues (1996), using hierarchical linear modeling analyses, found that negative transference reactions linearly decreased across sessions and had a significant quadratic slope in the U-shape. In addition, ISQ-rated expectations of mother significantly accounted for 43% of the base rate of negative transference reactions and for an additional 4% of the variance in the base rate of positive transference reactions. Pearson product-moment correlational analyses between each MITS subscale and each ISQ subscale demonstrated two significant findings. First, when the therapist perceived more negative transference reactions, the client similarly tended to see the therapist as more controlling and less sociable. Thus, the authors found partial support for the notion that parental schemas influence the extent of the transference displayed in a session, as observed by the counselor. A second, less powerful, but still significant finding was that the more positively the mother's responding is perceived, the more likely are positive transference reactions. Alternately, the more the client sees the mother as controlling, untrustworthy, unfriendly, and unsociable, the more likely negative transference reactions will arise by the middle of treatment. Expected responses of fathers were unrelated to negative or positive transference ratings, thus suggesting that clients' maternal schemas are a "stronger template for transference phenomena" (p. 251).

If transference is influenced by the patient's representations of relationships, could other components of the therapeutic relationship be strained or enhanced depending on parental schemas? The working alliance, or reality-based relationship with the therapist, one of the most robust predictors of outcome in psychotherapy to date (Horvath & Symonds, 1991; Orlinsky, Howard, & Bergin, 1986), has been positively associated with complementarity between patients and therapists early in treatment (Kiesler & Watkins, 1989). Thus, the alliance may be similarly strained or enhanced depending on patients' pretreatment interpersonal schemas.

Soygut, Nelson, and Safran (2001b) investigated the relationship between ratings on the ISQ and the Working Alliance Inventory (WAI;

Horvath & Greenberg, 1989) with 26 patients in individual cognitive therapy. Using partial correlation coefficients to control for symptom severity at intake, the authors found significant positive associations between expectations of submissiveness from others and agreement on tasks and goals with the therapist. They also found significant negative associations between expectations of dominant responding and the desirability of such dominance with agreement on goals in therapy.

Thus, patients who expected predictable, complementary (dominant) responding to their submissive behavior perceived greater agreement with their therapists on the tasks and goals of therapy. On the other hand, patients who anticipated submissive responses when they behave in a dominant fashion reported less agreement with therapists on the goals of treatment. Furthermore, patients who expected less desirable responses from others when they behaved in a dominant fashion also perceived less agreement on therapy goals. As Kiesler and Watkins (1989) suggested, the therapist typically assumes the role of a dominant-friendly caregiver whereas the patient behaves as a submissive-friendly help seeker. These roles may be even more salient in cognitive therapy, which tends to emphasize the directive, advising, and educative functions of therapists. Since cognitive-behavioral therapy depends heavily on collaboration and agreement, patients who expect to dominate others may have more difficulty working with the cognitive therapist (Rush, 1985; Safran & Segal, 1990). He or she may become embroiled in power struggles or refuse to accept advice or feedback, which in turn would lead to impasses in treatment.

CURRENT DIRECTIONS AND FUTURE RESEARCH

The resolution of impasses in treatment, particularly in ruptures in the therapeutic alliance, provides a model for investigating how transactions between patients and therapists are associated with improvements in therapy (Safran & Muran, 1996). *Ruptures* are defined as deteriorations in the relationship between therapist and patient that emerge when both unwittingly participate in maladaptive interpersonal cycles. Whereas in discussion of transference, the focus is often on the patient's contribution, in this model the therapist's role is equally central:

> A therapist who responds to a hostile patient with counterhostility confirms the patient's view of others as hostile and obstructs the development of a good therapeutic alliance. The therapist who responds to a withdrawn patient by distancing confirms the patient's view of others as emotionally unavailable, thereby perpetuating a vicious cycle. (p. 447)

Ruptures that are exceptionally intense, enduring, frequent, or undetected may lead to treatment failure. However, when properly dealt with, they may provide the clinician and patient with a significant opportunity for exploration, discovery, and therapeutic change.

In order to manage a potentially destructive impasse, therapists must recognize their participation in the maladaptive cognitive-interpersonal cycle (Safran & Segal, 1990). By sustaining the emotional impact of the patient's interpersonal schemas and at the same time disengaging through mindfulness or empathy, they may provide a challenge to these rigid schemas (Safran, 1998; Kiesler, 1983, 1996; Safran & Muran, 2000). This challenge, in turn, may lead to core structural change. When clinicians become aware of their own emotional responses and action tendencies toward the patient, they better understand the reactions the patient tends to elicit in others. If therapists unhook from the cycle by not responding in the complementary fashion to the patient's pull, they may be better able to reflect on the interaction with the patient, or use "metacommunication" via nonjudgmental self-disclosure, in order to explore it in collaboration with the patient (Safran & Muran, 2000). In other words, by withholding potentially threatening responses, the therapist disconfirms schema expectations and thereby challenges them; by metacommunicating about the interaction, he or she offers the potential for a "corrective emotional experience" (Alexander & French, 1946).

In order to investigate the contribution of therapists to alliance ruptures in brief psychotherapy, preliminary data has been collected. Nelson (2002) used the ISQ to evaluate interpersonal expectations of 24 therapists in relation to their SASB-rated in-session behavior and to treatment outcome. Trained SASB raters viewed 15-minute segments of early and late treatment sessions that were described by patients as marked by tension with their therapists. Nelson found that therapists who expected to elicit hostile responses from their fathers on the ISQ also tended to engage in hostile behaviors with their patients, as rated by the SASB. Therapists' expectations of friendliness and warmth with their mothers did not predict in-session affiliation with patients, nor were their schemas of significant others associated with hostility or warmth toward patients. If therapists' paternal schemas interact with alliance-related behaviors and clients' maternal schemas influence transference phenomena (Multon et al., 1996), these findings in tandem reflect the interpersonal impact of differential therapeutic roles: the therapist is the more dominant helper, and the patient the more submissive help seeker (Kiesler & Watkins, 1989).

Contrary to Nelson's (2002) prediction, friendly and affiliative therapists did not have better outcomes with their patients than hostile therapists. This finding seems counterintuitive, unless one considers the possibility that the hostile therapists in this study also made substantial and successful attempts to resolve ruptures in the alliance, and it was this ongoing effort that contributed to good outcome. To test this hypothesis, studies analyzing the therapeutic alliance before and after tension-filled sessions—not just during—are needed. Nelson's results also suggest that fathers are more influential in the interpersonal domain than expected; prior studies offer some support for this notion. Hill and Safran (1994) found that students expected more hostile responses from their fathers and more friendly responses from their mothers. Boyacioglu and Savasir (1995) found that depressed Turkish students expected more hostile responses from their fathers than from mothers in hostile situations. Although the latter attributed their finding to possible cultural differences, further research is needed to more fully understand fathers' role in attachment experiences and the formation of interpersonal schemas.

SUMMARY

As the recent empirical literature shows, the ISQ offers a method of assessing generalized representations of the self in relation to others that has solid psychometric properties and can be flexibly tailored to the context of any close relationship. Researchers may employ it to address many important theoretical issues—from the rules and patterns of relational behavior to the interpersonal styles of particular groups, cultures, or populations; from the interaction of gender on relationship expectations to how attachment style intersects with interpersonal schemas in adulthood. The interpersonal schema construct in general, and the ISQ in particular, can increase attention to the individual and contextual factors within which complementary (and noncomplementary) exchanges take place.

The clinical and research implications are profound for understanding what triggers interpersonal schemas, as well as for helping people change or control their activation. In fact, assessment of the content and structure of interpersonal schemas provides a basis for differentiating among various forms of psychopathology and for evaluating both normal development and therapeutic change. Future research is needed as to how the therapeutic process leads to modification of these cognitive–affective schemas. At the same time, the construct may also prove to be a useful tool in the clinical training and research education of future psychotherapists as they learn to assess their own interpersonal schemas and identify the individuals, relationship beliefs, stages of treatment, and other contexts that predict transference reactions or alliance ruptures across different treatment approaches. Better yet, increased explicit knowledge of implicit relationship expectations may guide therapists in adopting relational stances that facilitate rather than hinder good therapeutic outcomes.

Taken together, the various research findings with the ISQ support the notion that internal working models of relationship interactions are developed early and are evoked repeatedly in life, as individuals attempt to maintain emotional contact with others. While often adaptive in childhood, these interpersonal schemas can prove maladaptive in new, subsequent relationships as they are implicit structures and thus are not readily apparent, not easy to articulate, nor open to modification and feedback. In essence, the interpersonal schema construct enables greater interchange between basic social cognition research and clinical theory and practice, as it builds on interpersonal and attachment theories to emphasize the social origins of mental life and of mental distress.

REFERENCES

Ainsworth, M. D. S., Blehar, M. E., Waters, E., & Wall, S. (1978). *Patterns of attachment: A psychological study of the Strange Situation.* Hillsdale, NJ: Erlbaum.

Alexander, F., & French, T.M. (1946). *Psychoanalytic psychotherapy.* New York: Ronald Press.

Andersen, S. M., & Cole, S. W. (1990). "Do I know you?": The role of significant others in general social perception. *Journal of Personality and Social Psychology, 59*, 384–399.

Baldwin, M. W. (1992). Relational schemas and the processing of social information. *Psychological Bulletin, 112*, 461–484.

Baldwin, M. W., & Keelan, J. P. R. (1999). Interpersonal expectations as a function of self-esteem and sex. *Journal of Social and Personal Relationships, 16*, 822–833.

Bartholomew, K., & Horowitz, L. (1991). A four category model of attachment. *Journal of Personality and Social Psychology, 61*, 226–241.

Bartlett, F. (1932). *Remembering: A study of experimental and social psychology.* London and New York: Cambridge University Press.

Beck, A. T. (1967). *Depression: Clinical, experimental and theoretical aspects.* New York: Hoeber.

Beck, A. T. (1978). Beck Depression Inventory. In K. Corcoran & J. Fischer (Eds.), *Measures for clinical practice* (pp. 107–110). New York: Free Press.

Beck, A. T., & Freeman, A. (1990). *Cognitive therapy of personality disorders.* New York: Guilford Press.

Benjamin, L. S. (1974). Structural analysis of social behavior. *Psychological Review, 81*, 392–425.

Benjamin, L. S. (1996). *Interpersonal diagnosis and treatment of personality disorders.* New York: Guilford Press.

Blatt, S. J., D'Afflitti, J. P., & Quinlan, D. M. (1976). Experiences of depression in normal young adults. *Journal of Abnormal Psychology, 85*, 383–389.

Blatt, S. J., & Maroudas, C. (1992). Convergence of psychoanalytic and cognitive behavioral theories of depression. *Psychoanalytic Psychology, 9*, 157–190.

Blatt, S. J., & Zuroff, D. C. (1992). Interpersonal relatedness and self-definition: Two prototypes for depression. *Clinical Psychology Review, 12*, 527–562.

Bordin, E. (1979). The generalizability of the psychoanalytic concept of the working alliance. *Psychotherapy: Theory, Research, and Practice, 16*, 252–260.

Bowlby, J. (1969). *Attachment and loss: Vol. 1. Attachment.* New York: Basic Books.

Bowlby, J. (1973). *Attachment and loss: Vol. 2. Separation: Anxiety and anger.* New York: Basic Books.

Boyacioglu, G., & Savasir, I. (1995). The standardization, validity and reliability study of the Interpersonal Schema Questionnaire (ISQ) for Turkish university students. *Turkish Journal of Psychotherapy, 35,* 40–58.

Bretherton, I. (1987). Security, communication, and internal working models. In J. Osofosky (Ed.), *Handbook of infant development* (pp. 1061–1100). New York: Wiley.

Bucci, W. (1985). Converging evidence for emotional structures: Theory and method. In H. Dahl, H. Kachele, & H. Toma (Eds.), *Psychoanalytic process research strategies* (pp. 22–49). New York: Springer.

Burns, D. D., Sayers, S. L., & Moras, K. (1994). Intimate relationships and depression: Is there a causal connection? *Journal of Consulting and Clinical Psychology, 62,* 1033–1043.

Carnelley, K., Pietromonaco, P., & Jaffe, K. (1994). Depression, working models of others, and relationship functioning. *Journal of Personality and Social Psychology, 66,* 127–140.

Carson, R. C. (1969). *Interaction concepts of personality.* Chicago: Aldine.

Carson, R. C. (1982). Self-fulfilling prophecy, maladaptive behavior, and psychotherapy. In J. C. Anchin & D. J. Kiesler (Eds.), *Handbook of interpersonal psychotherapy* (pp. 64–77). New York: Pergamon Press.

Cloitre, M., Cohen, L., & Scarvalone, P. (2002). Understanding revictimization among childhood sexual abuse survivors: An interpersonal schema approach. *Journal of Cognitive Psychotherapy, 16,* 91–111.

Coady, N. F., & Marziali, E. (1994). The association between global and specific measures of the therapeutic relationship. *Psychotherapy, 31,* 17–27.

Coyne, J. C., Burchill, S. A. L., & Stiles, W. B. (1991). An interactional perspective on depression. In C. R. Snyder & D. R. Forsyth (Eds.), *Handbook of social and clinical psychology* (pp. 327–349). Elmsford, NY: Pergamon Press.

Crittenden, P. (1988). Relationships at risk. In J. Belsky & T. Nezworski (Eds.), *Clinical implications of attachment* (pp. 136–174). Hillsdale, NJ: Erlbaum.

Derogatis, L. R. (1977). *SCL-90 administration, scoring and procedure manual.* Baltimore: Johns Hopkins University School of Medicine.

Eagle, M. N. (1984). *Recent developments in psychoanalysis.* New York: McGraw-Hill.

Eagly, A. H. (1987). *Sex differences in social behavior: A social-role interpretation.* Hillsdale, NJ: Erlbaum.

Foa, U. G. (1961). Convergences in the analysis of the structure of interpersonal behavior. *Psychological Review, 68,* 341–353.

Freud, S. (1958). The dynamics of transference. In J. Strachey (Ed. & Trans.), *The standard edition of the complete psychological works of Sigmund Freud* (Vol. 12, pp. 97–108). London: Hogarth Press. (Original work published 1912)

Greenberg, L. S., & Safran, J. D. (1987). *Emotions in psychotherapy: Affect, cognition and the process of change.* New York: Guilford Press.

Greenson, R. R. (1967). *The technique and practice of psychoanalysis* (Vol. 1). Madison, CT: International Universities Press.

Henry, W. P., Schacht, T. E., & Strupp, H. H. (1986). Structural analysis of social behavior: Application to a study of interpersonal process in differential psychotherapeutic outcome. *Journal of Consulting and Clinical Psychology, 54,* 27–31.

Huebner, R. A., & Thomas, K. R. (1996). The relationship between attachment, psychopathology, and childhood disability. *Rehabilitation Psychology, 40,* 111–124.

Heubner, R. A., Thomas, K. R., & Berven, N. L. (1999). Attachment and interpersonal characteristics of college students with and without disabilities. *Rehabilitation Psychology, 44,* 85–103.

Hill, C., & Safran, J. (1994). Assessing interpersonal schemas: Anticipated responses of significant others. *Journal of Social and Clinical Psychology, 13,* 366–379.

Horowitz, M. J. (1991). *Personal schemas and maladaptive interpersonal patterns.* Chicago: University of Chicago Press.

Horvath, A. O., & Greenberg, L. (1989). Development and validation of the Working Alliance Inventory. *Journal of Counseling Psychology, 36,* 223–233.

Horvath, A. O., & Symonds, B. D. (1991). Relation between working alliance and outcome in psychotherapy: A meta-analysis. *Journal of Counseling Psychology, 38,* 139–149.

Kiesler, D. J. (1982). Confronting the client–therapist relationship in psychotherapy. In J. C. Anchin & D. J. Kiesler (Eds.), *Handbook of interpersonal psychotherapy* (pp. 274–295). New York: Pergamon Press.

Kiesler, D. J. (1983). The 1982 interpersonal circle: A taxonomy for complementarity in human transactions. *Psychological Review, 90,* 185–214.

Kiesler, D. J. (1987a). *Checklist of Interpersonal Transactions–Revised.* Richmond: Virginia Commonwealth University.

Kiesler, D. J. (1987b). *Research manual for the Impact Message Inventory.* Palo Alto, CA: Consulting Psychologists Press.

Kiesler, D. J. (1992). Interpersonal circle inventories: Pantheoretical applications to psychotherapy research and practice. *Journal of Psychotherapy Integration, 2,* 77–99.

Kiesler, D. J. (1996). *Contemporary interpersonal theory and research: Personality, psychopathology and psychotherapy.* New York: Wiley.

Kiesler, D. J., & Watkins, L. M. (1989). Interpersonal complementarity and the therapeutic alliance. *Psychotherapy, 26,* 183–194.

Leary, T. (1957). *Interpersonal diagnosis of personality.* New York: Ronald Press.

Leventhal, H. (1984). A perceptual–motor theory of emotion. In L. Berkowitz (Ed.), *Advances in experimental social psychology* (pp. 117–182). New York: Academic Press.

Main, M., Kaplan, N., & Cassidy, J. (1985). Security in infancy, childhood and adulthood: A move to the level of representation. In I. Bretherton & E. Waters (Eds.), Growing points in attachment theory and research. *Monographs of the Society for Research in Child Development, 50,* 66–104.

Marcus, D. K., & Nardone, M. E. (1992). Depression and interpersonal rejection. *Clinical Psychology Review, 12,* 433–449.

Markus, H. (1977). Self-schemata and processing information about the self. *Journal of Personality and Social Psychology, 35,* 63–78.

Martin, C. L., & Paulhus, D. L. (1984, August). *A new approach to assessing interpersonal flexibility: Functional flexibility.* Paper presented at the 92nd annual meeting of the American Psychological Association, Toronto.

Martin, J., & Sugarman, J. (1997). The social-cognitive construction of psychotherapeutic change: Bridging social constructionism and cognitive constructionism. *Review of General Psychology, 1,* 375–388.

Millon, T. (1983). *Million Clinical Multiaxial Inventory manual* (3rd ed.). Minneapolis, MN: National Computer Systems.

Mitchell, S. A. (1988). *Relational concepts in psychoanalysis: An integration.* Cambridge, MA: Harvard University Press.

Mongrain, M. (1998). Parental representations and support-seeking behavior related to dependency and self-criticism. *Journal of Personality, 66,* 151–173.

Multon, K. D., Patton, M. J., & Kivlighan, D. M. (1996). Development of the Missouri Identifying Transference Scale. *Journal of Counseling Psychology, 43,* 243–252.

Najavits, L. M., & Strupp, H. H. (1994). Differences in the effectiveness of psychodynamic therapists: A process-outcome study. *Psychotherapy, 31,* 114–123.

Nelson, L. (2002). *Predicting therapist hostility.* Unpublished doctoral dissertation, New School University, New York.

Orlinsky, D. E., Howard, K. I., & Bergin, A. E. (1986). The relation of process to outcome in psychotherapy. In S. L. Garfield (Ed.), *Handbook of psychotherapy and behavior change* (3rd ed., pp. 283–330) New York: Wiley.

Rogers, T. B., Rogers, P. J., & Kuiper, N. A. (1979). Evidence for the self as a cognitive prototype: The "false alarms effect." *Personality and Social Psychology Bulletin, 5,* 53–56.

Rush, J. (1985). The therapeutic alliance in short-term directive therapies. *Psychiatry Update: American Psychiatric Association Annual Review, 4,* 562–572.

Safran, J. D. (1990). Towards a refinement of cognitive therapy in light of interpersonal theory: I. Theory. *Clinical Psychology Review, 10,* 87–105.

Safran, J. D. (1998). *Widening the scope of cognitive therapy: The therapeutic relationship, emotion, and the process of change.* Norvale, NJ: Jason Aronson.

Safran, J. D., & Muran, J. C. (1996). The resolution of ruptures in the therapeutic alliance. *Journal of Consulting and Clinical Psychology, 64,* 447–458.

Safran, J. D., & Muran, J. C. (2000). *Negotiating the therapeutic alliance: A relational treatment guide.* New York: Guilford Press.

Safran, J. D., & Segal, Z. V. (1990). *Interpersonal process in cognitive therapy.* New York: Basic Books.

Safran, J. D., Segal, Z. V., Hill, C., & Whiffen, V. (1990). Refining strategies for research on self-representations in emotional disorders. *Cognitive Therapy and Research, 14,* 143–160.

Schutz, W. (1978). *FIRO Awareness Scale manual.* Palo Alto, CA: Consulting Psychologists Press.

Segrin, C., & Abramson, L. Y. (1994). Negative reactions to depressive behaviors: A communication theories analysis. *Journal of Abnormal Psychology, 103,* 655–668.

Seligman, M. E. P. (1980). A learned helplessness point of view. In L. Rehm (Ed.), *Behavior therapy for depression* (pp. 123–142). New York: Academic Press.

Soygut, G., Nelson, L., & Safran, J. D. (2001a). The relationship between interpersonal schemas and personality characteristics. *Journal of Cognitive Psychotherapy, 15,* 99–108.

Soygut, G., Nelson, L., & Safran, J. D. (2001b). The relationship between pretreatment interpersonal schemas and therapeutic alliance in short-term cognitive therapy. *Journal of Cognitive Psychotherapy, 15,* 59–66.

Soygut, G., & Savasir, I. (2001). The relationship between interpersonal schemas and depressive symptomatology. *Journal of Counseling Psychology, 48,* 359–364.

Stein, D. J. (1992). Schemas in the cognitive and clinical sciences: An integrative construct. *Journal of Psychotherapy Integration, 2,* 45–60.

Stein, J. A., Newcomb, M. D., & Bentler, P. M. (1992). The effect of agency and communality on self-esteem: Gender differences in longitudinal data. *Sex Roles, 26,* 465–483.

Stern, D. N. (1985). *The interpersonal world of the infant.* New York: Basic Books.

Sullivan, H. S. (1940). *Conceptions of modern psychiatry.* New York: Norton.

Sullivan, H. S. (1953). *The interpersonal theory of psychiatry.* New York: Norton.

Sullivan, H. S. (1970). *The psychiatric interview.* New York: Norton. (Original work published 1954)

Swann, W. Jr., & Reade, S. J. (1981). Acquiring self-knowledge: The search for feedback that fits. *Journal of Personality and Social Psychology, 41,* 1119–1128.

Tronick, E. Z. (1989). Emotions and emotional communication in infants. *American Psychologist, 44,* 112–119.

Wachtel, P. (1997). *Psychoanalysis, behavior therapy, and the relational world.* Washington, DC: American Psychological Association.

Wiggins, J. S. (1982). Circumplex models of interpersonal behavior in clinical psychology. In P. C. Kendall & J. N. Butcher (Eds.), *Handbook of research methods* (pp. 183–221). New York: Wiley Interscience.

Wiggins, J. S. (1991). Agency and communion as conceptual coordinates for the understanding and measurement of interpersonal behavior. In D. Cicchetti & W. Grove (Eds.), *Thinking critically in psychology: Essays in honor of Paul E. Meehl* (pp. 89–113). Minneapolis: University of Minnesota Press.

Zajonc, R. B., & Markus, H. (1984). Affect and cognition: The hard interface. In C. E. Izard, J. Kagan, & R. B. Zajonc (Eds.), *Emotions, cognition and behavior* (pp. 73–102). Cambridge, UK: Cambridge University Press.

15

Self as a Society

The Dynamics of Interchange and Power

HUBERT J. M. HERMANS

An influential Vygotskian (1978) thesis says that the relationship of the mind with itself is preceded by the relationship of the mind with other minds. This thesis implies that the self is not functioning as a self-contained entity, but as part of an interchange between self and others, with the other not located outside but constructed and reconstructed within the self. The central idea I promote in this chapter is that the experience of self and even mind (the process of thinking) is not isolated, unitary, and primarily logical (as is often assumed), but is more essentially dialogical. This dialogical process is not only taking place between self and others but also within the self. The self functions as a minisociety at the same time it is participating in society at large.

Some centuries ago Montaigne (1580/1603) characterized the human self in a striking way: "We are all framed of flappes and patches, and of so shapelesse and diverse a contexture, that everie piece, and everie moment playeth his part. And there is as much difference found betweene us and our selves as there is betweene our selves and others" (pp. 196–197). With this thesis, Montaigne suggests a basic similarity between the functioning of self and society. I elaborate on this view by arguing that the self can be understood as consisting of a multiplicity of positions that are interconnected in ways that are similar to the dynamics usually found in a society of people. Two processes are of particular importance: the interchange between particular positions or groups of positions and the interplay of power resulting in the relative dominance of some positions over others. I illustrate these processes by discussing some clinical applications, anthropological phenomena, cultural characteristics, and various phenomena involving the shifting among positions.

FROM RELATIONAL SCHEMA TO DIALOGICAL SELF

The processes of dialogical interchange and relative dominance can be illustrated by giving two examples from everyday life. The first example, taken from Baldwin (1992), concerns a teenage boy who wants to borrow the keys to his mother's car. The boy is aware that his mother's goal is to make sure that he and the car are returned safely. If she is reluctant, he knows that the required behavior is to reassure his mother that he will behave in a responsible way. So he verbalizes phrases that have been successful in the past, such as "I'll drive carefully" and "I'll be home before 1:00!" Proceeding this way, he expects that his mother will give him the keys. If he is not immediately successful, he may employ different routines, such as expressing his urgent need for transport or complaining about the unfairness of his mother's behavior. Along these lines "multiple if–then sequences" are organized into a complete production system for guiding behavior. As a result of these predictable sequences, the mother finally gives the teenager the keys.

Before the mother makes a decision, she vacillates between two opposing forces. Because she is concerned about the well-being of her son, she is hesitant and perhaps fearful to give him the keys. At the same time she is sympathetic to his desires, as he wants to enjoy a fine day. So she switches between two positions: the fearful mother and the helpful mother. From the first position she would say: "I am afraid that . . . ," from the second: "I can imagine that. . . . " After a process of negotiation in which she is moving to and fro between the two positions, she finally decides to give her son the keys. As long as the mother is involved in this process of negotiation, she is "distributed" between two positions. She is finally able to make a decision when one of the positions becomes dominant over the other.

The example of borrowing the keys illustrates several aspects of a dialogical self: its multivoiced nature, the interchange between the several positions or voices, and their relative dominance or power. However, the example reflects a repetitive sequence of positions that are part of a predictable chain of events. Prior interactions are patterned in repetitive ways on the basis of expected sequences. Such stereotypical interactions, which Baldwin (1992) describes in terms of "relational schemas," can certainly be understood as dialogical, but they lack a central ingredient that is crucial to the understanding of the dialogical self: the element of novelty. Let us, therefore, present a second example, this one from Hermans (1996a), which leads us to the heart of the dialogical self.

An author submits a manuscript to a scientific journal for publication. After some time, she receives three helpful but critical comments, with the encouraging advice to correct her text and resubmit it. After reading and rereading the reviews, the author is challenged by entirely new information and new problems to resolve. These problems can only be resolved by taking the positions of the reviewers into account in relation to her own position. This requires the author to move to and fro between the several reviewers in order to check them on consistencies and inconsistencies. Moreover, the author has to move between the reviewers' points of view and her own position as represented by the original manuscript. At first all these positions sound like a "cacophony of voices," but after several rounds of intensive dialogical interchange a new structure emerges. In an act of juxtaposition, the several views become simultaneously present, so that new, sometimes suddenly emerging, relationships between the diversity of insights arise. Finally, the author writes a thoroughly revised manuscript, in which her original position, as presented in the first manuscript, is significantly altered. It represents a position that has become more convincing than the original one and, at the same time, more dominant in the light of the multiplicity of alternative voices. The new manuscript can be seen as the sediment of a process, in which the opposing positions of the author and the reviewers, and the repositioning of the author, are part of a highly open, dynamic, multivoiced self. This highly complex process is potentially innovative as a result of the introduction of new voices, their dialogical interchange, and changes in their relative dominance.

In order to deepen the nature of the dialogical self, the present chapter is divided into three parts. First, the historical roots of the theory are explained. Second, several empirical applications are described in the light of specific theoretical questions. Third, a future perspective is briefly sketched.

HISTORICAL ROOTS: JAMES AND BAKHTIN

James's Extended Self

In order to understand the dialogical self, it is necessary to go back to James's (1890) distinction between *I* and *Me*, which according to Rosenberg (1979) is a classic contribution to the psychology of the self. The I–Me distinction is based on the consideration that the self is not simply a "unity in itself," but rather a process that implies a highly dynamic relationship between two parts of the self. In James's view, the *I* is equated with the self-as-knower and has three features: continuity, distinctness, and volition. The continuity of the self-as-knower is characterized by a sense of personal identity, that is, a sense of sameness through time. A feeling of distinctness from others, or individuality, also belongs to the subjective nature of the self-as-knower. Finally, a sense of personal volition is reflected in the continuous appropriation and rejection of thoughts by which the self-as-knower proves itself as an active processor of experience (see also Damon & Hart, 1982).

For James, the *Me* is equated with the self-as-known and is composed of the empirical elements considered as belonging to oneself. Crucial for the understanding of the self is that James observed a gradual distinction between *Me* and *Mine*. He concluded that the empirical self is composed of all that the person can call his or her own, "not only his body and his psychic powers, but his clothes and his house, his wife and children, his ancestors and friends, his reputation and works, his lands and horses, and yacht and bank-account" (James, 1890, p. 291). As this quotation suggests, people and things in the environment belong to the self, as far as they are felt as "mine." In agreement with this definition, James observed that not only "my mother" but even "my enemy" belongs to the self. In this view the self is not restricted to experiences within the skin but rather extended to the environment. The extended self can be contrasted with the Cartesian self, which is based on a dualistic conception, not only between self and body but also between self and other (Fogel, 1993; Hermans, 2003; Straus, 1958). With his conception of the extended self, and his view of the self as a dynamic opposition between *I* and *Me*, James (1890) paved the way for later theoretical developments in which contrasts, oppositions, and negotiations are part of a multivoiced, dialogical self.

Bakhtin's Polyphonic Novel

Multivoicedness and dialogicality are explicitly elaborated in the metaphor of the "polyphonic novel" proposed by Bakhtin in his book *Problems of Dostoevsky's Poetics* (1929/1973). Bakhtin's main thesis is that in Dostoyevsky's works there is not a single author at work—Dostoyevsky himself—but *several* authors or thinkers. These include characters such as Raskolnikov, Myshkin, Stavrogin, Ivan Karamazov, and the Grand Inquisitor. Such characters are not treated as obedient slaves in the service of one author-thinker, Dostoyevsky, but are put forward as independent thinkers, each with his or her own view of the world. There is a plurality of consciousnesses and worlds instead of a multitude of characters and fates within an *unified* objective world, organized by Dostoyevsky's individual consciousness. As in a polyphonic musical work, a multiplicity of voices accompany and oppose one another in dialogical ways. As part of this polyphonic construction, Dostoyevsky creates a variety of fascinating perspectives, portraying characters conversing with the Devil (Ivan and the

Devil), with their alter egos (Ivan and Smerdyakov), and even with carica-
tures of themselves (Raskolnikov and Svidrigailov).

Bakhtin argues that the notion of dialogue has the potential of differentiating the inner world of one and the same individual in the form of an
interpersonal relationship. When an "inner" thought of a particular character is transformed into an utterance, a dialogical relation is instigated to
occur between this utterance and the utterance of imaginal others. For example, in Dostoyevsky's novel *The Double*, the second hero (the double) is
portrayed as a personification of the interior thought of the first hero
(Golyadkin). A polyphonic construction is realized by externalizing an interior thought in a spatially separated opponent and, as a result, a fully developed dialogue between two relatively independent parties is created.
Such a dialogical narrative is not only structured by space and time, but
temporal relations can even be translated into spatial relations. As part of
this construction, temporally dispersed events are contracted into spatial
oppositions that are simultaneously present. In Bakhtin's terms, "This persistent urge to see all things as being coexistent and to perceive and depict
all things side by side and simultaneously, *as if in space rather than time*,
leads him [Dostoyevsky] to dramatize in space even the inner contradic-
tions and stages of development of a single person" (p. 23; emphasis
added).

The Difference between Logical and Dialogical Relationships

Dialogical relationships can only be properly understood when the notion
of space is taken into account. This can be illustrated by examining the difference between logical and dialogical relationships. Bakhtin gives the following example (see also Vasil'eva, 1988). Take two phrases that are completely identical, "life is good" and again "life is good." From the
perspective of Aristotelian logic, these two phrases are connected by a relationship of *identity*; they are, in fact, one and the same statement. From a
dialogical perspective, however, they are different because they can be seen
as two sequential remarks following each other in time and coming from
two spatially separated people in communication, who in this case entertain a relationship of *agreement*. The two phrases are identical from a logical point of view, but they are different as utterances: the first is a statement, the second a confirmation of that statement. The confirmation adds
something that was not included in the original statement. The original utterance is not finalized in itself. Instead, it is dialogically expanded.

In a similar way the statements "life is good" and "life is not good"
can be analyzed. In a logical sense, one is a *negation* of the other. However,
when the two phrases are taken as utterances from two different speakers,
a dialogical relation of *disagreement* can be seen to exist. In Bakhtin's
worldview, the relationship of agreement and disagreement are, like ques-

tion and answer, basic dialogical forms. In other words, dialogue can only be understood in terms of voices that are spatially located in actual, remembered, or imagined relationships.

James's Rivalry of Different Selves

As we have seen, James portrayed the *I* (self-as-knower) as a unifying principle that is responsible for organizing the different aspects of the *Me* as parts of a continuous stream of consciousness. In this part of his work, he seems to emphasize the continuity of the self more than its discontinuity. In other parts, however, James refers explicitly to the "rivalry and conflict of the different selves":

> I am often confronted by the necessity of standing by one of my empirical selves and relinquishing the rest. Not that I would not, if I could, be both handsome and fat and well dressed, and a great athlete, and make a million a year, be a wit, a bon-vivant, and a lady-killer, as well as a philosopher; a philanthropist, statesman, warrior, and African explorer, as well as a "tone-poet" and saint. But the thing is simply impossible. The millionaire's work would run counter to the saint's; the bon-vivant and the philanthropist would trip each other up; the philosopher and the lady-killer could not well keep house in the same tenement of clay. Such different *characters* may conceivably at the outset of life be alike possible to man. But to make any one of them actual, the rest must more or less be suppressed. (James, 1890, pp. 309–310; emphasis added)

As this quotation suggests, James certainly was aware of the multiplicity of the self and of the mutual rivalry and domination of its parts. His use of the term "character" to denote the different components of the self is very much in agreement with the multiplicity of characters implied in Bakhtin's notion of the polyphonic novel.

The Dialogical Self: A Dynamic Multiplicity of I Positions

Inspired by James's treatise on the self and Bakhtin's polyphonic novel, we conceptualize the self in terms of a dynamic multiplicity of relatively autonomous *I* positions in the landscape of the mind, intertwined as this mind is with the minds of other people (Hermans, 2002; Hermans, Kempen, & Van Loon, 1992). In this conception, the *I* has the possibility to move from one spatial position to another in accordance with changes in situation and time. The *I* fluctuates among different and even opposed positions, and has the capacity to imaginatively endow each position with a voice so that dialogical relations between positions can be established. The voices function like interacting characters in a story, involved in a process of question and answer, agreement and disagreement. Each of them has a story to tell about their own experiences from their own stance. As different voices, these characters exchange information about their respective *Me's*, resulting in a complex, narratively structured self. As part of this dialogical process, some voices are more influential or have more social power than others. (For a more elaborate discussion of this conception of the dialogical self, see Barresi, 2002; Bertau, 2004; Hermans, 1996a, 1996b; Josephs, 2002; Lewis, 2002; Valsiner, 2002).

As implied in the preceding analysis, an important feature of the dialogical self is its combination of temporal and spatial characteristics. Sarbin (1986), Bruner (1986), Gergen and Gergen (1988), and McAdams (1993), main advocates of a narrative approach, have extensively discussed the temporal dimension of narratives. Unquestionably, the temporal dimension is a constitutive feature of stories or narratives. Without time, there is no story. However, following Bakhtin's emphasis on the spatial dimension, time and space are seen as equally important for the narrative structure of the dialogical self. The spatial nature of the self is expressed in the words "position," "positioning," and "repositioning," terms that suggest, moreover, more dynamic and flexible referents than the traditional term "role" (Harré & Van Langenhove, 1991).

APPLICATIONS OF DIALOGICAL-SELF THEORY

In the following section I present a review of studies that are guided by some notions that are central to dialogical-self theory. It is my purpose not only to give an impression of the kind of empirical work but also of the questions that can be posed when taking this theory as a starting point.

The Case of Richard: Significant Changes in His Self

It is my intention to present in this section an example of a client in psychotherapy. I do so with the conviction that the psychotherapeutic situation provides a well-suited context for the study of changes in the self, and of innovation within the self in particular. Moreover, psychotherapy implies an interpersonal relationship in which two parties, psychotherapist and client, work closely together with the purpose of promoting the client's well-being.

The position repertoire of the client to be presented in this section was strongly dominated by a "perfectionist" as one of the main characters in his self-system. This position was so strongly established in his repertoire that the client was almost "immobilized" in his everyday life activities. I will demonstrate how this position was initially dominant but later received an answer from a new position that was gradually entering his repertoire: his self-accepting position. This case study, including a specific assessment method, is more extensively discussed by Hermans (2003). The case is discussed here in a summarizing way in order to demonstrate how some central theoretical notions in dialogical-self theory function in the life of an individual.

The client was Richard, a 38-year-old man, who contacted a psychotherapist (Els Hermans-Jansen in cooperation with me as a co-therapist) after many years of general dissatisfaction with his life. In the first conversation with the psychotherapists, he complained that he was not able to make any choices on important matters in his life. He worked as a part-time administrator but this work was unsatisfactory for him: he felt he was working far below the level of his capacities, and he blamed himself for not finishing his university studies. He also had intense feelings of guilt because he had not chosen to stay with his girlfriend, with whom he had lived for a long time. He considered himself a "failure" and was often overwhelmed by feelings of shame, guilt, and doubt about his own qualities.

One of the most important discoveries in the beginning phase of the therapy was the client becoming aware that most of his problems had to do with the devaluating influence of a "perfectionist" in himself who worked closely together with another influential position, the "dreamer":

> "I tend to see them as a pair [the perfectionist and dreamer]. The dreamer is the one who proposes things. The perfectionist then has a critical look at what has been made of it. The dreamer is the phantast, without any limitation by reality. The dreamer is very free and active. He is strongly developed. The perfectionist is more like a gatekeeper. He looks ahead: 'This will be nothing.' He also looks back and sees what has come out of all those dreams. He knows how it should be done. The perfectionist looks compassionate, shakes his head. . . . "

As this excerpt suggests, Richard recognizes the two positions (perfectionist and dreamer) as playing a significant role in his life and indicates that they tend to alternate. Whereas the dreamer is continuously building castles in the air that are never realized, the perfectionist is used to giving a merciless and harsh judgment indicating that Richard is a failure. This leads the dreamer, in turn, to build new castles in the air as a compensation for Richard's unsatisfactory accomplishments.

Although Richard admitted the relevance of the perfectionist in his life, he felt, at the same time, a resistance to admit the influential role of this position:

> "The perfectionist: I approach this with much caution. I tend to make movements around this topic. I shrank from giving this a place. It is an arrogant figure: this passionate shaking his head: 'This is not noteworthy.' This perfectionism has taken the form of expectations which have

formed my personality since long. Memories are transformed into expectations. As a truck driver I once caused an accident. Finally, there
was not more than material damage. But at that moment I thought:
'This is what you have made of your life.' It was something that went
beyond that situation: It was an expectation. It was the feeling that I
was not a person on myself. It was rather a movement by other people,
some kind of melting of my parents and myself. My grandfather had
very negative expectations of me, that nothing would become of me,
that I had no persistence. I was afraid of his depreciation. At the same
time I'm very wary of putting the problem in my grandfather or my
parents."

As the last sentences in the above excerpt suggest, Richard did not see the
position of the perfectionist in isolation, but in close connection with the
role that some significant others had played in his past. Although he was
hesitant to admit the significance of all these positions in their mutual relationship, he became aware of the connection between the voices of his parents and grandfather, on the one hand, and the emergence of the dreamer
and the perfectionist, on the other hand.

Given the unattainable standards of the perfectionist, the three of us
decided that Richard would start with some "innocent" activities, which
were, in the eyes of the perfectionist, scarcely noteworthy. The purpose
was to explore a space in the self that was somewhere beyond the reach of
the dictatorial perfectionist. Expecting that these activities would give him
at least *some* pleasure, he engaged in some relaxing activities like running,
cycling, and watching birds together with some friends. The idea behind
this plan was to stimulate Richard to do things at a very low-expectation
level, without the pressure of any "standards of excellence," in order to
keep the perfectionist "silent."

Some weeks later, Richard told us that his mood was somewhat improved. He explained that while doing these "innocent" activities he noticed that there were moments when he could accept the possibilities that
he had: "In these activities, not much progress is needed, there is less self-
blaming and there are less obstacles, and less energy is spoiled." He continued: "By this acceptance I experience somewhat more lightness in my
existence. I often continue to ruminate, yet I have created some islands of
well-being." After he had told us about his new activities, he spoke about
our role, the psychotherapist and me, as related to his slightly changing
view of himself: "You accept me and that's okay; I pick up ordinary activities and you agree with that; there is not the pressure to take it very
seriously. And these activities work: They provide an antidote to my self-
image. I make space for doing these things and also my friends give me that
space. This also liberates me from isolation."

For a proper understanding of the innovation of Richard's position repertoire, it should be stressed that the new activities were linked with our position as external helpers, and this linkage created a route to a new internal position that seemed to be of particular importance for his future self-development: "I as accepting." He developed this position as a significant part of his internal domain, stimulated as it was by the accepting attitude of his therapist. It seemed to have the potential to form a realistic counterweight to the hitherto dominant perfectionist.

Because we wanted to know how the new position (accepting) functioned in his everyday life, we invited Richard to describe a relevant situation and consider it from two opposite positions: the accepting position and the perfectionist position. The idea was to examine the actual difference between the two positions with attention to their dialogical relationship. Two weeks later, Richard presented us with the following description:

Acceptance

"This event, attending a lecture, the inspiring environment and the presentation, evoke a lot of memories about earlier times, how I hoped and wrestled; the dream to develop myself, to achieve much. Always I felt the disappointment and the failure and all these things came together in a source of aversion and accusation. Now I'm sitting here and cautiously I explore the possibility of acceptance. . . . I feel relaxation, lightness very directly, a cheerful feeling almost, like in a play . . . why not? Look forward, you get this free, consider your possibilities which are available and be content which what you have. The richness of sitting here and letting you inspire, after the beautiful walk along the old buildings, by a presentation from which you may learn something . . . this is free."

Perfectionism

"The feeling of sitting here so freely doesn't stay long enough. The space which was formed by the play of optimism is pulled away by a much deeper desire, a desire as deep as the source that always distributes contempt to and about myself. Besides that, acceptance is not possible and not sufficient. The past should be banished and forgotten by a great future. Reproach must be transformed into pride . . . contempt into admiration.

"On my way home, I succeed in keeping myself somewhat outside these poles or roles. Acceptance, optimism, perfectionism . . . walking along the enormous autumn trees, I can consider them with a smile: a puppetry with the shy and modest accepting, the ruddy, excited optimist and the perfectionist as the angry caricature pessimist. Not a bad day."

As these diary notes show, Richard focuses on a particular scene and relates his experiences from two positions, the accepting and the perfectionist. It is remarkable that, talking from the perspective of the "accepting," he starts with referring to his bad feelings associated with the perfectionist (" . . . the dream to develop myself, to achieve much . . . ") and then moves to the accepting position ("I explore the possibility of acceptance . . . "). Instead of dealing with the two positions in isolation, he shifts, in a rather flexible way, from the one to the other so that the acceptant position functions as a meaningful dialogical response to the perfectionist. Elements from one position are introduced as elements into the other so that, moving from the one to the other, their relational contrasts, oppositions, conflicts, and integrations are made visible.

Some of the main positions in Richard's case are summarized in Figure 15.1. At the same time this Figure can be used to illustrate some of the key elements of dialogical-self theory.

The Extension of the Self in Contemporary Society

James (1890) proposed that the self can be depicted as a circle. Elaborating on James's proposal, Figure 15.1 represents the self as a space composed of a multiplicity of positions distributed in two concentric circles. The inner

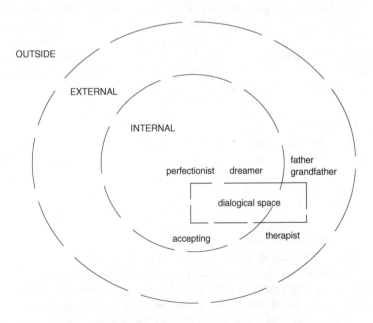

FIGURE 15.1. Domains of the self: Richard's main positions.

circle represents the *internal* domain of the self. It includes positions that are felt by the individual as belonging to him- or herself (e.g., "I as a perfectionist," "I as a dreamer"), whereas the outer circle refers to the *external* domain, that is, the extended self in terms of James (e.g., "my grandfather," "my therapist"). The parts of the circles where current positions are located represents a field of activity that functions as an arena for dialogue (Valsiner, 2000), where internal and external positions meet in processes of negotiation, cooperation, opposition, conflict, agreement, and disagreement. This arena is represented by the rectangle in Figure 15.1.

The circles in Figure 15.1 are partly open, suggesting that the boundaries between the different domains are highly permeable. The self is not an entity that is limited to internal positions only, but is extended to other positions in the extended domain. In more dynamic terms: the individual positions him- or herself in relation to one or more other positions or groups of positions. It should be noted that the process of positioning is not an activity that is always under the control of the individual. Dialogical activities among people imply that an individual is also "positioned" by other individuals or by the society to which the individual belongs. For example, Richard was positioned by his grandfather as "a child without any persistence."

The area in Figure 15.1 that is indicated as "outside" indicates a universe of people and groups of people that include "possible positions" for the self. They are somewhere outside the horizon of the individual self, but they can, depending on change of situations and time, become part of it. For example, before Richard asked for therapeutic assistance, the therapist was somewhere outside the boundaries of the self. As soon as he contacted her and regularly visited her, she became, as "my therapist," part of the extended (external) domain of the self.

From a more general point of view, it is important to note that contemporary society requires a more open self than ever. The increase of education level, international contacts, intercultural exchanges, media information, and Internet communication (Appadurai, 1990; Castells, 1989; Clifford, 1997; Hermans & Kempen, 1998; Pieterse, 1995) provides the self with a vast amount of positions and corresponding values that may enter the self in an increasing rate. In our present era, often labeled as "postmodern," we witness an unprecedented intensification of the flow and flux of positions entering the self-space and leaving it within relatively short time periods. Some challenging questions can be posed here, such as: Does this flow and flux lead to an empty self (Cushman, 1990) or to a saturated self (Gergen, 1991), or does it lead to a reorganization of the self so that an intensified flow of positions is counteracted by an increasing need for more stable positions in order to guarantee a minimal consistency of the self system?

An interesting point is made in a study by Kaufman (1991) on "newly-Orthodox Jewish women." Many women who grew up in secular Jewish homes in the United States found that secular values provided an inadequate foundation for their lives. In their teens or 20s they converted to Orthodox Judaism, despite the limitations it placed on women. They did so because the Orthodox Jewish belief system offered them the feeling of having a definite place in the world and of being rooted in a long, durable tradition. In a recent review of the psychology of globalization, Arnett (2002) refers in this context to the emergence of various kinds of fundamentalist movements in both Western and non-Western societies. He and other theorists (e.g., Giddens, 2000) argue that many of these movements arose in the late 20th century as a direct reaction to the changes caused by globalization. Apparently, such a worldview provides the self with a stable religious position that is based on a belief in a sacred past and a hierarchy of authority with men over women, adults over children, and God over all (Arnett, 2002; Marty & Appleby, 1993).

In summary, the open circles of the self, as depicted in Figure 15.1, allow an intensified transaction between the internal and external domains of the self and between the self and the outside world. The process of globalization implies an increasing transaction between self and world, challenging the boundaries of the self and populating it with a greater variety of positions than ever before in the history of humankind. This increasing "multiplicity of the self" (Hermans & Kempen, 1998; Rosenberg, 1997) poses the question of how the self responds to this increasing openness. Three reactions are possible: (1) the self becomes an arena of moving and mixing positions entering the self at a high speed and leading to a turbulent lifestyle; (2) the self returns to stable positions to compensate for the increasing fluctuation and instability of the social and cultural environment; and (3) the self reorganizes on the basis of a mixture of rapidly changing positions and a number of stable positions that enable the self to be open to the fluctuating environment, while at the same time establishing a sufficient degree of stability in order to maintain a basic sense of continuity.

Moving between External and Internal Positions

The Vygotskian (1978) thesis that the relationship of the mind with itself is preceded by the relationship of the mind with other minds can also be observed in Richard's case. The development of the accepting position was not restricted to the internal domain of the self. Rather, it first emerged from the dialogical relationship between Richard and the therapist and then was introduced into his internal domain. Certainly, the possibility can never be excluded that somewhere in the background of the self-space there was a "sleeping" accepting position before Richard contacted the therapist. Even if this was the case, however, this position was actualized as a result of the interaction between the two parties. It was the therapist who triggered the position in question. Apart from the question whether the crucial change was instigated by the introduction of a new position or by the foregrounding of an already existing position, the open nature of the self allows a position to move from the external to the internal domain, that is, the accepting position, originally located in the person of the therapist, moves from the external to the internal domain of the self and is incorporated as a more or less established part of the internal domain.

An informative example of the movement between domains in the self was recently presented by Gieser (2004) in a cultural-anthropological analysis of a form of radical identity change known as "shape shifting." Practiced by the Kuranko people of Sierra-Leone, shape shifting can be described as the culturally supported ability of a man to transform into an animal so that it can give him a sense of power, control, meaning, healing, and identity. Gieser, drawing on an earlier study by Jackson (1989), described the phenomenon of shape shifting as closely connected to a particular feature of the Kuranko people: their tendency to externalize and even spatialize internal events. For example, for the Kuranko, memory is seen as happening somewhere else, personhood resides in social relationships rather than in individuals, and the unconscious is represented by going into the bush. So, shape shifting is described as an inward change from the conscious into the unconscious, expressed as an exterior movement from town to bush. The typical ritual is that a man who wants to transform himself goes into the bush and identifies with the totem animal of the clan (e.g., an elephant), which then empowers him to extend his possibilities beyond the ordinary. When he returns to the village, he is respected by the other members of the clan and may even receive the status of a hero because he has proven the power of the Kuranko to tap the powers of the wild and confirmed the moral bond between his clanspeople and their totem animal.

In an insightful analysis, Gieser (2004) has discussed the process of shape shifting from the perspective of dialogical-self theory. An external position (the animal as object of shape shifting) is transformed into an internal position (I as animal). As soon as the external position is internalized, it becomes so dominant that it suppresses all other positions in the internal domain. In this phase of the transformation, the power asymmetries between the positions are pushed to the extreme. This asymmetry represents a dialogical form, which is described by Valsiner (2002) as "expropriating the other," a subclass of instability-bound forms of dialogical relations. The voice of the internalized character is so dominant that it leads to "monologicalization": there is only one voice, the voice of the person-as-animal, and all other voices are suppressed. The shape-shifter believes that he has transformed himself into the reality of another being. However, the effect is temporary. After the period of shape shifting, the new position loses its dominance and becomes a normal dialoguing partner in a multivoiced self. Gradually, it stabilizes itself in the repertoire together with all the characteristics the shape-shifter attributes to it (power, control, and healing). Although the new position loses its absolute dominance in the self after the shape shifting, it still has the power to subordinate earlier positions that were associated with marginality and powerlessness (Gieser, 2004).

The phenomenon of shape shifting not only exemplifies the increasing interest of cultural anthropologists in the "multiplicity of identity" (see Van Meijl & Driessen, 2003, for a review), it also elucidates the process of positioning and repositioning, typical of a radical identity change in a particular culture. The process of shape shifting can be summarized by two subsequent movements: (1) from an external to an internal position (an animal in the world becomes internalized) and (2) from an internal to an external position (the animal recedes and takes its place in the external world again). The result is a thorough reorganization and innovation of the position repertoire of the shape-shifter.

Although there are significant cultural differences between the phenomenon of shape shifting and the example of therapeutic change, there is a basic similarity in the latent structure of the change process. Not only the shape shifting, but also the therapeutic process as illustrated by Richard's case, can be described as an external–internal–external movement. Initially, the therapist was represented by Richard as an external position, but, as far as he identifies with her and her accepting attitude, she is introduced in his internal domain, so that Richard becomes more acceptant of himself. After the therapy, when the contact with the therapist is reduced or finished, she moves again to the external domain but leaves her traces in a reorganized internal domain.

Compensatory versus Complementary Relationship between Positions

The term "position" is chosen because it is a spatial term that by its nature suggests that there are always one or more other positions involved. Between different or opposed positions, dialogical relationships may develop in a field of tension emerging between the positions involved.

Because positions are always part of a position repertoire and always related to other positions, the nature of these relationships requires special attention. A distinction, proposed by Benjamin (1997), between compensatory and complementary relationships, seems to be of particular importance to a flexible functioning of the self: The difference between the two kinds of relationship can be illustrated by the example of Richard. The relationship between the dreamer and the perfectionist is typically of a *compensatory* nature. By ineffective fantasizing and building air castles, the dreamer is continuously filling a gap that is created by the dictatorial perfectionist. Because Richard does not feel able to fulfill the high standards of the perfectionist, he escapes into unproductive fantasies. However, in this way, the dreamer is never able to present an effective counterweight to the perfectionist, who maintains his position of power in spite of the futile efforts of the dreamer to fulfill the demands of the perfectionist.

The relationship between the accepting position and the perfectionist position is more of a *complementary* nature. Instead of functioning as a slave of the perfectionist, the accepting position introduces a quality that directly addresses the extravagant demands of the perfectionist. In one of the excerpts presented earlier in this chapter, Richard addressed the perfectionist from the perspective of the accepting position in this way: "Look forward, you get this free, consider your possibilities which are available and be content with what you have." In this sentence Richard directly addresses the extreme demands of the perfectionist, and along these lines tries to provide a real counterweight to the superpower who hitherto ruled the entire self system. Whereas the dreamer can only continue to confirm the established position of the perfectionist, providing no more than transient relaxation in the best case, the accepting position has the potential to limit the expansion of the perfectionist by giving, instead of a compensating, a correcting answer.

The phenomenon of shape shifting can also function as an example of a complementary relationship. Although the totem animal functions as a superpower during the process of shape shifting, it entertains a complementary relationship after the transformation has taken place. The internalized animal functions as a culturally supported and productive promoter of health and contributes to the status and respect the shape-shifter receives as a member of the clan. In this sense, the new position provides a healthy counterweight to experiences of powerlessness and social insignificance. That is, the accepting position in Richard's case and the new identity in the case of the shape-shifter have in common that they both have the potential to function as counterforces that are sufficiently different, opposed and, at the same time *fitting* to the nature of the perfectionist and the marginalized clan member, respectively.

As illustrated by Richard's case and the phenomenon of shape shifting, complementary relationships assume a certain heterogeneity and variety of the position repertoire and, as such, they contribute to its flexibility. Both the perfectionist in Richard's case and the powerless figure in the shape shifting are faced with a counterposition (Leiman, 2002) that offers a new possibility for action. Different positions have different memories, motivations, and goals, and, along these lines, different implications for a person's actions (Josephs, 2002; Hermans, 2001a, 2001b). A complementary position allows the individual to follow a track that is intrinsically different than the hitherto dominant position, in this way contributing to the adaptive capacities and flexibility of the system as a whole (Hermans & Hermans-Jansen, 1995).

Coalition of Positions: Shifting Loyalities in the Self

In this chapter it is argued that the self functions like a society of people. In the preceding section, we saw that some positions can compensate for or complement other positions. The same relationships can also be observed in a group of people in which, for example, one of the members takes the role of the joker, compensating for the unpleasant atmosphere created by an authoritarian leader. We are all familiar with situations where two team members are working together, with one having particular qualities that complement the qualities of the other. Together, however, they excel in highly effective and productive teamwork. Along the same lines, it can be argued that positions can also cooperate with each other in order to form coalitions that have a common purpose in the self system. Moreover, positions, like team members, can look for new partners so that shifting coalitions may emerge over the course of time.

The case of Fred, a 50-year-old man, who described himself as a "persistent doubter," offers an example of changing coalition. I was his counselor for 18 months. In order to follow his changes in detail, I applied a Personal Position Repertoire (PPR) method that allows one to study not only the content of personal positions but also their organization (see Hermans, 2001b, for a more detailed description of the method and the present case).

In Fred's case, it was found that three positions were particularly significant in his present life: the doubter, the perfectionist, and—somewhat at the background but very important to him—the enjoyer of life. The last position was certainly an enduring feature of his personal history, but seemed to be suppressed by the combination of the doubter and the perfectionist, with the latter position compensating for the anxiety aroused by the former.

In the course of the sessions, we discovered that the perfectionist could be tackled by learning to delegate tasks to other people at the right moment. Instead of completing a task in full detail, Fred learned to contact other people in order to cooperate on some of the tasks. He even delegated some tasks before he started the job. After more than a year of practicing this new style of working, we decided to investigate his position repertoire again. The most significant finding was that the perfectionist and the enjoyer had formed a coalition, one strong enough to push the doubter to the background of the self system. Whereas in the first investigation the perfectionist formed a coalition with the doubter, in the second investigation the perfectionist changed camps and joined the enjoyer of life, leading to a new coalition. This enabled Fred to work with more pleasure and to cooperate more easily with other people.

In order to study the new coalition (the perfectionist and the enjoyer) in more depth, I decided to study Fred's repertoire on the basis of a posi-

TABLE 15.1. Fred's Positions of the Doubter, Perfectionist, and Enjoyer of Life at Investigation 1 and Investigation 2

Investigation 1: Doubter and perfectionist versus enjoyer of life
Investigation 2: Enjoyer and perfectionist versus doubter

Correlation between enjoyer and perfectionist and "deep-down inside": .81
Correlation between enjoyer and "deep-down inside": .32
Correlation between perfectionist and "deep-down inside": .41

Valuation linking the doubter, the perfectionist, and the enjoyer:
"I accept the perfectionist in myself; I'm convinced that this is something which has grown in me, probably as a result of fear of failure; at the same time, the enjoyer cannot exist without the perfectionist; however, I don't let the perfectionist destruct me any more; they should learn to deal with each other and to make compromises; when something is performed well, I can enjoy it."

Note. Data from Hermans (2001b).

tion matrix in which the rows represent the internal positions and the columns the external positions. Each cell of the matrix represented the extent to which a particular internal position was prominent in relation to a particular external position. One of the internal positions was "I as deep-down inside," which was introduced into the matrix as a standard internal position. The investigation was organized in such a way that the separate positions (the perfectionist and the enjoyer apart) could be compared with their coalition (the perfectionist and the enjoyer as a team). The coalition showed a high correlation ($r = .81$) with "deep-down inside," higher than the correlations of the separate positions with "deep-down inside" ($r = .32$ and $r = .41$, respectively, see Table 15.1). This finding suggests that the coalition was not simply an addition of the separate positions but rather had the nature of a Gestalt with a surplus value above its constituents.

Metaposition as Committee Work

It should be noted that, although dialogical-self theory acknowledges the relative independence of positions, the several positions as part of an organized repertoire do not work in isolation of each other. In order to get more insight into the linkages between the separate positions, a participant or client can be invited to formulate the nature of their relationship in his or her own terms. In order to examine the relationship between the three positions (doubter, perfectionist, and enjoyer) from the perspective of the client, Fred was invited to phrase his insight in the relationship between the three positions at the end of the second investigation. He then formulated a personal meaning ("valuation") regarding the connections between the

three positions (see Table 15.1). In this valuation he emphasized the importance of cooperation between the enjoyer and the perfectionist and, moreover, placed the several positions in the broader context of his personal history. This formulation suggests that the client is able to consider the
linkages between a variety of positions in a way that is personally meaningful.

Fred's valuation in Table 15.1 can be considered the expression of a
metaposition, a perspective from which he phrases the linkages between
several significant positions in a self-reflective way. Several researchers
have proposed to introduce the notion of a metaposition or observing position (e.g., Georgaca, 2001; Hermans, 2003; Leiman, 2002) as a welcome
theoretical contribution to dialogical-self theory.

What is a metaposition? This question can be answered by imagining
a tennis player who is involved in a game. As long as he is in the game, the
best he can do is to concentrate fully on the task at hand. Any distraction
or any self-doubt would interfere with his performance. As long as he is
fully engaged at the moment of action, he is just *in* the position of the
player. As soon as he finishes the game, he may reflect on his own achievement, that is, he may think *about* his position as player. He is then on a
second level. At this level he may evaluate his play as good or bad or may
be satisfied or dissatisfied about some of his specific accomplishments. As
an *I* he evaluates his *Me* in this particular position and, as a result of this
evaluation, he may take a decision to follow a different strategy next time.
The player moves to a third level when he is faced with a question about
his future career. Will he continue to invest his best efforts in tennis? Does
he want to make tennis his career? Does he go for Wimbledon or not? At
this level of self-reflection, he explores the connection between his position
as tennis player and some other significant positions, for example, he as a
father, as a husband, or as a student who is very good in math. After he has
thought about this broader array of positions and talked about it with
some wise advisors, he has the feeling that he can make the right decision.
In sum, the tennis player can be at three levels: (1) being purely in a position; (2) reflecting on the position itself; and (3) reflecting on the specific
position as part of an interconnected web of other positions. The term
"metaposition"' is reserved for the last level.

A metaposition has some specific qualities: (1) it permits a certain distance toward the other positions, although it is attracted, both cognitively
and emotionally, toward some positions more than others; (2) it provides
some overarching view so that several positions can be seen simultaneously; (3) it leads to an evaluation of the several positions and their
organization; (4) it enables an individual to see the linkages between positions as part of his or her personal history (or the collective history of the
group or culture to which the individual belongs); (5) the individual
becomes aware of the differences in the accessibility of positions; (6) the

importance of one or more positions for future development of the self becomes apparent; and (7) it facilitates the creation of a dialogical space in which positions and counterpositions entertain significant dialogical relationships (Hermans, 2003).

A metaposition is not to be considered the "center" of the position repertoire or an agentic force that guarantees the unity and coherence of the self in advance. In order to avoid this confusion, it should be remembered that a metaposition is always bound to one or more internal and external positions that are actualized at a particular moment and in a particular situation. Moreover, depending on time and situation, different metapositions can emerge. Finally, as each position has its horizon, a metaposition, although it may permit meaningful linkages between a variety of positions, has a limited point of view and is far from a "God's eye view." These limitations are the consequence of the basic assumption that multiplicity precedes any unity or synthesis of the self. Unity and coherence are considered an achievement rather than a given (Hermans & Kempen, 1993).

A metaposition can be compared with a meeting of a committee in which representatives of a particular community discuss issues that are relevant to the well functioning of the community at large. Within the committee there are frequent interchanges in which different points of view are related and compared. Some representatives may be more influential than others and have more impact on the decision process. Finally, the committee reaches a conclusion, with one of the representatives having the most influence on the end result. In the beginning of Richard's therapy, it was the perfectionist who was discovered to be the most influential representative. However, in the course of the therapy, the accepting position played an increasingly important role and developed himself as a serious counterforce to the perfectionist. Each of the positions depicted in Figure 15.1 play a specific role in Richard's everyday life depending on the situation in which they are actualized. However, as soon as they are represented at the metalevel, they are brought together in an arena of dialogue as indicated by the rectangle in Figure 15.1.

Dominance Reversal as Radical Change

In everyday conversations the notion of "dialogue" is often depicted as a group of people sitting at a round table and discussing topics in a power-free way, with the expectation that they understand each other perfectly. I consider this conception of dialogue as a romantic ideal. In fact, dialogue is more power-laden than the romantic version suggests. Stronger, dialogue is intrinsically asymmetric and can only be realized when differences in the relative dominance of the interaction partners are taken into account.

In a study of participants in conversation, Linell (1990) argued that asymmetry exists in *each* individual act–response sequence. When participating in a process of turn taking, speakers can only communicate in meaningful ways if they are able to take initiatives and display their views in turn. As part of a reciprocal process, the actors continually alternate the roles of "power holder" and "power subject" in the course of their conversation. There are a variety of ways in which one of the parties can be said to control the "territory" to be shared by the interactants in communication. One party may take the most initiatory moves (interactional dominance), introduce topics and the perspective on topics (topic dominance), make the most strategic moves (strategic dominance), or just talk more than the other party (amount of talk as dominance). As these examples suggest, power is an intrinsic feature of turn taking and not something that is in contradiction with dialogue or alien to its nature. Verbal and even nonverbal dialogue needs some organization, implying that relative dominance is indispensable (see also Minsky, 1985, for a comparable view).

Apart from intrinsic differences between the partners in conversation, there are, moreover, institutional factors that contribute to power differences in dialogical processes. Such factors, present in institutional and societal structures, may enhance the power differences between the interaction partners. In an interrogation, for example, dialogue is usually strongly asymmetrical because one of the parties, the suspect, is forced into a yes-or-no answer frame and is hardly allowed to take initiatives. Or, in another example, parents are in a societal position to use extensively the dominance aspects of the dialogue, so that children do not have much opportunity to express their views themselves. In a study of pediatric consultations, Aronsson and Rundström (1988) observed that parents routinely step in as the spokespersons for their children. Even when the doctor addresses the child directly, mothers simply take their children's turn, reinforcing what the children said and explaining what they meant, so that the children do not get the opportunity to express it properly themselves (Linell, 1990, p. 162). Certainly, power differences can be reduced—for example, in an intimate conversation between friends—but they never disappear entirely.

Dominance reversals among positions can also be found in the case of radical change of the self. In a study of changes of the self through time, Hermans and Kempen (1993) compared the stories told by a research participant, Alice, as emerging from two opposed positions, described by the participant as "my open side" and "my closed side." From her open position she told stories that centered mainly around her unproblematic relationship with her mother, whereas from her closed side she related events that referred largely to her problematic relationship with her father. After the investigation, Alice was requested to rate her stories on two variables: relative dominance ("How dominant was this aspect of your life during the past week?") and meaningfulness ("How meaningful was this aspect of your life during the past week?"). It was found that, over the 3-week period, story parts of her closed position became more dominant than the story parts of her open position, whereas the elements of the latter position receded to the background. This change represents a clear example of a "dominance reversal," also found in another study (Hermans, 1996b). At the same time the meaningfulness of the stories from Alice's closed position increased strongly with a simultaneous decrease of the meaningfulness of the stories from her open position. Apparently, the increasing dominance of her closed position was experienced as highly meaningful, although this position was associated with a great deal of negative emotions. From her diary notes it could be concluded that the increase of meaning of her closed position could be understood as bringing hitherto neglected or suppressed experiences to the surface and as helping her to improve the relationships with her father and other family members. This study suggests that dominance may play a facilitating role for change of the self and is a necessary condition for bringing valuable forces to the surface that were hitherto neglected or suppressed. Dominance becomes a debilitating factor only if the position repertoire becomes rigidly organized and impedes an ongoing dialogue, as can be observed in the persistent neglect, suppression, or silencing of positions in a community of selves (Dimaggio, Salvatore, Azzara, & Catania, 2003).

The sudden rise of neglected or suppressed positions was already observed by James in his *Varieties of Religious Experience* (1902/1982). In this work James was interested not only in religious conversions of historical figures, but also in instances of sudden change in the selves of ordinary people. An informative example is his description of a case of "falling out of love" (p. 179). It was about a man who suddenly stopped his relationship with a girl with whom he had fallen in love 2 years earlier. Looking back at this period, the man described how he had fallen violently in love with a girl who had "a spirit of coquetry." He secretly knew that the girl was not the right person for him, but he could not stop the relationship as he regularly fell into a fever and could think of nothing else. After a long period of being plagued by jealousy and contempt for his own uncontrollable weakness, there was a sudden change:

> The queer thing was the *sudden and unexpected* way in which it all stopped. I was going to my work after breakfast one morning, thinking as usual of her and of my misery, when, just as if some outside power laid hold of me, I found myself turning round and almost running to my room, where I immediately got out all the relics of her which I possessed, including some hair, all her notes and letters, and ambrotypes on glass. The former I made a fire of, the latter I actually crushed beneath my heel, in a sort of fierce joy of revenge and punishment. I now loathed and despised her altogether, and as for myself I felt as if a load of disease had suddenly been removed from me. That was the end. (James, 1902/1982, p. 180; emphasis added)

James (1902/1982) considers this case an example of an "unstable equilibrium" of the self: on the surface the relationship with the woman seems stable for a long time, but there is a hidden force somewhere beneath the surface that creates an unstable field of tension: "At last, not gradually, but in a sudden crisis, the unstable equilibrium is resolved" (p. 180). What James describes in terms of a reversal of two layers after a period of unstable equilibrium corresponds with a dominance reversal of two positions in the framework of the dialogical self (Hermans, 1996b).

There is also a significant difference between James's description of the man in love and Alice's case of dominance reversal. Whereas James's subject shows a radical change in a *spontaneous* crisis, our subject initiates a dominance reversal in a period of explicit and systematic self-reflection from a metaposition, arranged in a cooperative project of psychologist and subject. The data of our study suggest that, if one pole of a pair of opposites is subordinated or suppressed in a particular period, the same pole may become strongly dominant at some later point in time when the person is engaged in an intensified self-reflection. Although we do not understand very much *what* precisely determines the reversal of dominance, *when* it takes place, and by *whom* it takes place, its empirical description points to the relevance of dynamic psychological conceptions of the self, in which the possibility of radical change of oppositional poles in a seemingly stable self-organization requires attention in future research of the self. (For a discussion of radical changes from the perspective of chaos theory, see Schwalbe, 1991.)

A dominance reversal in the self is like a political revolution in a society. A seemingly stable society can arrive at a period of radical change, with hidden or suppressed forces taking the lead, resulting in a new social structure. In political revolutions it can be observed that the rise of a particular force in society often implies the subordination of the old forces in a reorganized structure (Clarke & Foweraker, 2001).

CHALLENGE FOR THE FUTURE

Several decades ago, Greenwald (1980) described the self as an analogue to a totalitarian state. He argued that the organization of the self is characterized by cognitive biases that are strikingly analogous to totalitarian information-control strategies. In developing his thesis, Greenwald was drawing on extensive bodies of empirical research into "egocentricity" (i.e., the self as the focus of knowledge), "beneffectance" (i.e., perception of responsibility for desired, but not undesired, outcomes), and "cognitive conservatism" (i.e., resistance to cognitive change). His purpose was to illustrate the striking similarity between these cognitive biases governing the self and the propaganda devices that are defining characteristics of a totalitarian political system.

A comparison between this totalitarian self and the dialogical self suggests that the two views of the self represent two partly contrasting perspectives. The totalitarian view presupposes a strongly hierarchical organization of the self with one highly centralized *I* position governing the self in an authoritarian, unidirectional way. Dialogical-self theory certainly supports the importance and even the necessity of power and social dominance in the organization of the self. However, it deviates from the metaphor of the authoritarian state in that it acknowledges and even aims to promote a structural organization in which the different forces or positions are mutually complementary. A society in which different, relatively autonomous, parties complement and control each other has the potential to function in democratic ways.

When self and society have some basic commonalities, it makes sense to study both of them in terms of two basic concepts: dialogical interchange and relative dominance. It is precisely the combination of these concepts that enables both society and self to become engaged in a continuous process of innovation.

REFERENCES

Appadurai, A. (1990). Disjuncture and difference in the global cultural economy. In M. Featherstone (Ed.), *Global culture: Nationalism, globalization and modernity* (pp. 295–310). London: Sage.

Arnett, J. J. (2002). The psychology of globalization. *American Psychologist, 57,* 774–783.

Aronsson, K., & Rundström, B. (1988). Child discourse and parental control in pediatric consultations. *Text, 8,* 159–189.

Bakhtin, M. (1973). *Problems of Dostoevsky's poetics* (2nd ed., R. W. Rotsel, Trans.). Ann Arbor, MI: Ardis. (Originally published in 1929 under the title *Problemy tvorchestva Dostoevskogo* [Problems of Dostoevsky's Art]).

Baldwin, M. W. (1992). Relational schemas and the processing of social information. *Psychological Bullletin, 112,* 461–484.

Barresi, J. (2002). From "the thought is the thinker" to "the voice is the speaker": William James and the dialogical self. *Theory and Psychology* (Special issue: The dialogical self), *12,* 237–250.

Benjamin, L. S. (1997). Human imagination and psychopathology. *Journal of Psychotherapy Integration, 7,* 195–211.

Bertau, M. C. (2004). Introduction: The theory of the dialogical self. In M. C. Bertau (Ed.), *Aspects of the dialogical self: Extended proceedings of a symposium on the Second Conference on the Dialogical Self (Ghent, October 2002).*

Bruner, J. S. (1986). *Actual minds, possible worlds.* Cambridge, MA: Harvard University Press.

Castells, M. (1989). *The informational city: Information technology, economic restructuring, and the urban–regional process.* Oxford, UK: Blackwell.

Clarke, P. B., & Foweraker, J. (2001). *Encyclopedia of democratic thought.* New York: Routledge.

Clifford, J. (1997). *Routes: Travel and translation in the late twentieth century.* Cambridge, MA: Harvard University Press.

Cushman, P. (1990). Why the self is empty: Toward a historically situated psychology. *American Psychologist, 45,* 599–611.

Damon, W., & Hart, D. (1982). The development of self-understanding from infancy through adolescence. *Child Development, 4,* 841–864.

Dimaggio, G., Salvatore, G., Azzara, C., & Catania, D. (2003). Rewriting self-narratives: The therapeutic process. *Journal of Constructivist Psychology* (Special issue: The dialogical self), *16,* 155–181.

Fogel, A. (1993). *Developing through relationships: Origins of communication, self, and culture.* Hertfordshire, UK: Harvester Wheatsheaf.

Georgaca, E. (2001). Voices of the self in psychotherapy: A qualitative analysis. *British Journal of Medical Psychology, 74,* 223–236.

Gergen, K. J. (1991). *The saturated self: Dilemmas of identity in contemporary life.* London: Sage.

Gergen, K. J., & Gergen, M. M. (1988). Narrative and the self as relationship. *Advances in Experimental Social Psychology, 21,* 17–56.

Giddens, A. (2000). *Runaway world: How globalization is reshaping our lives.* New York: Routledge.

Gieser, T. (2004, August). *Witchcraft, shapeshifting and the dialogical self: An anthropological application.* Paper presented at the Third International Conference on the Dialogical Self, Warsaw, Poland.

Greenwald, A. G. (1980). The totalitarian ego: Fabrication and revision of personal history. *American Psychologist, 35,* 603–618.

Harré, R., & Van Langenhove, L. (1991). Varieties of positioning. *Journal for the Theory of Social Behaviour, 21,* 393–407.

Hermans, H. J. M. (1996a). Voicing the self: From information processing to dialogical interchange. *Psychological Bulletin, 119,* 31–50.

Hermans, H. J. M. (1996b). Opposites in a dialogical self: Constructs as characters. *Journal of Constructivist Psychology, 9,* 1–26.

Hermans, H. J. M. (2001a). The dialogical self: Toward a theory of personal and cultural positioning. *Culture and Psychology* (Special issue: Culture and the dialogical self: Theory, method and practice), *7,* 243–281.

Hermans, H. J. M. (2001b). The construction of a personal position repertoire: Method and practice. *Culture and Psychology* (Special issue: Culture and the dialogical self: Theory, method and practice), *7,* 323–365.

Hermans, H. J. M. (2002). The dialogical self as a society of mind: Introduction. *Theory and Psychology* (Special issue: The dialogical self), *12,* 147–160.

Hermans, H. J. M. (2003). The construction and reconstruction of a dialogical self. *Journal of Constructivist Psychology* (Special issue: The dialogical self), *16,* 89–130.

Hermans, H. J. M., & Hermans-Jansen, E. (1995). *Self-narratives: The construction of meaning in psychotherapy.* New York: Guilford Press.

Hermans, H. J. M., & Kempen, H. J. G. (1993). *The dialogical self: Meaning as movement.* San Diego, CA: Academic Press.

Hermans, H. J. M., & Kempen, H. J. G. (1998). Moving cultures: The perilous problems of cultural dichotomies in a globalizing society. *American Psychologist, 53,* 1111–1120.

Hermans, H. J. M., Kempen, H. J. G., & Van Loon, R. J. P. (1992). The dialogical self: Beyond individualism and rationalism. *American Psychologist, 47,* 23–33.

Jackson, M. (1989). The man who could turn into an elephant. In M. Jackson (Ed.), *Paths toward a clearing: Radical empiricism and ethnographic inquiry* (pp. 102–118). Bloomington: Indiana University Press.

James, W. (1890). *The principles of psychology* (Vol. 1). London: Macmillan.

James, W. (1982). *The varieties of religious experience: A study in human nature* (Gifford Lectures on Natural Religion, delivered at Edinburgh, 1901–1902). New York: Penguin Books.

Josephs, I. E. (2002). "The hopi in me": The contruction of a voice in the dialogical self from a cultural psychological perspective. *Theory and Psychology* (Special issue: The dialogical self), *12,* 161–173.

Kaufman, D. (1991). *Rachel's daughters: Newly-Orthodox Jewish women.* New Brunswick, NJ: Rutgers University Press.

Leiman, M. (2002). Toward semiotic dialogism: The role of sign-mediation in the dialogical self. *Theory and Psychology* (Special issue: The dialogical self), *12,* 221–235.

Lewis, M. D. (2002). The dialogical brain: Contributions of emotional neurobiology to understanding the dialogical self. *Theory and Psychology* (Special issue: The dialogical self), *12,* 175–190.

Linell, P. (1990). The power of dialogue dynamics. In I. Marková & K. Foppa (Eds.), *The dynamics of dialogue* (pp. 147–177). New York: Harvester Wheatsheaf.

Marty, M. E., & Appleby, R. S. (1993). *Fundamentalisms and society.* Chicago: University of Chicago Press.

McAdams, D. P. (1993). *The stories we live by: Personal myths and the making of the self.* New York: William Morrow.

Minsky, M. (1985). *The society of mind.* New York: Simon & Schuster.

Montaigne, M. de (1603). *The essayes; or, Morall, politike and millitarie discourses* (J. Florio, Trans.). London: Blount. (Original work published 1580)

Pieterse, J. N. (1995). Globalization as hybridization. In M. Featherstone, S. Lash, & R. Robertson (Eds.), *Global modernities* (pp. 45–68). London: Sage.

Rosenberg, M. (1979). *Conceiving the self.* New York: Basic Books.

Rosenberg, S. (1997). Multiplicity of selves. In R. D. Ashmore & L. Jussim (Eds.), *Self and identity: Fundamental issues* (pp. 23–45). New York: Oxford University Press.

Sarbin, T. R. (1986). The narrative as a root metaphor for psychology. In T. R. Sarbin (Ed.), *Narrative psychology: The storied nature of human conduct* (pp. 3–21). New York: Praeger.

Schwalbe, M. L. (1991). The autogenesis of the self. *Journal for the Theory of Social Behaviour, 21,* 269–295.

Straus, E. W. (1958). Aesthesiology and hallucinations. In R. May, E. Angel, & H. F. Ellenberger (Eds.), *Existence. A new dimension in psychiatry and psychology* (pp. 139–169). New York: Basic Books.

Valsiner, J. (2000, June 23–26). Making meaning out of mind: Self-less and self-ful dialogicality. Presentation at the First International Conference on the Dialogical Self, Nijmegen, The Netherlands.

Valsiner, J. (2002). Forms of dialogical relations and semiotic autoregulation within the self. *Theory and Psychology* (Special issue: The dialogical self), *12*, 251–265.

Van Meijl, T., & Driessen, H. (2003). Introduction: Multiple identifications and the self. *Focaal* (European Journal of Anthropology), *42*, 17–29.

Vasil'eva, I. I. (1988). The importance of M. M. Bakhtin's idea of dialogue and dialogic relations for the psychology of communication. *Soviet Psychology, 26*, 17–31.

Vygotsky, L. S. (1978). *Mind in society: The development of higher psychological processes*. Cambridge, MA: Harvard University Press.

16

An Integrative Review of Theories of Interpersonal Cognition

An Interdependence Theory Perspective

JOHN G. HOLMES *and* JESSICA CAMERON

The process of writing several integrative review papers (Holmes, 2000, 2002, 2004) has led the senior author to two conclusions about the field of close relationships. The first is that relationship cognition is the most important new direction for theory and research in the field, a direction that holds considerable promise for unraveling the mysteries of relationships. This conclusion certainly reinforces the benefits of collecting chapters covering the major perspectives into the current volume. The second conclusion is that the absence of a broad theoretical model capable of providing some integrative structure and "discipline" to the field of interpersonal cognition results in a variety of disparate points of view with seemingly little in common. This occurs in part as each midlevel theory introduces a new conceptual language that makes it difficult to fathom the points of similarity and distinctiveness among differing perspectives. This conclusion warns us of the risk of fragmenting the field by focusing on supposedly divergent, "competing" perspectives on relationship cognition.

In this chapter we first propose that tenets of interdependence theory could usefully serve as a broad framework for understanding both the content and structure of relational schemas. The theory essentially provides a prescriptive ideal detailing what social cognition is potentially "about," or the various elements that might comprise relational schemas. That is, the framework outlines the variety of *possible* distinctions that might be reflected in people's representations of their relationships based on a depiction of the "interpersonal realities" the representations were designed to capture. The theory can then be used as a template for evaluating and depicting various models of relational schemas, and for classifying and contrasting them according to the heuristic assumptions and social learning principles to which they seem to adhere.

After describing the interdependence theory framework, we use it to evaluate a number of prominent theories of relationship cognition, including Baldwin's (1992) relational schema model, the CAPS model of Mischel and Shoda (1995), attachment theory notions of working models (Mikulincer & Shaver, 2003), and the transference model of social cognition (Andersen & Chen, 2002). Our critique attempts to highlight both the strengths and weaknesses of the theories from the point of view of interdependence theory and to contrast their different virtues. Each theory has in our opinion unique core strengths that would not be lost by revisions that would enable the theory to contribute to a broader, more general integrative model.

Why have we chosen to focus on these particular theories? By attempting to identify the limitations of various theories we are not likely to increase our circle of friends. Thus we selected our favorite theories, theories that we believe are inoculated against criticism by the overall quality and richness of their ideas. Our goal is to spur a constructive discussion around four issues: the activation of schemas, the lawfulness of the content of relational cognition, individual differences and specific versus general models, and, finally, central themes in a normative process model of interpersonal cognition. Before we turn to a commentary on the theories, we first review prior work on the interdependence theory perspective as it relates to interpersonal cognition.

INTERDEPENDENCE THEORY

This distilled version of recent theoretical work on interdependence theory is adapted from a book by Kelley and Holmes (2003) that was being developed before Hal Kelley died in 2003. Some of the implications of this general theory for social cognitive processes have been developed in a paper by Holmes (2002). Generally speaking, interdependence theory (IT) expands the formula proposed by Lewin (1946) that behavior is a function of the person and the environment. In the context of a social relationship, the behavioral interaction (I) that occurs between persons A and B is a function of both persons' respective goal tendencies in relation to each other in the particular situation of interdependence (S) in which the interaction occurs.

Each "situation" specifies the ways in which two persons are dependent on and influence each other with respect to their outcomes (hence the term "interdependence"). The theory attempts to identify the kinds of interpersonal dispositions of persons A and B—their attitudes, motives, and goals—that are *functionally* relevant to dealing with decisions in each particular type of situation. Then the type of situation S, together with the relevant dispositions of A and B, determine the interaction I (in symbols, the SABI elements; Kelley & Holmes, 2003.) As this model implies, interdependence theory adopts a person-by-situation interactionist approach with a strong social-psychological focus on the nature of "situations." Each paradigmatic situation is viewed as presenting the two persons with a unique set of problems and opportunities.

The Person and the Situation

To give the reader some understanding of how a "situation" is defined in IT terms, an example of a 2 × 2 outcome matrix is presented in Figure 16.1a. This well-known situation involves "Exchange with Mutual Profit" (also known as the "Prisoner's Dilemma"). The particular numbers used to represent the consequences for the two persons of any pair of behavioral choices are intended to provide a symbolic representation of individuals' satisfaction or dissatisfaction with an interaction event, rather than concrete outcomes of any particular kind. The *abstract pattern* of numbers represents the essential social problem that a situation poses, the "dilemma" that individuals face. Thus the abstract features of a situation as in Figure 16.1a are intended to capture the essence of many concrete interdependence problems.

Figure 16.1a is classified as an exchange situation because each person has the ability to reward or help the other (by giving 10 units through choosing Option 1). If both individuals cooperate and conclude such a reciprocal exchange, they will both profit equally and benefit from "gains in trade" by dividing up a larger "pie" (20 units) than is available by any other pair of choices. What complicates the situation and leads to the "dilemma" is that each person's personal preference (of 5 units) favors the other behavioral choice, Option 2. Thus each person is tempted to defect from the cooperative exchange and to choose the second option, which could result in the most individual gain and the greatest competitive advantage (if the other person chooses Option 1). For example, a husband and wife both dislike cleaning the dishes, but if both pitch in, the task is quickly accomplished and they reap the benefits of cooperation. Of course, each would be sorely tempted, if the other started the job, to just let the partner finish the unpleasant task. That way, the dishes are done and the dreaded task is once again avoided!

A central idea in the theory is that situations differ in terms of the particular interpersonal dispositions relevant to coping with the specific prob-

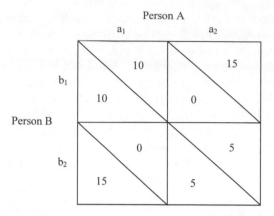

FIGURE 16.1a. Mutual exchange with profit situation.

lems they represent. Thus the linkages between the situation and the person domains are ones of logical relevance, or *affordance*. Essentially, interpersonal dispositions reflect people's preference ratings, or "valuations," of the different interaction possibilities afforded by a particular situation. We conceptualize this process of evaluating behavioral options and making choices as the application of *rules*. By distinguishing the valuation rules logically applicable to various situations, we essentially summarize the various attitudes, motives, and goals that guide interpersonal behavior.

For instance, the Exchange with Mutual Profit situation in Figure 16.1a provides the opportunity through the choice of a rule for "being" a certain type of person, but not other types. This situation provides the opportunity for expressing "cooperative" or prosocial goals, because selecting Option 1 would follow valuation rules to "maximize joint profit" or "achieve equality." Alternatively, a person might have a valuation rule that specifies "maximize one's own competitive advantage" or "maximize own outcomes." This situation does *not* allow people to express a variety of other possible interpersonal goals, such as being dominant or submissive, showing initiative, being loyal or dependable, and so on.

Thus the situation and the person domains exist in close, complementary relation to each other. One way to describe this relation is to say that each disposition can be defined abstractly as a tendency to psychologically *transform* one situation into another one, or using Lewin's (1946) concept, to "restructure the field." In our current example, a cooperative person would thus be someone who turned this inherently ambiguous (i.e., "mixed-motive") situation into a cooperative one by attaching particular value to the cooperative pair solution. From this perspective, one can only identify the "person" as a "figure" against the "ground" of the situation.

As we hope the reader will grasp intuitively from this example, how-ever, the actor's (A) choice of rules does not occur in a vacuum. The goal person A pursues is likely to depend heavily on expectations about the other's goals and motives (B). Indeed, Holmes (2002) has suggested that expectations about the other person's goals are the single most important and basic consideration in interpersonal relations, one that probably has evolutionary roots. Thus, not only may two partners be behaviorally inter-dependent, but they will frequently be *rule-interdependent* as well, espe-cially in long-term close relationships. That is, an actor's rule may be *con-tingent* on the rule he or she expects the other person to choose.

Put another way, the type of person one can "be" is often constrained by the type of person a partner is "expected to be." In Kelley and Stahelski's (1970) pioneering research exploring the social dilemma de-picted in Figure 16.1a, for instance, cooperative individuals typically held contingent rules for the goal they would pursue, following a cooperative rule only if they expected the other person to reciprocate. Faced with someone they believed had a competitive goal, they could not "be them-selves" and instead engaged in more competitive behaviors.

A Taxonomy of Situations

A group of scholars recently extended IT by developing a systematic taxon-omy of situations (*An Atlas of Interpersonal Situations*; Kelley et al., 2003). By applying analysis of variance logic to the 2×2 matrix depiction of situations, they demonstrated that each such situation can be character-ized by four dimensions. The first dimension involves the degree of interde-pendence between two persons, that is, the extent to which each has influ-ence over the other's outcomes. A high degree of interdependence defines one sense of the term "closeness" (Berscheid, 1983). The second dimension involves the extent to which dependence is mutual or unequal, with one person having less power than the other. The third dimension involves the degree of correspondence of the two persons' outcomes, ranging from cor-responding to conflicting interests. The fourth dimension involves the dis-tinction between exchange and coordination problems. These two types of problems constitute the "basis" of interdependence and differ as to whether the main "problem" people must deal with concerns justice in terms of who gets what, or instead, mutual control and initiative in coordi-nating actions.

The situation depicted in Figure 16.1b is an example of the important category of situations involving *coordination* (rather than exchange) prob-lems. Such situations are extremely common in close relationships. For ex-ample, the numbers in the matrix closely mirror the preference ratings from a study of dating couples deciding which movie to attend (Kelley, 1979). The large numbers in the diagonal make it clear that the two per-

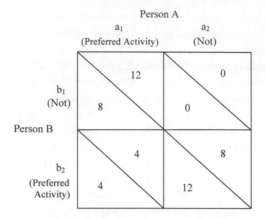

(Strong mutual desire to do same activity is
complicated by difference in preferred activity)

FIGURE 16.1b. A matching example of hero.

sons have a strong mutual desire to coordinate their actions so that they
can enjoy doing things together. However, they have different personal
preferences (of four units) for which movie to attend, and have to find a
way to determine whose preferred movie they will attend jointly.

This situational structure is typically given the name "Hero" because
it affords the opportunity for either person to show initiative and say,
"Let's do it your way," thereby exerting a type of leadership by stepping
forward and selecting the movie preferred by the partner. Though this initiative furthers joint goals, it is clearly considerate of the partner's feelings
and benefits the partner the most. On the other hand, behavioral preemp-
tion could also be used in a controlling fashion by selecting one's own preferred movie, either for somewhat selfish reasons or as a result of
egocentrically assuming the partner wants what you want.

In many situations, such as Hero, there is more than one way to satisfy a particular goal, which in this case is to share an activity together and
maximize pair outcomes. The rules "take the initiative" or "wait for the
other to act first" represent the particular *means* of achieving the person's
overall goals. Such situations permit the expression of one form of dominance or submission, a tendency to display assertiveness or passivity in decision making and action.

Kelley et al. (2003) extended their analysis to include two further dimensions. The fifth dimension involves the temporal structure of the decision process (which is represented by a "transition list"). Some interactions
have immediate consequences, whereas others are extended in time, such

that the problem to be solved—the "goal" in the situation—is reached only at the end of a required sequence of intermediate steps. Two prototypical examples are delay of gratification and investment situations. Finally, a sixth dimension involves the extent to which uncertainty about outcomes is an essential feature of the situation. Whereas many situations involve quite complete information, others involve incomplete information about the other's outcomes or uncertainty about what the future holds. The six dimensions are listed in Table 16.1.

An Interactionist Perspective on Dispositions

The analysis of situations by Kelley et al. (2003) suggests that there are approximately two dozen prototypical situations like Exchange with Mutual Profit or Hero that have distinctive and interesting properties in terms of the type of problem or opportunity that they pose for the persons. By analyzing each of these prototypical situations, Kelley and Holmes have attempted to logically derive the full set of rules relevant to making choices within all the situations in our taxonomy. Clusters of rules that appear to have a common interpersonal "theme" or function can then be identified. (Some of these decisions would of course be open to interesting debate.) A quite limited number of such rule clusters or "dispositions" seems necessary for describing the set of possible adaptations to the problems encountered in prototypical social situations. Thus through such functional analysis, we can essentially deduce an interactionist theory of interpersonal dispositions.

Such dispositions could be regarded as the dimensions of "personality" if they described people's consistent response tendencies across interaction partners. Or they could be regarded as "relational dispositions" if they were *limited* to a specific close relationship. (Interestingly, two partners' set of dispositions would be one way of describing the nature of their "relationship.") We believe that there is much value in being able to describe personality and relational dispositions in commensurate terms so that the association between the two can be explored.

Though this work is still in progress, Kelley and Holmes reached some tentative conclusions about a possible set of interpersonal dispositions. The dispositions, not surprisingly, have an analogical correspondence to the dimensions of situations themselves. We have tried to make this correspondence apparent by the cross-listing in Table 16.1. The reader will note that the six dimensions of personality derived from our analysis have a rough correspondence to an integrated version of the "Big Five" and the two attachment style dimensions (with the anxiety dimension of attachment roughly corresponding to an interpersonal version of the neuroticism dimension from the Big Five). When the exact rule clusters that are the ba-

TABLE 16.1. Dimensions of Situations and Interpersonal Dispositions

Dimension of situation	Function of rule	Interpersonal disposition
1. Degree of interdependence	Increase or decrease dependence on partner	Avoidance of interdependence/ comfort with dependence
2. Mutuality of interdependence		
3. Correspondence of outcomes	Promote prosocial or self-interested goals	Cooperative/competitive Responsive/unresponsive
	Expectations about partner's goals	Anxiety about responsiveness/ confidence or trust
4. Basis of control	Control through exchange (promise/threat) or coordination (initiative/follow)	Dominant/submissive Assertive/passive
5. Temporal structure	Promote immediate or distant goal striving	Dependable/unreliable Loyal/uncommitted
6. Degree of uncertainty	Cope with incomplete information or uncertain future	Need for certainty/openness Optimism/pessimism

sis for the dimensions are examined in detail, they include facets of the traits that are quite different from the existing literature, as well as novel interpersonal perspectives on the various dispositions.

In this chapter we are not trying to persuade the reader of the virtues of this particular taxonomic system. Rather, we are using it to illustrate two crucial points. First, we need to have some means of classifying the specific *content* of people's interpersonal goals. The dispositions listed in Table 16.1 can be used not only to classify the goals of an actor (A), but also the interpersonal themes central to the actor's expectations about the interaction partner's (B) goals. Second, the theory is built on the inter-actionist premise that situations and dispositions have a complementary relation. This suggests that features of situations should be responsible for selectively activating expectations about *relevant* dispositions. Situations are thus a key organizing principle for one's own goals as well as expectations about others' goal tendencies.

The SABI Model as a Prescriptive Framework

The SABI model described above can be viewed as a prescriptive ideal for understanding the *possible* distinctions that people might make among situations and among categories of dispositions. It describes the basic *building blocks* for constructing mental models, the SABI elements that are potentially available to be combined, like Lego pieces, into a variety of different structures. Of course, people's *actual* mental models may deviate from such templates, often for very functional reasons. For instance, very articulated mental models might not be optimal if they forfeit the benefits of more efficient conceptual systems that capture important shared variance across partners and situations. The SABI model thus gives researchers the conceptual tools to allow comparison of the idealized theoretical map with the actual character of people's interpersonal cognitions. We can identify the ways in which people's thinking may be "truncated," favoring aggregation in particular areas of their interpersonal life, as compared to richly textured and complex, favoring differentiation. The extent to which particular heuristics and cognitive shortcuts prove useful and efficient versus damaging and dysfunctional can then be investigated.

The SABI model can also be used as a theoretical template for comparing the different assumptions and distinctions made by various theories, the task that we will attempt in the current chapter. Of course, theorists, like real people, could make a case that certain distinctions are best ignored for the sake of parsimony or efficiency in the cognitive system. By identifying the "shortcuts" taken by the various approaches, we hope to motivate theorists to either defend the current version of their model, or instead, to incorporate new elements into their perspectives. In what follows, we organize our discussion around four central issues highlighted by the SABI model of interdependence theory and discuss how the different theories deal with each issue.

THE ACTIVATION OF RELATIONAL SCHEMAS

Relational Schemas

The SABI model has four different elements, each of them interrelated in a tangled web. How well is this cognitive network captured by current theories? In a seminal integrative article, Baldwin (1992) theorized that a "relational schema" generally has three components: (1) a self-schema that represents how the self is experienced in interaction with another; (2) a partner schema that represents attributes of the partner; and (3) an interpersonal script represented as expectations generalized from past interactions, specifying "if–then" contingencies (e.g., "If I depend on my partner for support, I will be let down."). He further suggested that the relational schema notion implies a cognitive organization that would result in *conjoint priming* effects, whereby if one or more element is primed, the remaining elements should become more accessible.

Though he ignores situations as an organizing feature, Baldwin's theoretical framework very nicely reflects important aspects of the interdependence point of view, capturing the idea of two persons (A and B) in *relation* to each other, and the social interaction they produce (I). It contrasts dramatically with most previous social-cognitive models, which conceived of social schemata as generalized representations of the self, *or* of other persons, in isolation from each other. In reviewing these ideas, Holmes (2000, 2002) has argued that the "self-in-relation-to-other" model of social cognition is a major breakthrough. Impressive empirical research has also illustrated each of the three different components of relational schemas.

In the tradition of Sullivan (1953), self-schemas are conceptualized as an identity that is socially embedded—that is, one experiences *who* one is only in relation to others (Baldwin, 1992). For instance, Baldwin and Holmes (1987) used priming procedures to activate images of others as having either an accepting or a "conditional" evaluative style. Participants who then failed a test felt more inadequate and self-critical when their primed "private audience" was more judgmental. The most compelling example of the self-in-relation-to-other conceptualization is a study by Hinkley and Andersen (1996). They showed that when a significant-other representation is primed by resemblance, it brings to mind the specific *aspects* of the self experienced in relation to the significant other. For instance, if the significant other was a mother, then the person felt like "self-with-mother" in the presence of a new person resembling the mother (e.g., "When I'm with _____, I feel quite dependent and immature").

An important recent example of self-schemas comes from the work of Fitzsimmons and Bargh (2003) on their "automotive model." In one example, they showed that if the thoughts of a friend were primed, people were more likely to be helpful to a stranger canvassing for a charity. Consistent with Holmes's (2002) arguments, this is evidence that self-*goals* (A) are automatically primed in relational contexts, and not simply behavior that mimics the other. For instance, Gunz, Sahdra, Holmes, and Kunda (2003) primed university students to think of a professor or a high-school student. When they expected to later interact with the target, *complementary* goals were activated, such that they described themselves as feeling submissive in the professor condition and dominant in the student condition. In contrast, the opposite, cognitive assimilation pattern occurred when there was no anticipation of interaction (e.g., Bargh, Chen, & Burrows, 1996). Apparently, goals *in relation* to the other become activated when action is required.

Andersen, Reznick, and Manzella (1996) also illustrated the influence of activating a "partner" schema using a very creative methodology. They demonstrated that once a significant-other schema is activated by features in a "new" person that indicate some degree of "resemblance," individuals react to the new person in various ways *as if* he or she were the significant other, similar to the clinical construct of *transference*. Participants' expectations about a new person's acceptance or rejection of them were tied to the activation of liked or disliked significant-other schemas. Consistent with the rule interdependence idea, expectations about the other's motivations toward the self (B) were then tied to reports of own liking toward the other (A), and even to nonconscious facial affect. This important evidence of schema-driven affect suggests a functional interpersonal regulation system, as we discuss later.

Overall, there is less research on interpersonal scripts than self- or other schemas, even though the study of abstract scripts holds considerable promise. Because interaction (I) is a consequence of all three (SAB) causal elements, scripts might have some special "summary" status in individuals' cognitive structures. Holmes (2002), for instance, speculated that people's "story skeletons" were important as overlearned heuristics, or strategies for dealing with "hot" issues or common problems. As an example, Andersen et al. (1996) found evidence that interpersonal scripts to either approach a new acquaintance or to avoid close contact depended importantly on whether the person resembled a liked or a disliked significant other.

Though the construct of relational schemas explored in the above work captures important aspects of the SABI model, the relevance of the "situation" concept is missing.

Situation Signatures in the Structure of Cognition

As we described earlier, interdependence theory is built on the interactionist premise that situations and dispositions have a complementary relation. This suggests that features of situations should be responsible for selectively activating expectations about *relevant* dispositions that are afforded by the circumstances. Situations are thus a key cognitive organizing principle for both one's own goals and one's expectations about others' interpersonal tendencies. Though both Baldwin (1992) and Andersen and Chen (2002) do not incorporate such a logic in their theories, it is very congruent with Mischel and Shoda's (1995) work on the "cognitive-affective personality system" (CAPS). The CAPS framework has had a tremendous influence on the field of personality psychology in recent years. Their conceptualization incorporates a person-by-situation interactionist perspective (Cantor & Kihlstrom, 1987; Endler & Hunt, 1969) into a more general social-cognitive interpretation of the meaning of "personality."

Mischel and Shoda (1995) present impressive evidence that an individual's "behavioral signature" is typically quite stable over time if behavior is examined within the context of specific situations. A person's signature is comprised of *if–then* patterns of situation–behavior associations. The CAPS model contends that specific *features of situations* activate subsets of cognitive mediating units, which in turn generate distinctive responses to the different situations. Mischel and Shoda suggest that "situations" need to be considered in abstract terms, redefining them "to capture their basic psychological features, so that behavior can be predicted across a broad range of contexts that contain the same features" (p. 248).

As is apparent from the previous discussion, we strongly agree with this principle (and indeed Holmes, 2002, developed it as a major theme in his paper on the structure of cognition). However, Mischel and Shoda's definition of the "situation, " the "if" in their if–then model, has not been particularly abstract, but instead has focused largely on the *other's behavior* as the context for the actor's behavior. For example, one "situation" in their famous summer camp study was "Adult warned the child." This perspective is certainly not unreasonable, given that focusing on what people "see and hear" in the social world, on the concrete "stimulus," is the most common usage of the term "situation" in social psychology (Ross & Nisbett, 1991).

From the SABI model perspective, however, the social problems people face (their situations of interdependence, to use our terminology) should be specified separately from characteristics of interaction partners B. Further, the weakest link in Mischel and Shoda's CAPS proposal is that it needs "a theory of situations" before it can be used in an *a priori* way to predict the organization and activation of particular cognitive–affective units in the interpersonal domain. As things now stand, "situations" are defined in an ad hoc and nominal way and focus on another person's behavior. Within the current perspective, the CAPS model needs a typology of situational features (S), as well as a (logically related) typology of possible dispositions (i.e., goals rather than behavior) of the interaction partner (B). This would specify the two elements in the "social situation" that comprise the "If" in the situation–behavior link. The SABI model, like the CAPS model, then predicts that people's own goals or dispositions (A) will be activated, resulting in actual interaction behavior (I).

A critical implication of the current model is that cues for situational features will often be responsible for activating people's "theories" about the other person's goals and motives that are *relevant* to and afforded by such situations. The cues should "select" the appropriate mental model for dealing with person B within circumstances S, for tuning in to relevant knowledge and emotions in that domain. "Theories" could be quite specific to a situation, or might cover more ground, dealing with "families" of situations that were similar. The taxonomy of situations and related "dispositions" described earlier suggests one possible template for cognitive organization. Sets of expectations would be selectively applied only to relevant classes of situations—they would exhibit an appropriate "*situation signature*," a context-wise application. For instance, situations involving conflicts of interest, such as the exchange example described earlier, would activate people's concerns about the extent of B's prosocial versus selfish motivations.

This logical connection between partner dispositions and particular situations suggests that people might often use cues about a partner in a way that could bias judgments about the type of situation they are in—a backward type of logic. For instance, if you knew another person is not dependable, that knowledge would make you more vigilant for situations where you could be let down. Worrying that others will reject you would result in a readiness to interpret situations as having the potential for rejection (Downey, Freitas, Michaelis, & Khouri, 1998), and so on.

Very few theories include any consideration of how interpersonal cognition might be organized by features of situations. The exception is attachment theory, which has provided some of the most thoughtful examples of what clinicians have called a "stress–diathesis" analysis. The analysis was prompted by Bowlby's (1982) contention that the attachment system will only be activated to deal with circumstances involving threat, fear, and interpersonal conflict. Studies on the effects of working models have thus most often focused on one of these three contexts. Most impressively, a number of studies have directly compared them to control conditions, and have demonstrated that insecure attachment styles involving a lack of trust have a "signature" closely linked to such "diagnostic" situations (e.g., Pietromonaco & Barrett, 1997; Simpson, Rholes, & Nelligan, 1992; Simpson, Rholes, & Phillips, 1996).

Psychological States as Situation Cues?

Although attachment theorists should be commended for their emphasis on critical situations, they have often focused on individuals' emotional reactions to situations rather than on the situations themselves. Such an approach clearly neglects the goal of identifying the key themes, the signature situations, behind the "threat and anxiety" posited to activate the system. Analyses focusing on the "*psychological states*" of the actor (e.g., anxiety or vulnerability) risk seriously confusing the issue of what constitutes "the situation." Interdependence theorists might agree that such affective states are an effective (even evolutionary) mechanism for "summarizing" experiences in situations and keying approach/avoidance behavior. But they would also contend that a focus on the "objective," abstract features of situations and their *relation* to psychological properties is important if one is to avoid an "all-in-the-head," social-constructionist point of view (Holmes, 2002). Further, as we argued earlier, a heightened readiness to "see" rejection threats and to experience anxiety can be viewed as part of "personality" itself (see Downey et al., 1998). We cannot simply assume that anxiety is an accurate reflection of some external situational "reality."

The attachment research by Simpson and his colleagues is exemplary in keeping the distinction between the objective situation and the subjective reaction very clear. Indeed, Simpson and colleagues actually utilized key dimensions of interdependence to define the situational context (perhaps because Simpson has a background in IT from working with Ellen Berscheid). They created experimental situations involving high conflict of interest to study anxiety (Simpson et al., 1992), and a high degree of interdependence to study vulnerability (Simpson et al., 1996). Similarly, both Downey et al. (1998) and Murray, Bellavia, Rose, and Griffin (2003) used an innovative *within*-subjects design to show that rejection-sensitivity dynamics were most apparent on days following marital conflicts reported in daily diaries. A fuller discussion of attachment-style situation signatures and the type of cognitive organization that would result is presented in Holmes (2002, pp. 14–15).

Recently, Chen (2003) suggested the innovative notion that people are likely to have lay theories about how the "psychological states" (the thoughts and feelings) of significant others relate to their behavior. In contrast to above, the distinctions made in the SABI model would certainly support Chen's claim that psychological states of *others* are crucial. This is because the states are a window to the intentions, the *goals*, of others (i.e., the B in the model, not the S). Thus, if the perceived psychological state influences expectations about the other's goals, it will consequently be important in determining an actor's *own* goals: as we discussed earlier, people are rule-interdependent. For example, a person in an interdependence situation where costly help was needed might think, "If my mother is angry at me, she is not likely to be responsive to my needs." In such circumstances, the person might then avoid relying on the mother for help.

THE METATHEORY: A FUNCTIONAL, ECOLOGICAL PERSPECTIVE

As discussed above, the SABI model contends that personality and the self have a correspondence with situational affordances, and thus there is a *lawful structure* to relationships that dictates the content and structure of relational cognition. In social psychology, MacArthur and Baron (1983) have most clearly articulated such an "ecological psychology" point of view, giving primacy to reality as the "engine" driving cognition. They criticize social perception researchers for telling us "much about the processing of information and little about what the stimulus information is" (p. 215). Indeed, social psychology has generally emphasized the subjective side of human affairs, favoring the view that "people engage in an active and motivated *construction* of their own social realities" (see Jost & Kruglanski, 2002, p. 173). The "power of construal" (Ross & Nisbett, 1991) has been the common working assumption. Cognitive psychologists, however, have been less equivocal, as is apparent in the writing of Anderson (expressed in the ACT acronym, which refers to the "*adaptive* control of thought"). In Anderson's words, "the mind has the structure it has because the world has the structure it has" (1991, p. 428).

The ecological approach requires a characterization of the "reality" of social situations. In the absence of objective benchmarks for the external structure of reality, we use interdependence theory as an imperfect proxy that provides some plausible assumptions about the reality of interpersonal phenomena. Indeed, our use of the SABI model as a prescriptive template makes just such a working assumption. Our metatheoretical assumption is that interpersonal cognition will be designed to adapt to and reflect the "realities" of interpersonal relations (see Holmes, 2004). This assumption is clear in our earlier discussion of the "interpersonal dispositions" (see Table 16.1) *necessary* for adapting to and coping with the structure of the interpersonal problems people face. For functional reasons, then, the nature of "situations" shapes the cognitive content of people's goals and the themes of their expectations about the goals of others.

To what extent do other existing theories take a functional approach and describe interpersonal cognition as having content that reflects the lawful nature of relationships?

Attachment Theory and Interdependence

Attachment theory has similar roots in an ecological perspective. Bowlby (1982) was an ethologist by training, and much of his thinking was based on the notion that attachment styles, and their associated "mental models," were adaptations by infants for dealing with the "realities" of their attachment figures' responsiveness to them (and ultimately, for ensuring survival itself). Our framing of the thrust of his argument is that the adaptations were in service of striking a balance in terms of providing an optimal level of safety or security *given the circumstances of their caregiving environment*. Essentially, the cognitive processes served to estimate a caregiver's responsiveness to needs (see Reis, Clark, & Holmes, 2003), and then to develop goal strategies to deal with the perceived exigencies.

This framework is very congruent with an IT perspective, though the latter makes no assumptions about the age at which dispositions develop. The IT argument is that people's experience of others as prosocial, dependable, and helpful across social situations develops into a generalization about what others "can" potentially provide. The positive or negative nature of their experience then leads them to develop valuation rules (i.e., dispositions) designed to control their degree of interdependence with others (i.e., an approach vs. avoidance dimension). Further, people's estimate of the extent that others value them *in particular* is important because it is the basis for predicting whether others "will" choose to respond to their needs (i.e., corresponding to the anxiety dimension). As in Bowlby's version of attachment theory, then, it is the combination of expectations about others' goals *and* how others value the self specifically that is the basis for predictions that another person will act in a prosocial way and be responsive to one's needs.

There are, of course, differences between the two theories. IT seems sterile in comparison to the richly textured story told by attachment theory, irrespective as to whether the story should focus on infant development or not. That is because IT is only intended as a broad analytical framework, an abstract theory that needs to be fleshed out and brought alive by the concrete and vivid problems people face in their interpersonal lives. In that sense, the two theories are very complementary.

Transference Model

In contrast to the above theories, most theories in the field of interpersonal cognition have been agnostic in their assumptions about the role of external realities in shaping cognition, with a strong tendency to focus largely on subjective construal (e.g., Baldwin, 1992). For instance, in their transference model of social cognition, Andersen and Chen (2002) note that "a key element of the if–then model is the idea that situations, or ifs, are subjectively rather than objectively defined" (p. 628). The authors go on to argue, somewhat differently, that "our theory converges with the broader if–then model [of Mischel and Shoda] in the idea that *idiographic psychological situations*, rather than objectively defined ones, mediate if–then relations" (p. 628; our italics). The latter implicitly suggests that there is an objective reality that needs mediating, but the point is that the emphasis is heavily on the power of construal and the uniqueness of the meaning that individuals will attach to situations.

As we discussed earlier, IT, with its Lewinian heritage, would not take issue at all with the idea that people differ in the "psychological meaning" they attach to situations. Indeed, the "transformation process" has been a central basis of the theory since Kelley (1979). As discussed earlier, transformations define the very nature of people's "valuation rules," that is, their personality itself. But the point in IT is that some*thing* was transformed, an objective reality was interpreted. And the nature of that reality must surely shape the interpretation, or we risk creating an "all-in-the-head" science where there are no external constraints on people's ability to construct their social worlds.

According to the SABI model, there are regularities in terms of the particular types of adaptational challenges that people encounter. Thus it would not be the case that everyone's interpretations would be, willy-nilly, "unique and idiosyncratic." Those people who encountered with some regularity similar social problems and similar interaction partners would develop characteristic ways of coping with them (i.e., "signatures"; see Holmes, 2002) that shared common predictable elements or themes.

Thus theories with an ecological perspective, such as IT or attachment theory, would take issue with the authors' lack of effort in defining the nature of the "reality" of the if-situation, which in this case Andersen and Chen (2002, p. 628) define as "the new person one encounters" and the "resemblance of the person to a significant other." But resemblance in terms of what types of features? In actual experiments on transference, people's written descriptions of their significant other are used to activate schemas by depicting aspects of the new person in exactly worded, overlapping language. In real interactions, though, what type of triggers for resemblance are operative? Surely, it's very possible that the major adaptive "lessons" that people learn in interaction with significant others have common themes across people who had similar "objective" experiences?

That is, key features of resemblance might be quite abstract and thematic, and at least somewhat nomothetic in nature. Is it possible, for instance, that if a person had a rather judgmental parent and developed anxiety about being accepted by that parent, then actual features of a new person, or situation, that activated concerns about rejection would result in a transference reaction? And critically, is the very nature of such a "rejection-sensitive person" not revealed in studies that demonstrate that such a person perceives rejection on the basis of ambiguous "objective" cues as rated by observers (Downey et al., 1998)? In part, it is the *disjunction* between the current "reality" of a situation and the "idiographic psychological situation" that reveals crucial themes related to experience with the significant other. Indeed, this disjunction is the very basis for attribution theory: a person's dispositions are revealed by the discrepancy between the "mands of a situation" and a person's behavior in it.

Mischel and Morf (2003) recently applied the logic of the CAPS model to understanding the self and identity. Their views are more consistent with the IT functional perspective on the issue of nomothetic trends resulting from situational affordances than Mischel's earlier view. They suggest that the "ability to make subtle discriminations between different types of social situations, so that behavior can be adapted to the specific affordances, appears to have functional value" (p. 32). They further contend that "self-construction *types*," or contextualized midlevel personality dispositions, will develop in people who have similar goals and processing dynamics as elicited in particular types of situations. As they put it, "A self-construction type consists of people who have a common organization of relations among mediating units in the processing of self-relevant situation features" (p. 34). The authors suggest that the narcissistic and rejection-sensitive prototypes are good examples of this type of logic.

Given that most theories of interpersonal cognition say little about the ecological underpinnings of cognition, or the functional nature of cognitive processes, this criticism of the transference model is unfair in that sense. Our goal, however, is to suggest that efforts at incorporating such concepts could enrich even a theory as rich and interesting as the transference model. As we speculated, transference reactions may be predicated on recognizing in a new person seminal "interpersonal themes" from one's relationship with a significant other.

INDIVIDUAL DIFFERENCES: LEVEL OF ABSTRACTION ISSUES

As we suggested earlier, IT raises the important question of the extent to which relational experiences are best represented, in terms of adaptive effectiveness, in an articulated, finely grained way, or truncated into more abstract models. Indeed, we contend that level of abstraction per se can be considered a crucial aspect of individual differences, along with the specific content aspects we discussed earlier. A discussion of levels of abstraction must deal with how we represent our episodic experiences with particular people, and, as well, how our mental models might generalize *across* different people in our lives.

Episodic versus Semantic Models

Baldwin (1992) and Mischel and Shoda (1995) have typically described the interaction partner in *behavioral* terms. In the current framework, descriptions of the other person are at two different "levels": at the more concrete level of behavior in the interaction itself (I) and at the more abstract level of the other person's goals or dispositions (B). In the SAB component analysis, the "person" factors refer to B's goals and motives that are directly relevant to dealing with the particular situation encountered. To apply SAB analysis to the Mischel and Shoda (1995) camp study, the question is not only the behavior, that the "adult issued a warning," but whether the adult is seen by the boy as trying to be helpful in coordinating things or instead trying to show "who's boss." Similarly, a peer who teases could be viewed as inviting cooperative play or as displaying hostile intent that requires a response in kind (e.g., Dodge, 1993).

There is considerable gain for an actor developing expectations about person B's motives and goals (what Kelley and Holmes, 2003, call "rules") rather than B's expected behavioral patterns. The reason for this is that abstract goals such as cooperation are typically relevant across a wide variety of prototypical situations. For example, cooperative, prosocial motivation is obviously relevant in the many types of mixed-motive encounters involving some conflict of interest. Further, we suggested earlier that a quite limited number of such goals is sufficient to describe the variety of motivations relevant to dealing with a multitude of situations (especially when the range of concrete instantiations is considered). Thus, the parsimony and power of framing expectations about others in terms of their rules or goals is substantial.

Perhaps it is not surprising then that evidence from research on attributions suggests that people often spontaneously perceive dispositions (and the goals or rules they imply) as a basic element of perception (see Gilbert, 1998). Further, Park (1986) and others have found that people increasingly use abstract traits (instead of specific behaviors) to describe an acquaintance as they gain experience with the person. Moreover, Klein, Loftus, Trafton, and Fuhrman (1992) found that when judges had "extensive experience" with someone, behavioral exemplars were not even retrieved from memory when judgments were being made about how well a trait described the target.

Similarly, recent research on memory systems suggests that when the amount of experience with another person is high, abstract summary representations about the person are directly accessed without also activating memories of the evidence on which the conclusions were based (Klein, Cosmides, Toobey & Chance, 2002). Indeed, there is evidence that summary representations do not even preserve a record of the episodic evidence from which they were inferred: the semantic and episodic memories are essentially dissociated, independent systems. Only evidence of situations in which *trait-inconsistent* behavior occurred is retained, to provide boundary conditions for the scope of the generalization. In this formulation, situations serve as "tags" or markers in memory to signal when more specific knowledge is required.

Research by Fleeson (2001) aptly illustrates why such markers would be necessary. He demonstrated that even highly extraverted people show considerable variation across situations in the extent to which they actually act in an outgoing manner. This variation was reduced dramatically when he took into consideration the extent to which the situational context "afforded" extraverted behavior, consistent with our ideas and the Mischel and Shoda (1995) thesis.

The implications of these current models of memory for interpersonal relations have not really been explored. However, it is interesting to speculate about the potential inertial or "frozen" properties of conclusions that would seem to be implied by the claim that the evidence on which a conclusion is based is stored separately and not easily accessed. For instance, when people with low self-esteem experience an interpersonal success and are supposedly "upgrading" their self-conclusions, do they have ready access to past successes, or instead, is their tendency to simply tag the new success as an exception?

The Generality of Models of Self and Others

Apart from whether expectations about others center more on their abstract goals or on their behaviors, a very critical issue remains as to the level of generality in representations of self and others. Collins and Read (1994) presented one of the most thoughtful analyses of this issue. They pointed out that attachment theorists have generally been rather vague about how abstract models are organized in cognitive networks that might also contain representations of specific relationships. Indeed, most theorists have simply portrayed people as having a single set of models and a unique attachment style.

Collins and Read (1994) proposed a hierarchical framework with different levels of abstraction, ranging from general working models, to generalizations about particular significant others, to differentiated representations of specific others in specific roles or situations. They described the general model as the "default option," a global style that develops from early experience with caregivers. They suggested that a connectionist framework could accommodate the varying levels of complexity and generality within a single network (e.g., Kunda & Thagard, 1996). This is in contrast to the much more typical view that general models exert top-down, assimilative pressures on perceptions in specific new attachment relationships (e.g., Hazan & Shaver, 1987).

At the theoretical level, attachment theorists have almost always treated attachment orientations as individual differences or traits, that is, as general models. Indeed, much of the fascination with the theory has been based on that assumption, and it has surely been central to its identity. The term "styles" or the phrase "secure individuals" certainly implies it, as does research linking the global dimensions to a wide variety of health and life outcomes. Indeed, Mikulincer and Shaver (2003) discuss styles in terms of general systems of emotion-regulation processes. And even though the phrase "working models" suggests the possibility of the evolution of models, the metaphor has been one where later experience with new "attachment figures" such as good friends or romantic partners is expected to be importantly shaped by the "foundation" set by early experience.

Other social-cognitive models, such as Baldwin's (1992) pioneering work on relational schemas, have been more agnostic on such issues as the role of early experience and even the notion that people have relatively unitary, global attachment models. Baldwin, Keelan, Fehr, Enns, and Koh-Rangarajoo (1996), for instance, asked people to classify each of their 10 closest relationships in terms of the three Hazan and Shaver

(1987) attachment-style categories. They found that close to half the people used all three models, though the most frequently mentioned model corresponded on average to their self-described general style.

They suggested that people might have multiple abstract representations of a variety of different types of relationships. The relative availability and accessibility of such knowledge structures would determine thinking about relationships in particular instances, and the mark of a "general" style might be that it is more chronically accessible. Andersen et al.'s (1996) social-cognitive model of transference relies on similar activation principles. Their demonstration that subtle priming of a particular significant other representation colors social perceptions suggests that central figures in a person's interpersonal life will often have distinctive representations.

Research by Cook (2000) provides an excellent example of the benefits of exploring distinctions about the generality of expectations. He studied individuals' ratings of attachment security in over 200 families with two teenaged children. Because each person could rate his or her sense of security with each of the other family members, the round-robin format permitted the use of Kenny's (1988) Social Relations Model to partition variance as to the source of felt security or insecurity. Importantly, Cook found consistency in attachment security across relationships, indicating that actors' *general* working models indeed do have an influence on their expectations about specific relationships. If a mother felt insecure about the affections of one member of her family, she tended to report the same concerns with other family members.

He also found evidence for "partner effects," meaning that certain people tended to *induce* insecurity (or security) in most others. Interestingly, this finding supports the view that interpersonal expectations typically are not simply "all-in-the-head" constructions, but rather reflect objective (or at least intersubjective) aspects of the social environment, that is, qualities of the specific partner. Further, Cook also found that a person's reported attachment security had a component uniquely tied to a particular partner, a relationship-specific or dyadic effect. These "interpersonal chemistry" effects were just as strong as the individual difference effects.

Cozzarelli, Hoekstra, and Bylsma (2000) and Pierce and Lydon (2001) measured both general models and partner-specific models in romantic relationships. In both cases, they found that associations between these models were only modest. They also found that specific models were much stronger predictors of relationship quality than the general models. Indeed, in the impressive Pierce and Lydon study, specific models generalized to global ones over time (as in Murray & Holmes, 2000), but the reverse link was much weaker, contrary to any notions about the assimilative, "foundational" pull of the global models.

What does all this mean? On the positive side of the ledger, the

Baldwin et al. (1996) and Cook (2000) results are at least supportive of the idea that people indeed have a "core" general model involving global interpersonal themes that tie a common thread across the fabric of relationships. However, the very modest correlations between specific and general models in the above results and the lack of strong predictive validity for the general measures for relationship functioning also raise some disturbing questions, both on the theoretical and the methodological fronts.

Convergent and Divergent Validity Problems in Attachment Research

One plausible reason for the weak correlations between general and specific models in the Cozzarelli et al. (2000) and Pierce and Lydon (2001) studies is that both sets of authors quite reasonably asked people to use the scales to evaluate their relationships with attachment figures in *general*, including parents, siblings, close friends, and dating partners. This is not common practice. Investigators often do not report their instructions at all, but when they do, they usually involve rating "your general style in *romantic* relationships." The heavily used Fraley, Waller, and Brennen (2000) scales even mix in questions about dating relationships generally ("I worry a lot about my relationships") with questions that appear to refer to the current partner ("I often worry *that my partner doesn't love me*" (italics ours; note present tense).

The risk of seriously compromised and contaminated measures would seem high if one were then to turn around and ask people to rate the qualities of their current relationship. The claim that people would remember to respond "generally" seems an empty one given current research on priming and memory. Indeed, Cameron and Holmes (2003) found in a large sample of university students that the item means for specific-partner questions from the Fraley measure were significantly more secure than for general questions. They also found that on average about half of the 19- or 20-year-old sample had had only one other serious relationship, making the notion of their considering "relationships in general" quite tenuous.

Similarly, Overall, Fletcher, and Friesen (2003) attempted to create a latent variable out of separate specific reports about styles with current and past dating relationships. They found that the ratings did not cohere and that current relationship ratings were most strongly correlated with a "general" close relationship attachment measure. They also found that ratings across family members and across friends were more coherent and that all three "domains of attachment" were best represented in factor models as separate domains nested under higher level global models. Such findings are encouraging, but why would the authors suggest that the "findings provide support for the common use of general scales to assess attachment *within domains*" (p. 1491)? If so, why are there not careful studies documenting how the quality of people's *past* dating experiences links to their "style" in the close relationships "domain"?

Given the history of attachment theory, and the fact that almost all studies on close relationships discuss early childhood experience as the basis for styles, how can one reasonably recommend domain-specific measurement? What exactly is the theoretical rationale for that? Further, within the close-relationship domain, the overlapping method variance with the current relationship makes such an approach very misleading. In fact, we believe that the above results actually suggest that general attachment styles be measured in studies of close relationships by uncontaminated scales focusing on nonromantic relationships, such as *family and close friends*. Such a historical approach is more consistent with Bowlby's thinking. It is also encouraged by impressive recent evidence on the predictability of people's behavior with a romantic partner from ratings of their parents' nurturance and hostility toward them when they were seventh graders 8 years earlier (Conger, Cui, Bryant, & Elder, 2000). This evidence certainly suggests a process of social learning, but one not captured in current scales.

Cameron and Holmes (2003) developed new scales to examine self and other models (SOMS), using Bartholomew and Horowitz's (1991) logic, within each of the three domains (Overall et al., 2003, used the three-category Hazan and Shaver, 1987, measures). They found that the three domains cohered nicely for models of self (with correlations of .57, .50, .64), providing support for the model suggested by Overall et al. The Fraley et al. (2000) anxiety scale was most strongly related to the romantic relationship model (.64), but encouragingly, also to self-models with family and friends (.41, .50). Interestingly, model of other did not cohere well at all (.30, .19, .35), and a factor analysis indicated separate domain models. Also, the Fraley et al. (2000) measure of avoidance *only* related strongly to romantic partners (.73), not to family or friends (.17, .35).

These results remind us that many authors contend that the "self" is a common mental thread that organizes together a wide variety of self-relevant cognitions (e.g., Klein et al., 2002). But is there any good functional reason why representations of *others'* goals and motivations should be undifferentiated? In this vein, Holmes (2002) proposed that an important marker of a "healthy" functional mental organization is the extent to which images of significant others are differentiated and *"person-wise,"* even if they share a modicum of common variance. Put another way, when the other person B is viewed as one aspect of the "social situation," variation in expectations about significant others represents one type of "signature" of the sort identified in the Mischel and Shoda (1995) model—a signature that suggests that the actor is "adapting" to differences among interaction partners. Andersen and Chen (2002) make a similar assumption about people having unique mental models for significant others.

Surely, exploring the degree of articulation in memory of models of others is an important task for research on interpersonal cognition. Further, this differentiation aspect of cognition is not captured at all by current measures.

The idea that insecure people with less "healthy" personalities are most likely to see others as more uniformly untrustworthy and unkind was explored in the classic paper by Kelley and Stahelski (1970). They illustrated that cooperative communal individuals expected others to vary considerably in their prosocial communal orientations. Their own communal goals were set to be contingent on perceiving similar goals in specific other people. In stark contrast, individuals who were competitive, especially those high on authoritarianism, tended to have little variance in their images of others, seeing people as basically selfish and unkind. The result of this belief was typically a self-fulfilling prophecy that produced poor outcomes but also insulated their dysfunctional expectations from being revised.

Model of Self and Self-Esteem

Cameron and Holmes (2003) also explored the idea that cognitive models of the self as "worthy of love" have a close theoretical resemblance to the sociometer model logic that the self is "socially constructed" from reflected appraisals of how the self is viewed by others (Leary & Baumeister, 2000). While Leary and Baumeister have taken a view similar to those who support attachment theory that there is a core sense of self across domains, Kirkpatrick and Ellis (2001) have argued for the idea of "multiple sociometers" on the evolutionary, functional grounds that the attributes valued in different kinds of relationships are not the same. Thus, for instance, family and friends might represent different kinds of adaptation problems. In exploring this issue, Cameron and Holmes (2003) found that when models of self for family, close friends, and romantic partner were regressed onto the Rosenberg self-esteem measure, a multiple R of .66 resulted, without any correction for attenuation, and each domain contributed unique variance.

That struck us as a very substantial association, especially given that Rosenberg (1965) created a very North American, individualistic measure ("I am a person of worth. ... ") that makes no mention of how *others* value the self. The results would seem consistent with both Leary and Baumeister's (2000) notion of a general sociometer *and* Kirkpatrick and Ellis's (2001) contention that different domains contribute separate variance. Of course, it is unclear whether feelings of worth were actually derived from feeling cared for and valued by significant others, as Leary and Baumeister (2000) would contend, or whether core feelings about the self are projected onto close others (see Murray & Holmes, 2000), or both, as we suspect. It is interesting to note that the Fraley et al. (2000) romantic anxiety measure correlated .56 with Rosenberg (1965), even though it only indexes anxiety in one domain. The reader can probably read our minds: it is not at all clear that "attachment anxiety" has sufficient discriminant validity from self-esteem, and especially its sociometer counterpart, certainly not enough to warrant the two large literatures completely ignoring each other (see Griffin & Bartholomew, 1994).

In this vein, Murray and her colleagues have identified self-esteem as a major predictor of relationship-*specific* perceived regard (i.e., attachment anxiety) in a wide variety of studies. People with low self-esteem have been shown to project their poor sense of self-worth onto their partners, and this projection typically results in a large dose of unwarranted insecurity. Crucially, though, Murray has demonstrated that the most important variable in predicting reactions to relationship events, such as married individuals' perceptions in daily diaries, is relationship-specific perceived regard (Murray et al., 2003). This focused relationship "sociometer" is strongly predictive across a variety of studies even when *controlling* for self-esteem and satisfaction.

Recently a number of studies referencing the Murray and Holmes (2000) dependence-regulation model have partialled self-esteem out of their measure of so-called general romantic attachment anxiety. Their goal is to demonstrate that anxiety is more than "just" self-esteem. But, in our opinion, this goal is not achieved at all. We would suggest that in actual fact such results directly mimic those of Murray because of the measurement problems in the Fraley and other scales indexing romantic anxiety. That is, we believe the scales in good part measure worry and anxiety in relation to the *current* partner, demonstrating, just as Murray does, that the proximal, relationship-specific index is predictive even when self-esteem is controlled.

Does this then mean that we support Andersen and Chen's view (2002, p. 621) that the "self" is comprised of a set of *distinct* possible "relational selves," each representing the self-in-relation-to a different significant other? No. We are much more inclined to side with attachment theorists who believe that despite some important unique variance associated with specific relationships, there are core themes that people extract from across their most significant relationships, and that these core themes influence perception in new relationships. For instance, Cook's (2000) study of family members suggests people have themes that are common across significant others, themes that predict the key construct of perceived responsiveness to needs.

Indeed, we would suggest that a weakness of transference theory is that the principles of "transfer of training" are not spelled out. In a representation of a new romantic relationship, for instance, is transference controlled largely by ad hoc priming induced by concrete types of similarity with a particular significant other, as seems to be implied? Or instead, would that representation be shaped by elements from a variety of sources of abstract "resemblance," with some shared, convergent themes emerging across significant others? That is, how does social learning occur so that the "lessons" learned from important relationships can be integrated and applied to new ones so that the person doesn't have to adapt *de novo*?

A NORMATIVE PROCESS MODEL OF INTERPERSONAL COGNITION

It has been almost a matter of faith among attachment researchers that general individual difference models will reasonably determine people's "anxiety and avoidance" in their specific close relationships. This perhaps explains the startling fact that so few studies have even bothered to measure the more specific concepts in the romantic relationships they are studying so that core underlying assumptions could be tested. Further, the pull of individual difference thinking has been so strong among attachment theorists that they have seldom framed issues in terms of *normative processes*. As we explained earlier, interdependence theory suggests that the two attachment dimensions reflect basic processes that can be used to describe the *state* of any particular relationship. Bowlby (1982) and Baldwin (1992) have made similar arguments. However, the changing and idiosyncratic use of theoretical terms in current attachment theory has tended to obscure the fit with related work on basic processes.

Recently, for instance, attachment theorists have tended not to emphasize the more cognitive perspective of Bowlby in which self and other model together predict the degree of "felt security," or from our point of view, trust in another's responsiveness. In our opinion, there was much to gain from such a cognitive perspective on the sources of perceived responsiveness. One can make a persuasive argument that models of other and self, expectations about whether others "can and will" be responsive to one's needs, can be viewed as central elements in a functional theory of social adaptation (cf. Holmes, 2002; Reis, Clark, & Holmes, 2003).

Instead, theorists have tended recently to conceptualize an "anxiety" (i.e., self) dimension as an evaluative summary of the state of a "monitoring system" that tracks others' caring, and an avoidance (i.e., other) dimension viewed as a prototypical "strategic" or adaptive response to the state of affairs of the monitor (Fraley & Shaver, 2000). In our opinion, there is little evidence that the dimensions interact in this way (e.g., Murray et al., 2003; Collins & Feeney, 2000). This view also does not seem to have a clear touchstone with the cognitive models that were the conceptual basis of Bowlby's ideas. What's so unique about Bowlby's cognitive models is that they can be elaborated to serve as *explanatory organizing concepts* for people's interrelated cognitions, emotions, and behavioral adjustments *within* each dimension. In contrast, the labels "anxiety" and "avoidance" seem unidimensional and shift the focus between emotions and behavior.

To illustrate the benefits of focusing on cognitive models, anxiety or worry would be interpreted as an emotion that is the *consequence* of negative reflective cognitions about the self, of feeling unsure as to whether one is seen by a significant other as being worthy of his or her love and caring. This self-model, or sociometer, can easily be used to describe the state of a specific relationship. Moreover, this concept involves such a basic process that Tooby and Cosmides (1996) speculated that evolutionary pressures would actually have resulted in adaptations in which people's cognitive machinery would be very tuned to calibrating the extent to which they were valued by close others (see Kelley et al., 2003, Chapter 18, on Twists of Fate).

The *behavioral response* to feelings of insecurity about a specific other's regard, according to research on the "dependence-regulation model" (Murray & Holmes, 2000), is to self-protectively reduce closeness and interdependence. There is now substantial support for that principle, including evidence that married couples even regulate their everyday attachment on the basis of localized feelings of being valued and cared for (Murray et al., 2003). Note that the only behavioral items included in anxious attachment scales measure desire for merging or extreme closeness, which may reflect more of a wish or need than actual behavioral reactions.

The "avoidance" dimension seems to focus solely on behavior. As Mikulincer and Shaver (2001) describe it, however, avoidance reflects "the extent to which people distrust others' goodwill and strive to maintain emotional distance and remain independent from relationship partners" (p. 97). This reasoning makes it clear that avoidance is a strategic response to a negative model of the other, where others are seen as unresponsive and unkind. (In IT terms, a person's own goals are contingent on expectations about another's goals.) Moreover, the Fraley et al. (2000) scale also heavily features emotion items involving "discomfort" with closeness or with depending on others. Surprisingly, the scale neglects items about others' goodwill and responsiveness that are, as noted above, the likely basis for such feelings of vulnerability.

A comparable focus on independence (i.e., avoidance) versus interdependence has been a major theme in IT for many years, as we discussed earlier. But in that theory, goals or rules to regulate interdependence represent a normative process that can be specific to situations or to specific relationships. What's so beneficial about an elaborated version of Bowlby's cognitive models is that, taken together, they are a way of summarizing beliefs about a particular significant other's *motivations* or goals, consistent with how we portray the other person B in IT terms (and how we believe interaction partners are represented in memory systems).

This analysis has several implications. First, we believe there is much to gain by reframing attachment theory in terms of Bowlby's organizing principle of cognitive models of self and other, as was essentially done by Bartholomew (1990). This would clarify the theoretical relations among the three components and provide a better template for measurement. Second, Bowlby's notion that perceived responsiveness to needs is based on two distinct component expectations is surely a major insight, one that should serve as the foundation for cognitive models of relationships. It led Holmes (2002) to redefine trust in a *specific* relationship as a sense of "felt security" influenced by *both* model of self and model of other. Similarly, at the global level, Brennan and Shaver (1995) found that generalized trust was best understood as a joint function of both the anxiety and avoidance measures, essentially isomorphic with a secure "style."

Cameron and Holmes (2003) developed a measure of perceived responsiveness and found it was indeed predicted by both self and other models within each of the family, friends, and romantic relationship domains. As noted earlier, they also found that model of other was more sensitive to variations in the target person, consistent with Mischel and Shoda's (1995) model of context-sensitive adaptations. Cameron and Holmes discovered that "perceived regard" was also predicted by both self and other models and that it correlated strongly (.60–.70) with perceived responsiveness, a logical connection in hindsight given the shared link to felt security. Similarly, Murray (Murray et al., 2003) found that the association of perceived regard with the anxiety and avoidance dimensions in her large married sample exceeded 0.40 in each case.

These findings are intriguing when one considers the results from the extensive program of research on dependence regulation showing that insecurity in perceived regard predicts reduced closeness and relationship devaluation (see Murray & Derrick, Chapter 7, this volume). That raises the intriguing specter that it is not just the "avoidance" or "other" dimension that relates to the regulation of interdependence and closeness, but that the anxiety (self-esteem) dimension may play just as important a role as well. (Ironically, it appears that the term chosen to describe the avoidance dimension may mislead one into begging the question about which dimension is related to closeness.)

The integrating and central dynamic feature that may make sense of all this is the concept of perceived responsiveness. A tentative hypothesis is that insecurity in expectations of responsiveness that arise from *either* source, the model of self or expectations about the other, will result in people dealing with their vulnerability by self-protectively distancing themselves from the other and reducing dependence on the relationship. In summary, our biased opinion is that Bowlby's original concept of cognitive models brings a coherence to attachment theory that was missing in recent years as interpretations of the two dimensions were changed and debated.

CONCLUSION

The field of interpersonal cognition has made huge advances in the recent decade, with a number of impressive and fascinating theoretical viewpoints being articulated. The goal of the present chapter was to try to examine the working assumptions of these various theories from the point of view of the broad framework of interdependence theory. Our overview indicates that tremendous strides have been made, but that the theories conflict in important ways in terms of a number of core working assumptions. The resolution of these issues, or at least an extended debate about them, could foster integration across theories and add to the existing strengths of each point of view.

REFERENCES

Andersen, S. M., & Chen, S. (2002). The relational self: An interpersonal social-cognitive theory. *Psychological Review, 109,* 619–645.

Andersen, S. M., Reznik, I., & Manzella, L. M. (1996). Eliciting facial affect, motivation, and expectancies in transference: Significant-other representations in social relations. *Journal of Personality and Social Psychology, 71,* 1108–1129.

Anderson, J. R. (1991). The adaptive nature of human categorization. *Psychological Review, 98,* 409–429.

Baldwin, M. W. (1992). Relational schemas and the processing of social information. *Psychological Bulletin, 112,* 461–484.

Baldwin, M. W., & Holmes, J. G. (1987). Salient private audiences and awareness of the self. *Journal of Personality and Social Psychology, 52,* 1087–1098.

Baldwin, M. W., Keelan, J., Fehr, B., Enns, V., & Koh-Rangarajoo, E. (1996). Social-cognitive conceptualization of attachment working models: Availability and accessibility effects. *Journal of Personality and Social Psychology, 71,* 94–109.

Bargh, J. A., Chen, M., & Burrows, L. (1996). Automaticity of social behavior: Direct effects of trait construct and stereotype priming on action. *Journal of Personality and Social Psychology, 71,* 230–244.

Bartholomew, K. (1990). Avoidance of intimacy: An attachment perspective. *Journal of Social and Personal Relationships, 7,* 147–178.

Bartholomew, K., & Horowitz, L. M. (1991). Attachment styles among young adults: A test of a four-category model. *Journal of Personality and Social Psychology, 61,* 226–244.

Berscheid, E. (1983). Emotion. In H. H. Kelley, E. Berscheid, A. Christensen, J. H. Harvey, T. L. Huston, G. Levinger, E. McClintock, L. A. Peplau, & D. R. Peterson (Eds.), *Close relationships* (pp. 110–168). New York: Freeman and Company.

Bowlby, J. (1982). *Attachment and loss: Vol. 1. Attachment.* London: Hogarth Press.

Brennan, K., & Shaver, P. (1995). Dimensions of adult attachment, affect regulation, and romantic relationship functioning. *Personality and Social Psychology Bulletin, 21,* 267–283.

Cameron, J., & Holmes, J. G. (2003). *Domain-specific models of self and other: A critical examination of attachment theory measurement.* Unpublished manuscript, University of Waterloo.

Cantor, N., & Kihlstrom, J. (1987). *Personality and social intelligence.* Englewood Cliffs, NJ: Prentice-Hall.

Chen, S. (2003). Psychological state theories about significant others: Implications for the content and structure of significant-other representations. *Personality and Social Psychology Bulletin, 29,* 1285–1302.

Collins, N. L., & Feeney, B. C. (2000). A safe haven: An attachment theory perspective on support seeking and caregiving in intimate relationships. *Journal of Personality and Social Psychology, 78,* 1053–1073.

Collins, N. L., & Read, S. J. (1994). Cognitive representations of attachment: The content and function of working models. In K. Bartholomew & D. Perlman (Eds.), *Advances in personal relationships* (Vol. 5, pp. 53–90). London: Jessica Kingsley.

Conger, R., Cui, M., Bryant, C., & Elder, G. (2000). Competence in early adult romantic relationships: A developmental perspective on family influences. *Journal of Personality and Social Psychology, 79,* 224–237.

Cook, W. L. (2000). Understanding attachment security in family context. *Journal of Personality and Social Psychology, 78,* 285–294.

Cozzarelli, C., Hoekstra, S., & Bylsma, W. (2000). General versus specific models of attachment: Are they associated with different outcomes? *Personality and Social Psychology Bulletin, 26,* 605–618.

Dodge, K. (1993). Social-cognitive mechanisms in the development of conduct disorder and depression. *Annual Review of Psychology, 44,* 559–584.

Downey, G., Freitas, A., Michaelis, B., & Khouri, H. (1998). The self-fulfilling prophecy in close relationships: Rejection sensitivity and rejection by romantic partners. *Journal of Personality and Social Psychology, 75,* 545–560.

Endler, N., & Hunt, J. (1969). Generalizability of contributions from sources of variance in the S-R inventories of anxiousness. *Journal of Personality, 37,* 1–24.

Fitzsimons, G., & Bargh, J. (2003).Thinking of you: Nonconscious pursuit of interpersonal goals associated with relationship partners. *Journal of Personality and Social Psychology, 84,* 148–163.

Fleeson, W. (2001). Toward a structure- and process- integrated view of personality: Traits as density distributions of states. *Journal of Personality and Social Psychology, 80,* 1011–1027.

Fraley, R. C., & Shaver, P. R. (2000). Adult romantic attachment: Theoretical developments, emerging controversies, and unanswered questions. *Review of General Psychology, 4,* 132–154.

Fraley, C., Waller, N., & Brennan, K. (2000). An item response theory analysis of self-report measures of adult attachment. *Journal of Personality and Social Psychology, 78,* 350–365.

Gilbert, D. T. (1998). Ordinary personology. In D. T. Gilbert, S. T. Fiske, & G. Lindsey (Eds.), *The handbook of social psychology* (Vol. 2, pp. 89–150). Boston: McGraw-Hill.

Griffin, D. W., & Bartholomew, K. (1994). Models of the self and other: Fundamental dimensions underlying measures of adult attachment. *Journal of Personality and Social Psychology, 67,* 430–445.

Gunz, A., Sahdra, B., Holmes, J. G., & Kunda, Z. (2003). *Complementary and assimilative processes in automotive priming in relationship contexts.* Unpublished manuscript, University of Waterloo.

Hazan, C., & Shaver, P. (1987). Romantic love conceptualized as an attachment process. *Journal of Personality and Social Psychology, 52,* 511–524.

Hinkley, K., & Andersen, S. M. (1996). The working self-concept in transference: Significant-other activation and self-change. *Journal of Personality and Social Psychology, 71,* 1279–1295.

Holmes, J. G. (2000). Social relationships: The nature and function of relational schemas. *European Journal of Social Psychology, 30,* 447–496.

Holmes, J. G. (2002). Interpersonal expectations as the building blocks of social cognition: An interdependence theory perspective. *Personal Relationship, 9,* 1–26.

Holmes, J. G. (2004). The benefits of abstract functional analysis in theory construction: The case of interdependence theory. *Personality and Social Psychology Review, 8,* 146–155.

Holmes, J. G., & Rempel, J. K. (1989). Trust in close relationships. In C. Hendrick (Ed.), *Review of personality and social psychology: Close relationships* (Vol. 10, pp. 187–219). Newbury Park, CA: Sage.

Jost, J. T., & Kruglanski, A. (2002). The estrangement of social constructionism and experimental social psychology: History of the rift and prospects for reconciliation. *Personality and Social Psychology Review, 6,* 168–187.

Kelley, H. H. (1979). *Personal relationship: Their structures and processes.* Hillsdale, NJ: Erlbaum.

Kelley, H. H., & Holmes, J. G. (2003). *Interdependence theory: Situations, relationships, and personality.* Unpublished manuscript, University of Waterloo.

Kelley, H. H., Holmes, J. G., Kerr, N., Reis, H., Rusbult, C., & Van Lange, P. A. (2003). *An atlas of interpersonal situations.* Cambridge, UK: Cambridge University Press.

Kelley, H. H., & Stahelski, A. (1970). The social interaction basis of cooperators' and competitors' beliefs about others. *Journal of Personality and Social Psychology, 16,* 66–91.

Kenny, D. A. (1988). Interpersonal perception: A social relations analysis. *Journal of Social and Personal Relationships, 5,* 247–261.

Kirkpatrick, L., & Ellis, B. (2001). Evolutionary perspectives on self-evaluation and self-esteem. In G. Fletcher & M. Clark (Eds.), *The Blackwell handbook of social psychology: Interpersonal processes* (Vol. 2, pp. 411–436). Malden, MA: Blackwell.

Klein, S. B., Cosmides, L., Tooby, J., & Chance, S. (2002). Decisions and the evolution of memory: Multiple systems, multiple functions. *Psychological Review, 109,* 306–329.

Klein, S. B., Loftus, J., Trafton, J., & Fuhrman, R. (1992). Use of exemplars and abstractions in trait judgments: A model of trait knowledge about the self and others. *Journal of Personality and Social Psychology, 63,* 739–753.

Kunda, Z., & Thagard, P. (1996). Forming impressions from stereotypes, traits, and behaviors: A parallel-constraint-satisfaction theory. *Psychological Review, 103,* 284–308.

Leary, M. R., & Baumeister, R. F. (2000). The nature and function of self-esteem:

Sociometer theory. In M. P. Zanna (Ed.), *Advances in experimental social psychology* (Vol. 32, pp. 2–51). San Diego, CA: Academic Press.

Lewin, K. (1946). Behavior and development as a function of the total situation. In L. Carmichael (Ed.), *Manual of child psychology* (pp. 791–844). New York: Wiley.

MacArthur, L., & Baron, R. (1983). Toward an ecological theory of social perception. *Psychological Review, 90,* 215–238.

Mikulincer, M., & Shaver, P. (2001). Attachment theory and intergroup bias: Evidence that priming the secure base schema attenuates negative reactions to outgroups. *Journal of Personality and Social Psychology, 81,* 97–115.

Mikulincer, M., & Shaver, P. (2003). The attachment behavioral system in adulthood: Activation, psychodynamics, and interpersonal processes. In M. P. Zanna (Ed.), *Advances in experimental social psychology* (Vol. 35, pp. 53–152). New York: Academic Press.

Mischel, W., & Morf, C. (2003). The self as a psycho-social dynamic processing system: A meta-perspective on a century of the self in psychology. In M. Leary & J. Tangney (Eds.), *Handbook of self and identity* (pp. 15–46). New York: Guilford Press.

Mischel, W., & Shoda, Y. (1995). A cognitive-affective system theory of personality: Reconceptualizing situations, dispositions, dynamics, and invariance in personality structure. *Psychological Review, 102,* 246–268.

Murray, S. L., Bellavia, G., Rose, P., & Griffin, D. (2003). Once hurt, twice hurtful: How perceived regard regulates daily marital interaction. *Journal of Personality and Social Psychology, 84,* 126–147.

Murray, S. L., & Holmes, J. G. (2000). Seeing the self through a partner's eyes: Why self-doubts turn into relationship insecurities. In A. Tesser, R. B. Felson, & J. M. Suls (Eds.), *Psychological perspectives on self and identity* (pp. 173–198). Washington: American Psychological Association Press.

Overall, N., Fletcher, G., & Friesen, M. (2003). Mapping the intimate relationship mind: Comparisons between three models of attachment representations. *Personality and Social Psychology Bulletin, 29,* 1479–1493.

Park, B. (1986). A method for studying the development of impressions of real people. *Journal of Personality and Social Psychology, 51,* 907–917.

Pierce, T., & Lydon, J. (2001). Global and specific relational models in the experience of social interactions. *Journal of Personality and Social Psychology, 80,* 613–631.

Pietromonaco, P., & Barrett, L. (1997) Working models of attachment and daily social interactions. *Journal of Personality and Social Psychology, 73,* 1409–1423.

Reis, H., Clark, M., & Holmes, J. G. (2003). Perceived partner responsiveness as an organizing construct in the study of intimacy and closeness. In D. Mashek & A. Aron (Eds.), *Handbook of closeness and intimacy* (pp. 201–228). Mahwah, NJ: Erlbaum.

Rosenberg, M. (1965). *Society and the adolescent self-image.* Princeton, NJ: Princeton University Press.

Ross, L., & Nisbett R. E. (1991). *The person and the situation: Perspectives of social psychology.* Philadelphia: Temple University Press.

Simpson, J. A., Rholes, W. S., & Nelligan, J. (1992). Support-seeking and support-giving within couples within an anxiety provoking situation: The role of attachment styles. *Journal of Personality and Social Psychology, 62,* 434–446.

Simpson, J. A., Rholes, W. S., & Phillips, D. (1996). Conflict in close relationships: An attachment perspective. *Journal of Personality and Social Psychology, 71,* 899–914.

Sullivan, H. S. (1953). *The interpersonal theory of psychiatry.* New York: Norton.

Tooby, J., & Cosmides, L. (1996). Friendship and the banker's paradox: Other pathways to the evolution of adaptations for altruism. *Proceedings of the British Academy, 88,* 119–143.

Index